D1311805

Hello, My Name Is...

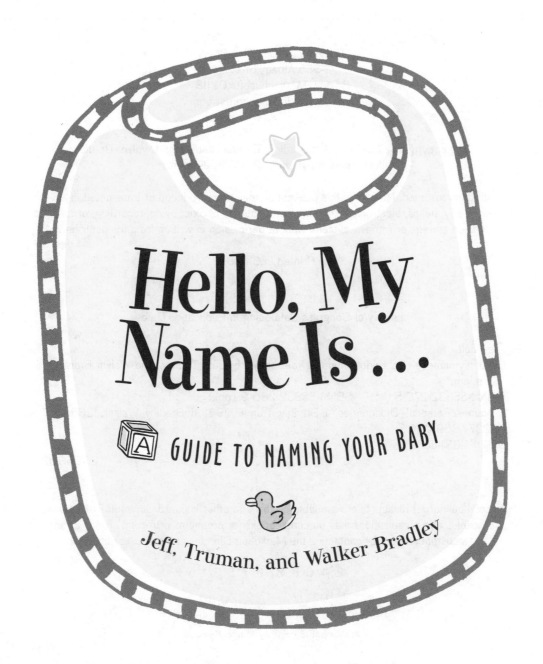

Hello, My Name Is . . .

GUIDE TO NAMING YOUR BABY

Jeff, Truman, and Walker Bradley

THE HARVARD COMMON PRESS
Boston, Massachusetts

The Harvard Common Press
535 Albany Street
Boston, Massachusetts 02118
www.harvardcommonpress.com

Printed in China

Library of Congress Cataloging-in-Publication Data

Bradley, Jeff.
    Hello, my name is-- : a guide to naming your baby / by Jeff, Truman, and Walker Bradley.
        p. cm.
    ISBN 1-55832-279-5 (hc) -- ISBN 1-55832-280-9 (pbk)
    1. Names, Personal--Dictionaries. I. Bradley, Truman, 1981- II. Bradley, Walker, 1985- III. Title.
    CS2377.B69 2005
    929.4'4'03--dc22

                                                                        2005002159

Special bulk-order discounts are available on this and other Harvard Common Press books.
Companies and organizations may purchase books for premiums or resale, or may arrange
a custom edition, by contacting the Marketing Director at the address above.

2 4 6 8 10 9 7 5 3 1

BOOK DESIGN & ILLUSTRATIONS BY JILL WEBER

Author photograph by Marta Turnbull

To Marta

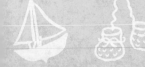
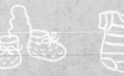
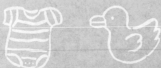

Acknowledgments

A great team put together *Hello, My Name Is . . . .* Truman Bradley and Walker Bradley researched and compiled the list of names that makes up the bulk of this book. Almost every page demonstrates their diligence and attention to detail. Few fathers these days have an opportunity to work on any significant project with their sons, much less a book, and I will never forget those weeks in which all three of us toiled together during a Colorado summer.

Linda Ziedrich capably edited *Hello, My Name Is . . . ,* the third book on which we have worked together. She is that rare person, a professional with high standards who challenges me and improves my prose, yet remains a good friend.

Bruce Shaw, publisher of The Harvard Common Press, signed me to my first book contract when the Press overlooked the town common of Harvard, Massachusetts. His faith in me launched my publishing career, and his support has sustained me through three books.

I am grateful as well to the many people who told me the stories of their names or their children's names, and to the organizations and individuals who allowed me to reprint other stories. Special thanks go to Cari and Wes Clark for sharing their wonderful collection of Utah names.

—Jeff Bradley

Contents

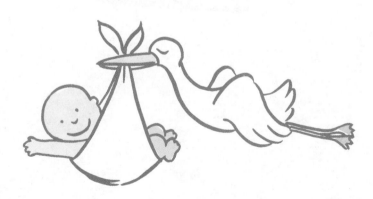

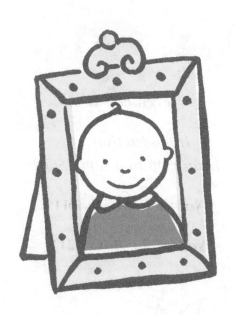
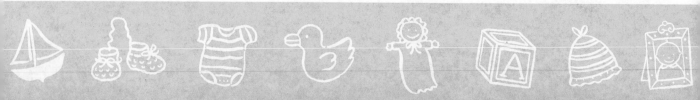

Preface

n May 1, 1898, during the Spanish-American War, Admiral George Dewey commanded a U.S. fleet that steamed into Manila harbor in the Philippines and destroyed the Spanish fleet. When word reached this country, he instantly became a national hero.

Four months after this triumph, a baby was born in Kingsport, Tennessee. The father had his heart set on a boy, and planned to name him *Dewey Manila* in honor of the admiral and his victory. The child turned out to be a little girl, but the parents named her *Dewey Manila* anyway.

This girl with the unusual name grew up to become my great-aunt, and Aunt Dewey became my introduction to the world of interesting personal names. My mother wanted to name me *George Ernest Bradley III*, but my father, George Ernest Bradley, Jr., would have none of it. Although known to family and friends as Son, he had suffered confusion with his father, George Ernest Bradley, Sr., and wanted my name to be something else. *Jeffrey*, I am informed by reliable sources, came from the son of a Washington, D.C., cab driver, and my parents picked up Vincent while visiting Hungry Mother State Park in Virginia. And so I became Jeffrey Vincent Bradley. I now go by *Jeff*.

I attended rural East Tennessee schools with kids who had all manner of unusual given names, revealed to one and all in the yearbook during our

senior year of high school. Some of the boys' first and middle names were *William Otto, Vivert Aaron, Rush Floyd,* and *Gale Omar.* The girls' names included *Cheryl Ruthita, Mary Alyce, Neda Jane, Eufaula Carole,* and *Rena Rebecca.*

Then there were the Anns. Like their counterparts today, parents of children starting school in the fifties found that many of their precious darlings shared names with classmates. In my senior class, we had Patty Ann, Elizabeth Ann, Marsha Ann, Linda Ann, Barbara Ann, Teresa Ann, Cynthia Ann, Shirley Ann, Judy Ann, Patricia Ann, and Mozella Ann. I didn't have to wait till the end of my senior year to learn some of these middle names, because Southerners have a tradition of calling people by both of their given names. I have a cousin whom we always called *Martha Ann,* and at school I addressed John Paul, Mary Alyce, and Jenny Sue by their two names.

My high school teachers had first names that I wish we could have used to their faces: Prezzle, Fern, Laurena, Ermalie, and Pietro. Lunch was served by Estelle, Naomi, Pearl, and Minerva.

After school and in the summers, I worked at my family's construction company, which employed men named *Royal, Fate, Shirley,* and *Jehovah.* I went off to college and later became a reporter, writing about the blind Baptist gospel disk jockey J. Bazzel Mull and interviewing Judge Sue K. Hicks, the real-life inspiration for Johnny Cash's hit song "A Boy Named Sue."

You can't come from a background like that and not have an interest in names.

A fellow East Tennessean, the late Richard Marius, hired me to teach writing at Harvard, and this led me into a world of student names, some of which I now see in articles in the *New York Times.*

After eight years in the classroom, I landed a job in Harvard's fundraising office, where I wrote about donors and well-preserved class chairmen from as far back as the class of 1910. I once put out an annual report listing

the more than twenty-seven thousand names of people who had made gifts in the past year to the Harvard College Fund. Many of those old boys had wonderfully WASPy first names: *Bancroft, Hamilton, Gardner, Hallowell, Malcolm, Francis, Whitfield, Bertram, Morris,* and *Wolcott.* Every now and then I would encounter one of them wandering around the office, in a navy-blue blazer, white Oxford-cloth shirt, and striped tie—a special Brooks Brothers one if the man had put his name on a check to Harvard for more than ten thousand dollars.

When my wife became pregnant for the first time, she and I bought several baby-name books. They were mind-numbing tomes with all the charm of a telephone directory. Like many parents-to-be, we wanted our baby to have a name that was distinctive but not weird. We had chosen not to know until birth whether our child was a boy or a girl. We picked out *Truman* for a boy's name and *Lydia* for a girl's.

The first names were the easy part. My wife, Marta, had kept her maiden name, *Turnbull,* and we had long discussions over which last name to give our child. Marta wanted to hyphenate our names, which would come out as either *Bradley-Turnbull* or *Turnbull-Bradley.* Our child would actually have four names instead of three.

I objected. Both combinations made me imagine a royal-family fop who sat around eating cucumber sandwiches at the Henley Royal Regatta. "And what if our kids marry someone else with a hyphenated name?" I asked.

"That's their problem," replied the love of my life.

Suppressing a roll of the eyes, I responded, "You can't just say that an odd name is someone else's problem. That's like naming a boy *Sue* and blithely claiming that he has to deal with the consequences."

On and on the discussion went, as Marta grew larger and the due date bore down upon us. Finally, we reached a compromise: We would stick with three names. If the child was a boy, his middle name and last name would be *Turnbull Bradley.* If the child was a girl, her middle and last names would be *Bradley Turnbull.*

Mercifully, we had boys. In 1981, Truman Turnbull Bradley was born, and he was followed four years later by Walker Turnbull Bradley. Both of them helped produce this book.

Hello, My Name Is … has the large quantity of names requisite in books of this sort. Because many of these names have ancient origins, our various sources sometimes disagreed about derivations. In each case, I used my best judgment. In assembling sample lists of names from other countries, I favored names that Americans could readily pronounce.

As anyone who has used a baby-name book can attest, looking through a seemingly endless list of names quickly gets boring. For this reason, *Hello, My Name Is …* contains an eclectic collection of supplementary material: accounts of how people received unusual names, lists of different kinds of names, and stories from real people reflecting about their names or the names of their children. These bits of naming lore occur throughout the book.

Giving a person a name–which with good luck and health he or she will bear for a hundred years–is a great responsibility, but it can also be a great deal of fun. It's an opportunity unlike any other, with a chance to do very well or very badly. If naming your child becomes an irresistible opportunity to show off your creativity or make some kind of statement, keep one thing firmly in mind: The person who bears the name will probably be the one who picks out your nursing home.

If you make a good choice, though, you will see a baby grow into the chosen name and become that name–to him or her, to you, and to the world. Through the years, you will see the name on kindergarten rolls, team rosters, Scout lists, diplomas, business cards, and more. The name you choose will become one of the sweetest words in your vocabulary.

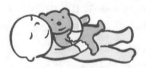

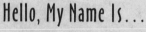

Introduction

GETTING OFF TO A GOOD START

A mother-to-be lay reading in bed while her husband was brushing his teeth and getting ready to join her. She had placed a baby-name book on his pillow. When he came to his side of the bed, he placed the baby-name book on his bedside table and picked up a Tom Clancy novel. She put her book down.

"When are you going to start looking at that baby-name book?" she asked.

"I have *looked* at it," he replied.

"I haven't seen you look at it."

"Believe it or not," he countered, "I think about names quite a bit—while I am at work, while I am driving home. I just don't want to do it right now."

Some people choose the names of their children years before they are born. Some even choose names for their babies while they are children themselves. But other people struggle to choose names. They want to find, out of what seems like an infinity of choices, the one name that perfectly suits the child they don't yet know. Some people just have a hard time making choices and living with a decision. If you struggle to choose from a menu or to select wallpaper or paint–all relatively minor matters–you can be in for a rough ride in choosing a name for your child.

Then there's the challenge of dealing with everyone else who wants in on the baby-name decision. You'll want to work with your partner, of course, but your parents, other family members, and friends can easily become overbearing with their suggestions. Getting ready for a new baby should be a wonderful experience, and choosing a name shouldn't detract from the pleasure. If you feel you're facing a challenging decision, you may first want to choose a process for coming up with a name. The process you use will reflect the kind of person you are, or the kind of relationship you and your partner have. Some parents-to-be get into a real production mode, with folders and spreadsheets and Post-its and highlighters. Others never write anything down; they just keep one or more names in mind until better ones replace them, in a kind of mental king-of-the-mountain effort.

If you are single, choosing a name is a little easier–you don't have someone else with whom you have to compromise. If you are like most people, however, you have to work with the other parent–someone whose ideas about naming and decision-making may be very different from your own. If you can agree on a process, you'll have a smoother time agreeing on a name.

Decide how to decide.

"Owning the process" is a phrase often used in business. It means taking responsibility for the sequence of actions that leads to achieving a goal. Say a couple is renovating a bathroom. If one person takes the initiative to go to building-supply stores and narrow the selections of tile and paint and fixtures so that the second person can make a choice, the first person owns the process.

As you and your partner get ready to pick a baby name, take a few minutes to think about how the two of you have made other big choices in your lives. Some people like to make decisions quickly, using instinct, whereas others like to assemble as much information as possible and carefully deliberate before making a choice. If you want to collect a lot of information, you are the best one to own the process of choosing a name. By taking the lead, you won't be spinning your wheels and getting frustrated while waiting for your spouse to move. If both of you are deliberative, flip a coin to select the person who will set the agenda. If both of you are impulsive, you really need a good process.

If you took the initiative to select and purchase this book, you have already begun to own the process of naming your baby. Owning the process does not mean dictating the way things go. It means making sure you get agreement on how to proceed and then keeping the process going. The following advice, and the stories scattered throughout the book of how other people have chosen names, will give you ideas to consider as you decide what process will work best for you.

You are naming more than a baby.

As you consider names for your baby, keep in mind that you are picking a name for a lifetime. You are naming a cuddly baby, to be sure, but you may also be naming a fourth-grade soccer player, a cast member of the eighth-grade play, a seventeen-year-old high school senior, a twenty-six-year-old applying for a job, and a young parent naming his or her own babies. You may be naming an executive, a senator, a professor, or a professional athlete. You may be choosing a name for a grandfather, an eighty-five-year-

old who does water aerobics, and, finally, a tombstone or memorial wall. Try to pick a name that works well in all stages of life.

Consider the order in which you'll choose names.

For most people, the last name of the baby is the easiest to determine. Many people then begin discussions on the first name, leaving the middle slot available for compromises, second choices, and so on.

Get everything out front in the beginning.

"I'm thinking we might name our son Sean,*" says an expectant father.*

"Never!" replies the mother-to-be. "One of my ex-boyfriends was a Sean. There's no way we can use that name."

It helps to get everything on the table at the beginning of the naming process.

Before deciding which name you want, it may be easier to decide which ones you don't want. List any names you cannot abide: those of ex-boyfriends and ex-girlfriends, relatives you detest, and so on. If one of your families has a naming tradition that you want to follow, bring that up as well. If you or your partner comes from a particular ethnic or religious group, do you want the name to reflect that background? Do you want to give each other an automatic veto on names, or do you want to allow one person to try to convince the other? This all sounds obvious enough, but a father who approaches parenthood with the thought that his baby boy is going to be Thurston Howell IV needs to know right away if his partner wants a name unique to that child.

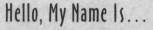

How much advice will you tolerate from relatives?

Whether or not your relatives express opinions about the name of the newest family member, believe us—they will have opinions. You cannot control this. But you *can* control the degree to which your parents and other family members get involved in the naming decision. It's a good idea to decide at the start which relatives, if any, you wish to consult with, and which ones to avoid.

It goes without saying that the people whose advice you want least are the ones with the most strident opinions. These are the same folks who ask, "How much weight have you gained?" and who delight in telling birthing-room horror stories. A couple must stand together against the efforts of others to name their baby. Don't ever blame your partner to avoid offending a family member. You have to stick together to get the name you want.

A good way to avoid arguments with relatives is never to tell them the name you have chosen before the birth. Tell them you're still deciding, and change the subject. When the child is born, put the name you have chosen on the birth certificate, and the deed is done. Relatives might gripe, but by then it is too late.

Should you use a family name?

If you want to honor your family in naming your child, consider casting a wide net for names. If a relative has collected genealogical information about your family, get copies of the documents. Talk to older relatives who can give you the names of their cousins or other family members you might not know. You may find a wonderful name that is already in your family.

Some parents honor a family member by using the initial letter of his or her name. For instance, you could take *E* from *Eliot* and use it in *Evan.* Your grandfather Eliot might wish you had chosen his name, but he will take some comfort in knowing that you were thinking of him in using that first letter.

Junior or Mini-Me?

Some couples choose to give their firstborn son the same name as his father, adding Junior on the end. Although this carries on the father's name and ties the two together for life, here are two thoughts to consider.

A person with the same name as his father may feel less like a distinctive individual and more like Mini-Me, the diminutive sidekick in the Austin Powers movies. Frank Sinatra, Jr., is a talented singer in his own right, but how can he ever live up to his name? If father or son ever becomes famous or infamous for any reason, the other is dragged into the spotlight as well.

Women have another reason to be leery of making their sons into Juniors. With the divorce rate in this country approaching 50 percent, a woman who gives her son her husband's name has a 50-50 chance of having to call him the name of her ex for the rest of her life.

Three or four names?

Choosing to give a baby four names can make the naming process easier; as you narrow your selection, there's one less name you have to cut. Your children will have three names from which to choose how they would like to be informally addressed. And having four names, at least in America, is distinctive.

The first President Bush has four names: *George Herbert Walker Bush.* It is interesting to note, however, that he gave his son, the second President Bush, only three names: *George Walker Bush.*

Most forms, particularly the online ones, allow for only three names. Many other forms have room only for first name, middle initial, and last name. How will your four-name offspring fill out these forms?

Test the name.

Think of all the ways a name might be used and how it will sound. Try the name out in different ways. Yell it out the back door. Use it in the following phrases:

_____, dinner is ready!

Now playing guard, _____.

This is my grandmother, _____.

All rise! Court is in session, the Honorable _____ residing.

Graduating with highest honors is_____.

And now, our headliner for the evening. Let's give a big welcome to

_____.

Is the name too popular?

Countless parents have taken a child to preschool or kindergarten only to find that two, three, or even four other children in the classroom share the child's name. The poor teacher then has to come up with a distinctive way of addressing each student, and usually winds up saying Jacob B. or Emily K. or using a child's entire last name–options that few kids like.

The Social Security Administration keeps lists of the most popular names given to babies. You can go to www.ssa.gov and search for "popular baby names." The latest listings are about a year out of date, but they still give a very good sense of the names you might want to avoid. For those with old-fashioned tastes, top-ten lists from sample years in the past century are scattered throughout this book.

Consider the tease factor.

Ask people how they were teased as a child and they can instantly tell you—the memories remain vivid. A woman named *Gabriella* acquired the nickname Gabby. In middle school, when she was mildly overweight, she was known as Flabby Gabby. The pain of that time is evident decades later.

Whereas many prospective parents, seeking to be creative, favor names that are far from the mainstream, children with odd names often just want to fit in. When you think about a name for your child, try to think how the little bullies in the fourth grade will handle it. Does it rhyme with any "bad" words or adjectives such as flabby? Is it hard to pronounce? Is it so strange that other children will laugh at it?

Should you spell it creatively?

Whether or not they choose an unusual name, some parents decide that they will bless their child with an unusual spelling. Thus, *Alice* becomes *Allyce* or *Alyce* or even *Alliss*. There are two ways of looking at this. First, giving your child a one-of-a-kind spelling will set him or her apart from others. Second, you will have condemned your child to having to spell the name aloud and correct other people's spelling of it for a lifetime. This can get old. Furthermore, some people assume that individuals with oddly spelled names come from uneducated, lower-class households in which the parents did not know the more common spelling of a name.

If you really want an offbeat spelling, a good compromise is to give your child a second name that is more conventionally spelled. Later, he or she can choose which name to use.

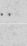

Consider the initials.

Although the days of monogrammed sweaters seem long gone, it's never a bad idea to make sure that your bambino's initials don't spell or stand for something inadvertently hilarious. Here are prime offenders: *SOB, DOG, CAT, BAD, TIT, DUD, TNT, SOS,* and *SAP.*

A girl becomes prone to wayward initials later in life if she takes her husband's last name. Giving a girl a first name beginning with a consonant and a second name beginning with a vowel is playing with fire. Just ask the Alexandra Helen Jones who married Sam Gerber.

What if you want to change the name later?

Laws vary from state to state, but generally states allow parents to make changes in their child's birth certificate for a year after birth without having to go to court. All that is needed is an affidavit from both parents—or from just one parent, if the child has only one. The birth certificate is marked as "Amended."

If it is too late to change the name with an affidavit, parents can change a child's name through a court procedure.

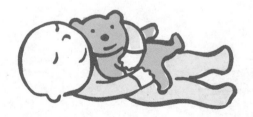

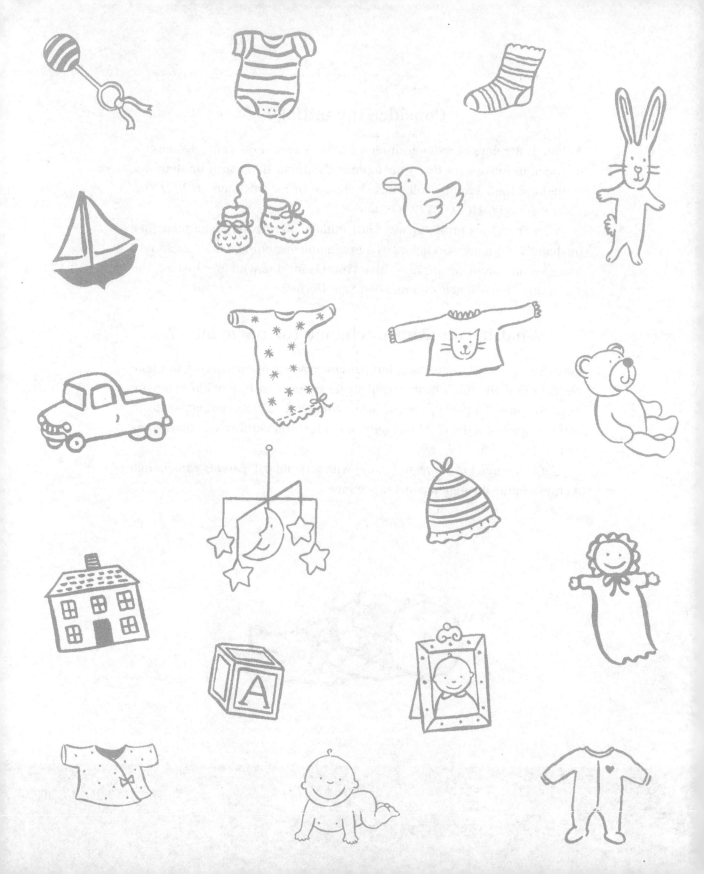

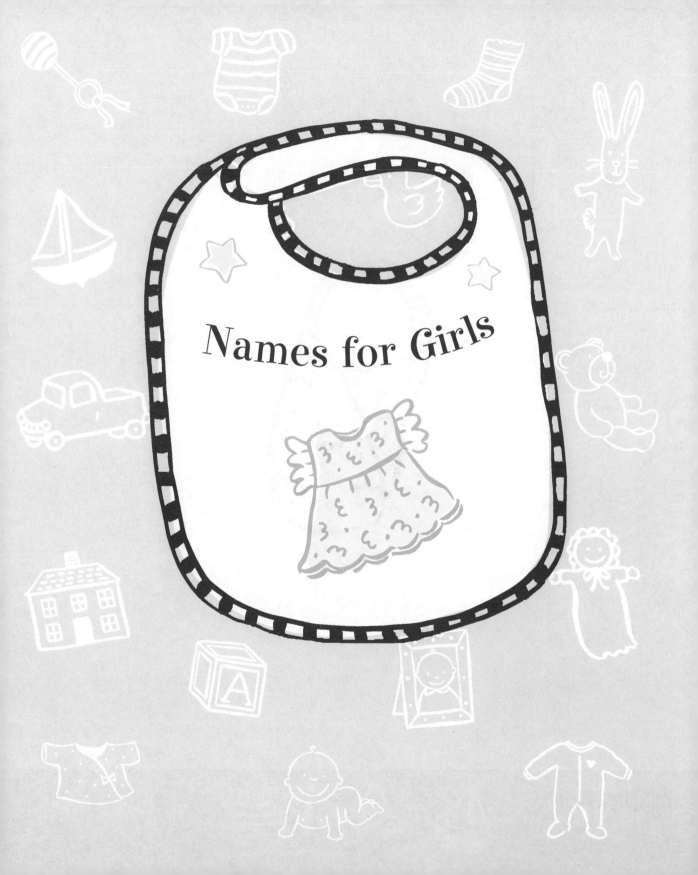

Names for Girls

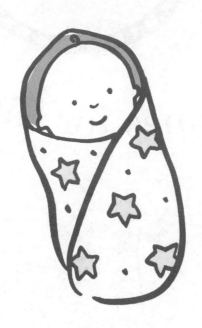

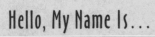 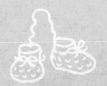

AALIYAH Arabic. "Tall, towering."

ABARRANE Basque. Feminine form of **Abraham.** Hebrew, "father of many." **Abame**

ABEBI Nigerian. "She came after asking."

ABELIA Feminine form of **Abel.** Hebrew, "sigh." **Abella, Abelle**

ABELLONA Feminine form of **Apollo.** Greek God of the sun. **Apolline** et al.

ABIA Arabic. "Great."

ABIDA Arabic, "She who worships." Hebrew, "My father knows."

ABIGAIL Hebrew. "My father is joyful." **Abagael, Abagail, Abagale, Abagil, Abaigeal, Abbe, Abbey, Abbi, Abbie, Abbigael, Abbigale, Abbigall, Abby, Abbye, Abigal, Abigael, Abigale, Abigayle, Abigil, Gail** et al.

ABIJAH Hebrew. "God is my father." **Abisha, Abishah**

ABIR Arabic. "Scent."

ABITAL Hebrew. "My father is dew." **Avital**

ABRA Feminine form of **Abraham.** Hebrew, "father of many." **Abrahana**

ABRIANA Feminine form of **Abraham.** Hebrew, "father of many." **Abrianna, Abree, Abrielle, Abrienne**

ACACIA Greek. A leguminous tree. **Cacia, Cacie, Casey** et al., **Casia, Cassie, Cassy, Kacey** et al., **Kassja, Kassy**

ACADIA Former French name for Nova Scotia.

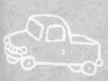

ACANTHA Greek. "Thorny."

ACCALIA Latin. The foster mother of Romulus and Remus, the founders of Rome.

ACELINE French feminine form of **Acelin**. "Highborn." **Asceline**

ACIMA Feminine form of **Acim**. Hebrew, "the Lord will judge." **Acimah, Achima, Achimah**

ADA German. "Noble." **Adan, Adda, Addi, Addiah, Addie, Addy, Adey, Adi, Adia, Adiah, Adie**

ADAH Hebrew. "Beauty." **Addah**

ADAIR Scottish. "Oak tree ford."

ADALIA Hebrew, "God is my refuge." Old German, "noble one." **Adal, Adala, Adalee, Adall, Adalie, Adalley, Addal, Addala**

ADAMINA Feminine form of **Adam**. Hebrew, "child of the red earth." **Ada, Adamine, Adaminna, Addie, Mina, Minna**

ADARA Greek, "beauty." Arabic, "virgin." **Adra**

ADDULA Teutonic. "Noble cheer."

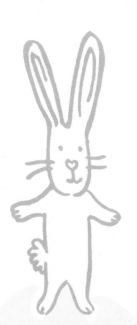

ADELAIDE Old German. "Noble." **Adal, Adale, Addala, Addalla, Addey, Addi, Addie, Addy, Adel, Adela, Adelaida, Adelais, Adele, Adelheid, Adelice, Adelicia, Adelis, Adey, Adi, Ado, Ady, Aline, Alline, Allosha, Del, Della, Delle, Delli, Deily, Heidi** et al., **Lady, Laidey**

ADELE Old German. "Noble." **Adeilah, Adelia, Adell, Adella, Adelle, Ahdella**

ADELINDA Teutonic. "Noble." **Adelind, Adelinde, Linda**

ADELINE Old German. "Noble." **Adalina, Adallina, Adelina, Aline, Dahlina, Dalina, Daline, Dallina, Delina, Deline, Dellina, Delly, Delyne, Edelie, Edeline, Eline, Lina**

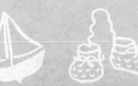

ADENA Hebrew. "Decoration." **Adene, Adina, Adinah, Denah, Dina, Dinah**

ADELPHA Greek. "Beloved sister."

ADEOLA Nigerian. "Crown." **Adola, Dola**

ADIBA Arabic. "Cultured, refined." **Adebah**

ADIELLA Hebrew. "The Lord's adornment."

ADIMA Teutonic. "Noble" or "renowned."

ADIN Hebrew. Disputed meaning. **Adeana, Adina**

ADIRA Hebrew. "Strong."

ADITI Sanskrit. "Abundance."

ADIVA Arabic. "Agreeable" or "gentle."

ADOLPHA Feminine form of **Adolph.** German, "noble wolf."

ADONCIA Spanish. "Sweet." **Doncia**

ADONIA Greek. Feminine form of **Adonis.** In myth, Adonis was a beautiful man and a lover of Venus.

ADORA Latin. "Adored." **Adorabelle, Adoray, Adore, Adorée, Adoria, Adorlee, Dora, Dori, Dorie, Dorri, Dorrie, Dorry, Dory**

ADRA Arabic. "Virgin." **Adara**

ADRIENNE French, from Latin. "From Adria," a city in northern Italy. **Adrea, Adreea, Adria, Adriah, Adriana, Adrianah, Adriane, Adrianna, Adriannah, Adrie, Adrien, Adriena, Adrienah**

AFINA Romanian. "Bilberry."

AFRA Arabic, "dust." Hebrew, "young deer." **Affera, Affery, Affra, Aphra, Aphrah, Ayfara**

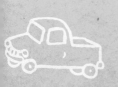

FROM BAD TO WORSE

Names that are perfectly fine in other countries or cultures sometimes cause problems when spoken in English. Such was the case with Lee Bum Suk, who was for a time the foreign minister of South Korea. When Korean officials began to notice badly concealed smirks when their leader's name was heard, they informed English speakers that the name should be pronounced "Pom Sok." This caused further problems, for Australians often refer to Brits as "poms." The problem was solved, alas, when the unfortunate Mr. Suk was blown up by a bomb planted by North Korean agents.

AFRAIMA Arabic and Hebrew. "Fertile."

AFRICA Latin. "Pleasant." **Affrica, Affrich, Affrika, Affrikah, Africah, Afrika, Afrikah, Aifric, Apirka, Apirkah**

AFTON Old English. A river in England. **Affton**

AGAPI Greek. "Love" or "affection." **Agape, Agappe**

AGATE Old French. A semiprecious stone.

AGATHA Greek. "Good." **Ag, Agace, Agafi, Agafia, Agafon, Agafta, Agapet, Agapit, Agata, Agathe, Agathi, Agatta, Aggi, Aggie, Aggy, Aggye, Agi, Agle, Agot, Agota, Agote, Agotha, Agotia, Agueda, Agy, Agye**

AGAVE Greek. "Illustrious" or "noble."

AGLAIA Greek. "Brilliant." **Aglae**

AGNES Greek. "Pure" or "virginal." **Ag, Aggi, Aggie, Aggye, Aghna, Agi, Agie, Agna, Agnah, Agnella, Agnellah, Agnelle, Agnesa, Agnese, Agnesse, Agneta, Agnetta, Agnettah, Agnola, Agnolah, Agy, Agye, Aignels, Aina, Ainah, Anals, Annals, Anneyce, Annis, Annisa, Annisah, Annise, Ina,**

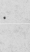

Inah, Inez et al., Ness, Nessa, Nessah, Nessie, Nessy, Nest, Nests, Nevsa, Nevesah, Neysa, Senga, Sengassa

AGNOLA Italian. "Angel." Agnoila, Agnolle

AGRAFINA Variant of Agrippa. Latin, "born feet first."

AGRIPPA Latin. "Born feet first." Agrafina, Agrippina, Agrippine

AHARONA Hebrew. Feminine form of Aaron. Hebrew, "exalted." Ahronit, Arni, Arnina, Arninit, Arona

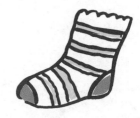

AHAVA Hebrew. "Loved one." Ahuda, Ahuva

AHIMSA Hindi. "Virtuous."

AHULANI Hawaiian. "Heavenly shrine."

AIBHLIN Irish variant of Helen. Greek, "bright one."

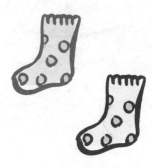

AIDA Old French. "To help." Aidan, Iraida, Zaida, Zenaida, Zoraida

A'IDA Arabic. "Guest" or "one who is returning."

AIDAN Irish. "Fire." Adan, Aden, Aiden

AIDEE Greek. "Modest." Aydee

AIKO Japanese. "Loved one."

AIFE Irish. In myth, the warrior queen of Alba with whom the hero Cuchulain had a son. Aoife

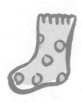

AILBHE Irish. "Noble" or "bright." Alvy, Elva et al.

AILEEN Scottish variant of Helen. Greek, "light." Ails, Ailee, Ailene, Ailey, Ailie, Ailli, Aleen, Alene, Aline, Alleen, Allene, Alline, Ilene et al., Lena et al.

AILITH Old English. "Seasoned warrior." Aldith

AILSA Scottish. "Pledge from God." Ailse, Elsa, Elsha, Elshe

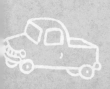

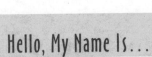

AIMÉE French. "Beloved." **Amy** et al.

AINA Scandinavian. "Forever."

AINE Celtic. "Happiness."

AINSLEY Scottish. "One's own meadow." **Ainslee, Ainsleigh, Ainslie, Ansley, Aynslee, Aynsley, Aynslie**

AIRLEA Greek. "Ethereal." **Airlia**

AISHA Arabic, "woman." Swahili, "life." The favorite wife of the Prophet Mohammed. **Aeesha, Aeeshah, Aesha, Aeshah, Aesiah, Aiesha, Aieshah, Aishah, Aisia, Aisiah, Asha, Ashah, Ashia, Asia, Asiah, Ayeesa, Ayeesah, Ayeesha, Ayeeshah, Ayeisa, Ayeisah, Ayeisha, Ayisa, Ayisah, Ayisha, Ayishah, Ieesha** et al., **Ylesha, Yleshah**

AISLINN Irish. "Dream." **Aisling, Ashlan, Ashlen, Ashling, Isleen**

AITHNE Feminine form of **Aidan.** Irish, "fire." **Aithnea, Eithne** et al., **Ena** et al.

AIYANA Native American. "Eternal blossom."

AKASMA Turkish. "White rose."

AKELA Hawaiian. "Noble."

AKILINA Greek, Russian. "Eagle." **Acquilina, Aquilina**

AKIKO Japanese. "Iris."

AKILA Arabic. "Smart." **Akili**

AKIVA Hebrew. "Shelter." **Kiba, Kibah, Kiva, Kivah, Kivi**

ALAIA Arabic. "Sublime."

ALAINE French feminine form of **Alan.** Irish, "rock."

ALALA Greek. "War goddess."

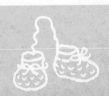

ALAMEA Hawaiian. "Precious."

ALANNA Feminine form of **Alan.** Irish, "rock." **Alaine, Alaina, Alana, Alannah, Alayna, Alayne, Aleine, Alenne, Aleyna, Aleynah, Aleyne, Alleen, Alleine, Allena, Allene, Alleynah, Alleyne, Allina, Allinah, Allyn, Lana** et al.

ALANZA Feminine form of **Alonzo.** Old German, "ready for battle."

ALAQUA Native American. "Sweet gum tree."

ALARICE Feminine form of **Alaric.** Old German, "noble king." **Alarica**

ALASTAIR Scottish feminine form of **Alexander.** Greek, "man's defender." **Alasdair**

ALAULA Hawaiian. "Light of daybreak."

ALBA Latin. "Dawn" or "white." Also a city in northwest Italy. **Albinia** et al., **Alva** et. al.

ALBERGA Latin, "white." Old German, "noble." **Alberge**

ALBERTA Feminine form of **Albert.** Old English, "brilliant." **Alberthine, Albertina, Albertine, Ali, Alit, Allie, Ally, Auberta, Auberte, Aubertha, Auberthe, Berrie, Berry, Bert, Berta, Berte, Berti, Bertie, Berty, Elberta** et al.

ALBINIA Latin, "white." **Alba** et al., **Albina, Alvina, Aubine**

ALBREDA Feminine form of **Aubrey.** Old German, "counsel from the elves."

ALCESTIS Greek. In myth, Alcestis gave her life for her husband.

ALCINA Greek. "Strong-minded." **Alcie, Alcine, Alcinia, Allcine, Allcinia, Alseena, Alsina, Alsyna, Alzina, Elsie**

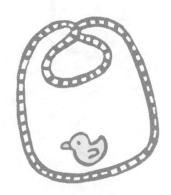

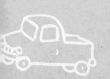

ALDA Feminine form of **Aldo.** Old German, "old." **Aldabella, Aldas, Aldea, Aldina, Aldine, Aldona, Aldonna, Aldya, Aldyne, Aldys, Allda, Alldina, Alldine, Alldona, Alldonna, Alldyne, Aude, Auld**

ALDARA Greek. "Winged gift."

ALDIS Old English. "Battle-seasoned." **Aldith, Allith**

ALEENA Arabic. "Silk of heaven." Also variant of **Alina.**

ALEEZA Hebrew. "Joy." **Aleezah, Aleezah, Alieza, Alista, Aliza, Alizah**

ALEGRIA Spanish. "Joy." **Allegria**

ALENA Variant of **Helen.** Greek, "light."

ALEPH Feminine form of **Aluph.** Hebrew, "leader." **Alufa, Alupha**

ALERIA Latin. "Eagle."

ALESHA Arabic. "Protected by God."

ALESIA Greek. "Help."

ALETA Greek. "Footloose." **Aletta, Alette, Alletta, Allette, Lettee, Lettie, Letty**

ALETHEA Greek. "Truth." **Alathia, Aleethia, Aleta, Aletea, Aletha, Alethia, Alithea, Alithia, Olethea** et al.

ALEXANDRA Feminine form of **Alexander.** Greek, "man's defender." **Alastrina, Alastriona, Alejanda, Alejandra, Alejandrina, Aleka, Aleki, Alesandare, Alesandere, Alessa, Alessanda, Alessandra, Alessandre, Alessandrina, Alessandrine, Alessi, Alessia, Alexandere, Alexanderia, Alexanderina, Alexanderine, Alexandre, Alexandrea, Alexandreana, Alexandrena, Alexandrene, Alexandretta, Alexandria, Alexandrina, Alexandrine, Alexea, Alexena, Alexene, Alexia, Alexina, Alexine, Alexis** et al., **Ali, Aliki,**

Naming for success?

In a study entitled "Are Emily and Brendan More Employable than Lakisha and Jamal?," researchers from the University of Chicago and MIT used names to measure the extent of race-based discrimination in the labor market in 2001 and 2002.

In the study, four resumes each were sent in response to more than 1,300 employment ads in Chicago and Boston newspapers. Half of the resumes had black-sounding names, among them *Latonya, Tyrone, Keisha,* and *Rasheed,* matched with surnames common among blacks, such as *Jones* or *Washington.* The other resumes—with the same level of qualifications—bore more white-sounding names, such as *Sarah, Allison, Neil,* or *Todd,* attached to last names such as *Walsh* or *Baker.*

The results? The fictitious prospective employees with white-sounding names were 50 percent more likely to be called in for initial interviews than those with black-sounding names. This means that job applicants who have white-sounding names have to send out only ten resumes to get a call, on average, while those with black-sounding names need to send fifteen resumes for the same result.

Is this a reason to avoid giving children black- or other ethnic-sounding names? Not according to the authors of the study. "Names are about identity," said Marianne Bertrand, a professor at the University of Chicago Graduate School of Business. "We do not advocate changing names to fit the system, and that is certainly not the point of our study."

Black parents who commented on the study had a range of reactions. Some claimed that, since blacks and other minorities will be discriminated against anyway, they should name their children whatever they want. Others said that the study underscores the wisdom of giving black children more conventional names, or, if parents want to honor their African-American heritage, of making the middle name the distinctive one.

Alissandre, Alissandrine, Alista, Alix et al., Alle, Allejandra, Allejandrina, Allessa, Allessandra, Allexandra, Allexandrina, Allexina, Allexine, Alit, Allie, Ally, Anda, Lesy, Lesya, Lexia et al., Ritsa, Sanda, Sande, Sandra et al., Sandrina, Sandrine, Sandy et al., Sasha et al., Shura, Shurochka, Sohndra, Sondra, Xandra, Zandra et al.

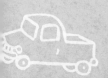

ALEXIS Greek. "Man's defender." **Alexa, Alexi, Alexia, Lexia** et al.

ALGOMA Native American. "Valley of flowers."

ALFONSINE Feminine form of **Alphonse.** Old German, "noble and ready for battle." **Alfonsia, Alonza, Alphonsine**

ALFREDA Feminine form of **Alfred.** Old English, "elf power." **Alfi, Alfie, Alfre, Alfredah, Alfredda, Alfreeda, Alfri, Alfried, Alfrieda, Alfryda, Allfie, Allfreda** et al., **Allfrie, Allfry, Elfrida** et al., **Freda** et al.

ALIA Hebrew. "Settler." **Alea, Aleah, Aliyah**

ALICE Old German. "Noble" or "nobility." **Adelice, Ailis, Ala, Alecia, Aleethia, Ali, Alica, Alicah, Alicea, Alicia, Alidde, Alika, Alikah, Aliki, Alis, Alisa, Alisah, Alisha, Alison** et al., **Alissa** et al., **Alitheea, Alitia, Aliz, Aliza, Alizz, Alla, Allecia, Alleece, Alles, Alless, Alli, Allice, Allicea, Allie, Allis, Ally, Allyce, Allyceea, Allys, Allyse, Allysia, Allysiah, Alyce, Alyceea, Alys, Alyse, Alysia, Alyss, Elissa** et al., **Elli, Ellie, Ellsa, Elsa, Illyssa, Ilysa, Ilysah, Ilyssa, Ilysse, Leece, Leese, Lissa, Lyssa**

ALIDA Latin. "Winged one." **Alaida, Aleda, Aleta, Aletta, Alette, Alidah, Alidia, Alita, Alldyne, Alleda, Allida, Allidah, Allidia, Allidiah, Allyda, Allydah, Alyda, Alydah, Dela, Della, Dila, Dills, Elida, Elita, Leda, Ledah, Lida, Lidah, Lita, Lyda, Lydah, Oleda, Oleta, Oletta, Olette**

ALIKA Nigerian. "Beautiful."

ALIMA Arabic. "Cultured."

ALINA Variant of **Helen.** Greek, "light." Arabic, "beautiful." **Aleen, Aleena, Alena, Alenah, Alene, Aline, Alleen, Allen, Alline, Allyna, Allynah, Allyne, Alyna, Alynah, Alyne, Lena** et al.

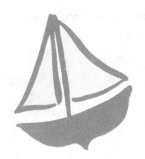

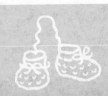

ALISA Hebrew. "Great happiness." Also variant of **Alice. Aleeza** et al., **Alisah, Alissa, Alissah, Aliza, Allisa, Allisah, Allissa, Allissah, Allysa, Allysah, Alyssa, Alyssah**

ALISHA Arabic. "Honest, truthful."

ALISON Variant of **Alice.** Old German, "noble" or "nobility." **Alicen, Alisann, Alisanne, Alisoun, Alisun, Allcen, Allcenne, Allicen, Allicenne, Allie, Allisann, Allisanne, Allison, Allisoun, Allisun, Allisunne, Allsun, Ally, Allysann, Allysanne, Allyson, Allysoun, Allysson, Alysan, Alysann, Alysanne, Alyson, Alysoun**

ALIX Old German. "Noble." Also short form of **Alexandra. Alex, Alexa, Allexa, Allix**

ALIYA Arabic. "Highborn." **Aliyah, Aliye**

ALIZA Arabic. The daughter of Prophet Ali.

ALLEGRA Italian. "Joyous." **Alegra, Legra, Leggra**

ALLENA Feminine form of **Allen, Alan.** Irish, "rock." **Alana, Alanna, Alena, Alene, Allene, Alleyne, Allynn, Allynne, Alynne**

ALLONIA Feminine form of **Alon.** Hebrew, "oak tree." **Allona, Alona, Alonia**

ALLYRIANE French, from Greek. "Lyre."

ALMA Latin, "giving nurture." Italian, Spanish, "soul." Arabic, "learned." **Allma, Almah, Aluma, Alumit, Elma**

ALMARINE Old German. "Work ruler." **Almeria**

ALMEDA Latin. "Ambitious." **Allmeda, Allmedah, Allmeta, Allmetah, Allmida, Allmidah, Allmita, Allmitah, Almedah, Almeta, Almetah, Almida, Almidah, Almita, Almitah**

ALMERA Feminine form of **Elmer.** Arabic, "aristocratic."

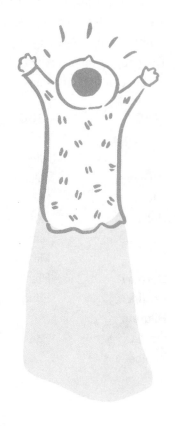

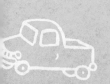

Cooking up names

The Pillsbury BAKE-OFF® is a challenge to amateur cooks to create original recipes for tasty dishes using one of a variety of the sponsor's products. The first names of the grand-prize winners through the years give a glimpse into the lives of the homemakers who cranked out dishes from No-Knead Water-Rising Twists, the first winner, all the way to 2004's Oats 'n Honey Granola Pie. The contest ran every year from 1949 through 1980, when it moved to a biennial schedule—hence the smaller lists of names from that year forward.

1949	1960s	1970s	1980s	2000s
Theodora	Leona	Nan	Millicent	Roberta
	Alice	Pearl	Elizabeth	Denise
1950s	Julia	Rose	Susan	Suzanne
Lily	Mira	Isabelle	Mary Lou	
Helen	Janis	Albina	Julie	
Beatrice	Mari	Bonnie		
Lois	Maxine	Francis	**1990s**	
Dorothy	Phyllis	Doris	Linda	
Bertha	Edna	Barbara	Gladys	
Hildreth		Luella	Mary Anne	
Gerda		Lois Ann	Kurt	
Eunice -		Lenora	Ellie	
		Esther		
		Linda		

BAKE-OFF® is a registered trademark of General Mills and is used here with permission.

Allmeera, Allmera, Allmeria, Almeera, Almeeria, Almeria, Almira, Almirah, Almire, Almyra, Elmira et al., **Meera** et al., **Mira** et al.

ALMINA Variant of **Elmina**, short form of **Wilhemina.** Old German, "Will-helmet." **Almeena, Almena**

ALMITA Latin. "Kind" or "caring."

ALODIE Old English. "Affluent." **Alodi**

ALMODINE Latin. "Precious stone."

ALOHA Hawaiian. "Love," "kindness," or "affection."

ALOISIA Feminine form of **Aloysius**. Old German, "famous fighter." **Aloisa, Aloise, Alouse, Aloys, Aloyse, Aloysia**

ALONA Hebrew. "Oak tree." **Allona, Allonia, Alonia**

ALONSA Feminine form of **Alonso**. Spanish, from Old German, "ready for battle." **Alonza**

ALPHA Greek. "First." **Alfa**

ALPHONSINE Feminine form of **Alphonse**. French, from Old German, "ready for battle." **Alfonsine** et al., **Alphonsina, Alphonzina, Alphonzine**

ALTA Latin. "Raised." **Allta, Altai**

ALTAIR Arabic. "Bird."

ALTHEA Greek. "Healthy." **Altha, Althala, Althia, Eltha, Elthea, Thea**

ALTHEDA Greek. "Like a blossom."

ALULA Arabic. "First."

ALURA Old English. "Divine adviser." **Allura, Alurea**

ALVA Variant of **Alba**. Latin, "dawn," "white." **Alba, Albinia** et al., **Alvah, Alvia**

ALVAR Old English. "Army of elves."

ALVERDINE Old English. "Counsel from the elves."

ALVINA Feminine form of **Alvin**. Old English, "of the elves." **Alveena, Alveene, Alveenia, Alvine, Alvineea, Alvinia, Alwinna, Alwyna, Alwyne, Elvina** et al., **Vina** et al.

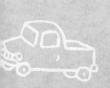

ALVITA Latin. "Lively."

ALYSIA Greek. "Entrancing."

ALYSSUM Greek. "Sane." Also a low-growing flowering plant. **Ilyssa, Lyssa**

ALZENA Persian. "Woman." **Alzeena, Alzina**

AMA Cherokee. "Water."

AMABEL Latin. "Lovable." **Ama, Amabell, Amabelle, Amabil, Amabilia, Amabilis, Amabilla, Amable, Amiable, Bel, Belle, Mabel** et al.

AMADA Latin. "Beloved." **Amadis, Amata**

AMADEA Feminine form of **Amadeus**. Latin, "God's beloved." **Amadée, Amedee**

AMADORE Italian. "Gift of love." **Amadora**

AMALA Arabic. "Hope." **Amahla**

AMALIA Hebrew. "God's word." Also a variant of **Amelia**. **Amaliah, Amalthea, Mali, Malia, Malika**

AMALIDA Old German. "Hardworking woman."

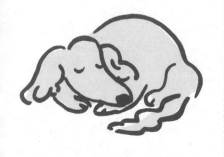

AMANDA Latin. "Much-loved." **Amandie, Amandine, Amandy, Manda, Mandaline, Mandy** et al.

AMANDLA African. "Power."

AMAPOLA Arabic. "Poppy."

AMARA Greek. "Lovely forever." **Amargo, Amargoe, Amargot, Amarinda, Amarra, Amarrinda, Mara, Marra**

AMARANTHA Greek. "Deathless." **Amarande, Amaranta, Amarante**

AMARIS Hebrew. "Pledged by God." **Amariah**

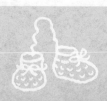

AMARYLLIS Greek. "Fresh." Also a bulbous perennial plant with showy flowers.

AMAYA Japanese. "Night rain."

AMBER Old French. "Amber." **Ambar, Amberetta, Amberly, Ambur**

AMBIKA Hindi. "Mother."

AMBROSINE Feminine form of **Ambrose.** Greek, "immortal." **Ambrosia, Ambrosina, Ambrosinetta, Ambrosinette, Ambrosiya, Ambrozetta, Ambrozia, Ambrozine**

AMELIA Old German, "hard-working." Arabic, "trustworthy" or "beautiful." **Aimiliona, Amalea, Amalee, Amaleta, Amalia, Amalie, Amalija, Amalina, Amaline, Amalita, Amaliya, Amalya, Amalyna, Amalyne, Amalyta, Amelie, Amelina, Ameline, Amelita, Ameliya, Amelyna, Amelyne, Amelyta, Amilia, Amy, Emeline** et al., **Emelita, Mali, Malia, Malika, Meline, Millie, Milly**

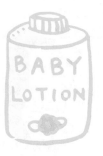

AMÉLIE French variant of **Amelia.** Old German, "hard-working." Also the name of a popular movie (2001) and its main character.

AMELINDA Spanish. Combination of **Amada** and **Linda.**

AMERICA Feminine form of **Amerigo.** Italian, from Old German, "home ruler."

AMETHYST Greek. Semi-precious wine-red jewel.

AMICA Latin. "Friend." **Amice**

AMILIA Latin. "Amiable."

AMINA Arabic. "Honest." **Aminah**

AMINTA Latin. "Protector." **Amynta, Minta, Minty**

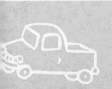

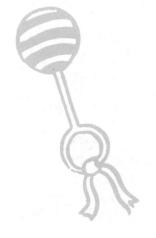

AMIRA Arabic. "Princess." **Ameera, Ameerah, Amera, Amerah, Amirah, Amyra, Amyrah, Meera** et al., **Mira** et al.

AMISA Hebrew. "Companion, friend." **Amissa**

AMITA Hebrew, "truth." Italian, "friendship."

AMITOLA Native American. "Rainbow."

AMITY Latin. "Friendship." **Amitie**

AMOR Spanish. "Love."

AMORETTE French. "Sweetheart."

AMY Latin. "Beloved." **Aimée, Aimey, Aimie, Amecia, Amey, Ami, Amia, Amiah, Amice, Amie, Amh, Amii, Ammie, Amye**

ANA Spanish variant of **Ann.** Hebrew, "grace." **Anita** et al.

ANAMOSA Sauk (Native American). "White fawn."

ANASTASIA Greek. "Resurrection." **Anastaise, Anastas, Anastase, Anastasie, Anastasija, Anastasiya, Anastassia, Anastay, Anasztaizia, Anasztasia, Anestassia, Anstass, Anstice, Asia, Nastasia** et al., **Nestia, Stacia, Stacy** et al., **Stasa, Stasiya, Stasya, Tansy** et al., **Tasenka, Tasha** et al.

ANATOLA Greek. "From the east."

ANDRA Old Norse. "Breath." **Anda, Andria**

ANDREA Feminine form of **Andrew.** Greek, "manly." **Aindrea, Andee, Andere, Anderea, Andi, Andie, Andra, Andre, Andreana, Andreas, Andree, Andreea, Andrei, Andresa, Andrewena, Andrewina, Andri, Andria, Andriana, Andy, Aundrea, Ondrea** et al.

ANDROMEDA Greek. In myth, an Ethiopian princess rescued from a sea monster by Perseus.

ANEMONE Greek. "Wind flower." **Ann-Aymone, Anne-Aymone**

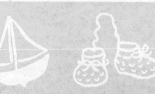

ANGAHARD Welsh. "Greatly loved." **Anchoret, Anchoretta, Ancret, Ancreta, Ancrett, Angharad, Ankerita, Ingaret, Ingaretta**

ANGELA Greek. "Messenger" or "angel." **Aingeal, Ange, Angel, Angele, Angeleta, Angelica** et al., **Angelina, Angeline, Angelita, Angelle, Angellina, Angie, Angil, Angiola, Angy, Angyola, Anjel, Anjela, Anngela, Anngil, Anngilla, Anngiola, Annjela, Gelya**

ANGELICA Latin. "Angelic." **Angelika, Algeliki, Angelique, Angyalka, Anjelica, Anjelika**

ANISAH Arabic. "Friendly." **Annissa**

ANITA Diminutive of **Ana.** Spanish, from Hebrew, "grace." **Anitra, Annita, Annitra, Annitta**

ANN Hebrew. "Grace." **Aine, Ana, Anci, Anechka, Ania, Anica, Anika, Aniko, Anissa, Anita** et al., **Anka, Anke, Anki, Anna, Annata, Anne, Annelle, Annelore, Annette** et al., **Anni, Annice, Annick, Annie, Annimae, Annina, Annora, Annuska, Anny, Anona, Anouche, Anouk, Anoushka, Anouska, Antje, Anushka, Anuska, Anya, Anyoushka, Anyshka, Anyu, Asya, Ayn, Hajna, Hanja, Hanka, Hannah** et al., **Hanneke, Hannelore, Nan** et al., **Nancy** et al., **Nanette** et al., **Netty** et al., **Nina, Ninette, Ninon, Ninor, Nita, Nona, Nonie**

ANNABELLE Combination of **Anne** and **Belle. Anabel, Anabela, Anabella, Anabelle, Anabill, Anabille, Anabul, Annabel, Annabell, Annabella, Annable, Annaple**

ANNABELINDA Combination of **Anna** and **Belinda.**

ANNAMARIA Combination of **Ann** and **Maria. Annamarie, Annemarie, Annmaria, Annmarie, AnnMarie**

ANNATA Italian variant of **Ann.** Hebrew, "grace."

Interview with the novelist

Anne Rice, whose literary character Lestat became the second-most famous vampire in the fictional world, has an interesting name story of her own. Her parents named her *Howard Allen O'Brien,* according to her Web site, www.annerice.com. She chose the name *Anne* herself when she was a young child.

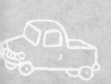

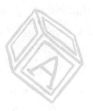

ANNELISE Combination of **Ann** and **Liese**. **Analeisa, Analiesa, Analiese, Analise, Anelisa, Anelise, Annaleisa, Annalie, Analiesa, Annaliese, Annalise, Anneliese, Annelisa**

ANNEMAE Combination of **Ann** and **Mae**. **Annamae, Annamay, Anemie**

ANNETTE Diminutive of **Ann**. Hebrew, "grace." **Anet, Anett, Anetta, Annetta**

ANNINA Variant of **Ann**. Hebrew, "grace." **Nina**

ANNIS Greek. "Completed." **Anissa, Annes, Annice, Annissa, Annys**

ANNORA Variant of **Honora**. Latin, "honor." **Anora, Anorah, Onora** et al.

ANNUNCIATA Latin. "Messenger." **Anonciada, Annunziate, Anunciacion, Anunciata, Anunziata, Nunciata, Nunzia**

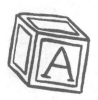

ANNOT Hebrew. "Light."

ANONNA Latin. "Born of the harvest." **Anona, Nona**

ANSELMA Feminine form of **Anselm**. Old German, "godly helmet." **Aselma, Aselmah, Selma, Sellma, Selmah, Zelma**

ANSONIA Feminine form of **Anson**. English, "son of Andrew."

ANTHEA Greek. "Flowery." **Annthea, Anthe, Anthia, Antia, Thia**

ANTHEMIA Greek. "In bloom." **Antheemia, Anthemya, Anthymia**

ANTJE German variant of **Ann**. Hebrew, "grace."

ANTIGONE Greek. In myth, the daughter of Oedipus; she accompanied him on his travels.

ANTOINETTE French feminine form of **Anthony**. Latin, "beyond price." **Antonetta, Antonia** et al., **Antonietta,**

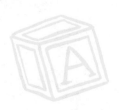

Netta, Netti, Nettie, Netty, Toinette, Tonechka, Tonette, Toni et al.

ANTONIA Feminine form of **Anthony.** Latin, "beyond price." **Antoinette** et al., **Antonie, Antonina, Antonine, Toni** et al., **Tonia, Tonie, Tony, Tonya, Tonye**

ANWEN Welsh "Very fair." **Anwyn**

ANWAR Arabic. "Light."

APHRA Hebrew. "Dust." **Affery, Afra**

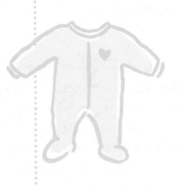

APOLLINE Feminine form of **Apollo.** Greek god of the sun. **Abbelina, Abbeline, Abellona, Appolinia, Apollonia, Apollyne, Apolonia** St. Apolonia.

APONI Native American. "Butterfly."

APRIL Latin. "Opening up." **Aprilete, Averel, Averell, Averil, Averill, Averyl, Averyll, Averylle, Avril, Avrril**

AQUILINA Feminine form of **Aquilino.** Spanish, "little eagle."

ARA Arabic. "Brings rain." **Ari, Aria, Arria**

ARABELLA Latin. "Answered prayer." **Ara, Arabel, Arabela, Arabele, Arabelle, Arbel, Arbela, Arbella, Arbelle, Bel, Bella, Belle, Orabel, Orabella, Orabelle, Orbel, Orbella, Orbelle**

ARACHNE Greek. "Spider." In myth, a peasant girl who wove so beautifully that she angered the goddess Minerva, who turned her into a spider. **Aranxe**

ARAM Persian. "Calm."

ARAMINTA Combination of **Arabella** and **Aminta.**

ARCADIA Greek. A pastoral region of ancient Greece regarded as a rural paradise. **Arcadie, Arkadia**

ARCELIA Spanish. "Treasure chest."

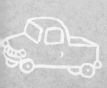

Hunting Season

Donna Devereux lives in Blowing Rock, North Carolina.

"I always liked the name *Elizabeth,* but my last name was *Taylor*, and I couldn't have a little girl named *Elizabeth Taylor*. When I was pregnant, I was watching a movie on television, and one of the actors was Season Hubley. I instantly liked the name. I wanted my daughter to have an usual name, and this one sounded just right.

"I waited until my daughter was born to see if she looked like a Season. She did, and so she got the name. For a middle name, I gave her *Marie*, so that if she later thought *Season* was too weird she would have a 'normal' name to use. She sometimes had a hard time when she was little, for teachers would think that she was trying to say *Susan,* but she got through that period and still goes by *Season*.

"Season's name helped an old friend of mine find me by Googling her. If I had named her Elizabeth Taylor, he would have gotten a million hits. By hunting Season, he got in touch with me."

ARDA Hebrew. "Bronze." **Ardah, Ardath**

ARDELLE Latin. "Burning with enthusiasm." **Arda, Ardelia, Ardelis, Ardella, Ardia, Ardis, Ardra**

ARDEN Latin. "Burning with enthusiasm." **Ardeen, Ardena, Ardene, Ardenia, Ardin, Ardine**

ARDITH Variant of **Edith.** Old English, "prosperity."

ARELLA Hebrew. "Messenger from God." **Arela**

ARETE Greek. "Woman of virtue." **Arethusa, Aretina, Aretta, Arette, Aritha, Oretta** et al.

ARETHUSA Greek. In myth, a hunter and follower of Artemis whose goddess changed her into a sacred spring. **Aretha, Aritha**

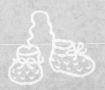

AREZOU Persian. "Desire."

ARGENTA Latin. "Silver."

ARIA Italian. "Melody."

ARIADNE Greek. "Holy one." In myth, Ariadne helped Theseus find the way out of the labyrinth. **Arene, Ariadna, Ariana, Ariane, Arianie, Arianna, Aryana, Aryane, Aryanie, Aryanna, Aryanne**

ARIANA Welsh, "like silver." Arabic, "full of life." **Ariane**

ARIEL Hebrew. "Lioness of God." The main character in Disney's *Little Mermaid.* **Aeriel, Aeriela, Aeriell, Ariell, Arielle**

ARINA Variant of **Irene.** Greek, "peace."

ARISTA Greek. "The best."

ARLENE Irish. "Pledge." **Arla, Arlana, Arlee, Arleen, Arlen, Arlena, Arlette** et al., **Arleyne, Arlie, Arliene, Arlina, Arlinda, Arline, Arluene, Arly, Arlyn, Arlyne, Arlynn, Lena, Lene, Lina**

ARLETTE French variant of **Arlene.** Irish, "Pledge." **Arlet, Arleta, Arletta**

ARLEY Variant of **Harley.** Old English, "long meadow." **Arlea, Arlee, Arleigh**

ARLISE Feminine form of **Arliss.** Hebrew, "pledge." **Arlyss**

ARMANI A contemporary fashion label.

ARMIDA Latin. "Armed one."

ARMILLA Latin. "Bracelet."

ARMINA Old German, "fighting maid." **Armantine, Armine, Arminie, Armyne**

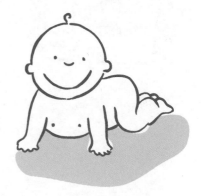

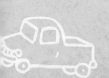

ARNALDA Feminine form of **Arnold.** Old German, "strength of an eagle."

ARNINA Feminine form of **Aaron.** Hebrew, "exalted." **Arona**

ARTEMIS Greek. Goddess of the hunt.

ARTHURETTA Feminine form of **Arthur.** Scottish, "rock." **Arthurina, Arthurine, Artice, Artina, Artis, Artrice**

ARUNA Hindi. "Dawn light."

ARVA Latin. "Countryside." **Arvella, Arvelle, Arvilla**

ASAKO Japanese. "Child of sunrise."

ASENATH Egyptian. "Owned by."

ASENCIÓN Spanish. "Ascension (into heaven)." **Asunción**

ASHANTI Ashanti. "Thank you." A West African people and former kingdom. **Asante, Ashanta, Ashante, Ashantee, Ashaunta, Ashaunte, Ashauntee, Ashaunti, Ashuntae**

ASHIRA Hebrew. "Rich."

ASHLEY Old English. "Ash-tree meadow." **Ashely, Ashlee, Ashleigh, Ashli, Ashlie, Ashly**

ASIA Contemporary American, from Greek. The continent. **Asiah**

ASIMA Arabic. "Guardian."

ASOKA Hindi. "Happy tree." **Ashok, Ashoka**

ASPASIA Greek. "Welcoming." **Spase**

ASPHODEL Greek. "Lily."

ASTA Greek. "Star."

ASTRA Latin. "Star." **Asters, Asteria, Astraea, Astrea, Astria**

ASTRID Old Norse. "Beautiful like a god." **Assi, Astrud, Astryr, Atti**

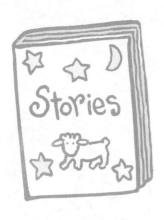

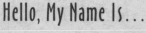

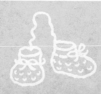

ASUNCIÓN Spanish. "Ascension (into heaven)." **Asención**

ATALANTA Feminine form of **Atlas.** Greek, "immovable."
Atlanta, Atlante

ATARA Hebrew. "Diadem," an ornamental headband. **Atera, Ateret**

ATHALIA Hebrew. "The Lord is exalted." **Atalee, Atalia, Atalie,
Athalee, Athalie**

ATHANASIA Feminine form of **Athanasius.** Greek, "immortal."

ATHENA Greek goddess of wisdom. **Athenais, Athene, Athie,
Attie**

ATIDA Hebrew. "The future."

ATIFA Arabic. "Empathy" or "affection."

AUBREY Old French. "Elf ruler." **Aubary, Aubery, Aubree,
Aubrette, Aubry, Aubury**

AUDA Old French. "Prosperous." **Aud, Aude**

AUDREY Old English. "Noble strength." **Audi, Audie, Audra,
Audre, Audree, Audreen, Audria, Audry, Audrye**

AUDRIS Old German. "Lucky."

AUGUSTA Feminine form of **Augustus.** Latin, "worthy of
respect." **Auguste, Augustina, Augustine, Augustyna,
Augustyne, Austina, Austine, Austyna, Austyne, Gus,
Gussie, Gusta, Gustel, Tina**

AUMI Japanese. "Peace." Pronounced "ah-you-me."

AURA Greek, "soft breeze." Latin, "gold." **Aure, Aurea, Auria,
Aurika**

AURELIA Latin. "Gold." **Auralla, Aurelee, Aureliana, Aurelie,
Aurelle, Aurita, Oralie** et al.

AURIEL Latin. "Golden." **Aural, Aurel, Aureola, Aureole,
Auriol, Oriole** et al.

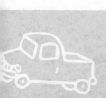

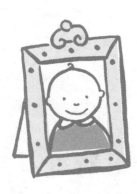

AURORA Latin. "Dawn." **Aurore, Ora, Rora, Rory** et al., **Zora, Zorica**

AUSTINE Feminine form of **Austin.** Latin, "worthy of respect."

AVA Latin. "Bird." **Avis**

AVALON Celtic. "Island of apples." In legend, the place where King Arthur's sword was forged and where he was taken after his last battle. **Avallon**

AVE Latin. "Hail."

AVENA Latin. "Field of oats."

AVICHAYIL Hebrew. "Strong father." **Abichail, Avigail**

AVIVA Hebrew. "Springlike," "fresh," or "dewy." **Avivah, Avivi, Avivit, Auvit, Viva** et al.

AXELLE Feminine form of **Axel.** Old German, "father of peace."

AYA Hebrew. "Bird." **Aiyana, Aiyanna, Ayana, Ayania, Ayanna, Ayannia, Iana, Ianna**

AYALA Basque place name.

AYESHA Persian. "Small one."

AZA Arabic. "Comfort."

AZADEH Persian. "Liberated."

AZALEA Latin. "Dry earth." Also a flowering shrub. **Azalee, Azalia**

AZELIA Hebrew. "Aided by God." **Azlyn, Azlin**

AZIZA Arabic, "beloved." Swahili, "precious."

AZUBA Unknown derivation. **Azubah, Zuba, Zubah**

AZURA Old French. "Blue." **Azor, Azora, Azure, Azurine, Azzura, Azzurra**

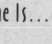

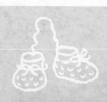

BAB Diminutive of **Barbara**. Greek, "foreign." **Babb, Babs**

BABETTE French diminutive of **Barbara**. Greek, "foreign."

BAILA Spanish. "Dance." Also variant of **Bilhah**. **Beyla, Byla**

BAILEY Old English. "Law enforcer, bailiff." **Ballee, Baily**

BAIRN Scottish. "Child."

BALBINA Latin. "Little stutterer." **Balbine**

BAMBI Short form of **Bambina**. Italian, "child." **Bambie, Bamby**

BAPTISTA Latin. "Dip." **Baptiste, Batista, Battista, Bautista**

BARA Hebrew. "To select." **Bari, Barra**

BARBARA Greek. "Stranger." **Bab, Baba, Babara, Babb, Babbett, Babbette, Babbie, Babe, Babett, Babette, Babita, Babs, Baibin, Bairbre, Barb, Barbary, Barbe, Barbee, Barbette, Barbey, Barbi, Barbie, Barbra, Barbro, Barby, Basha, Basia, Bauble, Bauby, Berbera, Berberia, Berberya, Berbya, Bobbie** et al., **Bonni, Bonnie, Bonny, Varvara**

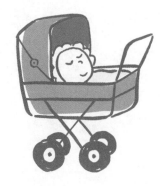

BARRIE Irish. "Sharp." Also a group of islands in Wales. **Bari, Barri**

BARTHA Old German. "Bright." **Barta, Bertha** et al.

BASHA Polish. "Stranger." **Basia**

BASILIA Feminine form of **Basil**. Greek, "royal." **Baseele, Baseelia, Baseelle, Basilisa, Bazeele, Bazeelia, Bazeelie, Basile, Basilie, Basille, Bazile, Bazille, Bazilia**

BATHILDA Old German. "Woman warrior." **Bathild, Bathilde, Berthilda, Berthilde, Bertilda, Bertilde**

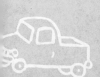

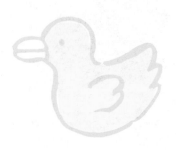

BATHSHEBA Hebrew. "Daughter of the oath." **Bathseva, Bathshua, Batsheba, Batsheva, Batshua, Bethsabee, Sheba** et al.

BATHSHIRA Arabic. "Seventh daughter."

BATYA Hebrew. "God's daughter." **Basya, Bethia, Bithia, Bitya**

BEATA Latin. "Blessed." **Beate**

BEATRICE Latin. "Bringer of gladness." **Bea, Beah, Beat, Beathy, Beatie, Beatrica, Beatrisa, Beatrix, Bebe, Bee, Beea, Beeatrice, Beeatris, Beeatrisa, Beeatriss, Beeatrissa, Beeatrix, Beitris, Beitriss, Trixie** et al.

BEBBA Hebrew. "God's pledge."

BECKY Diminutive of **Rebecca**. Hebrew, "joined."

BEDA Old English. "Battle maid."

BEDELIA Variant of **Bridget**. Irish, "strength." **Bedeelia, Bidelia**

BEE Diminutive of **Beatrice**. Latin, "bringer of gladness."

BEHIRA Hebrew. "Bright."

BELÉM Spanish. "Bethlehem."

BELINDA Combination of **Bella** and **Linda**. **Bel, Belle, Bellinda, Bellynda, Belynda, Linda, Lindie, Lindy**

BELITA Spanish. "Little beauty."

BELL Diminutive of **Isabel**; variant of **Bella, Belle**.

BELLA Latin. "Beautiful." Also short form of **Annabella, Isabella**, etc. **Bela, Belita, Bell, Belle, Bellette, Bellina, Billie** et al.

BELLANCA Italian. "Blonde." **Bianca, Blanca**

BELLE French variant of **Bella**.

BELLONA Latin. Roman goddess of battle.

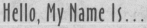
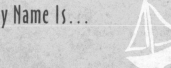
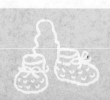

Women who heard the call

When most jobs were closed to women, religious organizations offered opportunities that could be found nowhere else. These women heard the call and answered.

Anne Ayers, who founded the first Episcopalian order for women

Antoinette Louisa Brown Blackwell, first ordained female minister in the U.S.

Evangeline Cory Booth, Salvation Army general

Olympia Brown, minister and social reformer

Frances Xavier "Mother" Cabrini, founder of Missionary Sisters of the Sacred Heart

Katharine Drexel, Roman Catholic nun and saint

Mary Baker Eddy, founder of Christian Science

Mary Hannah Fulton, physician and missionary

Anne Hutchinson, colonial religious leader

Joan of Arc, French saint and patriot

Leontine Kelly, African American bishop

Ann Lee, founder of the Shakers

Aimee Semple McPherson, evangelist

Elizabeth Ann Bayley Seton, first native-born American saint

Anna Howard Shaw, minister, doctor, feminist

Kateri Tekakwitha, Mohawk saint

Mother Teresa (born Agnes Gonxha Bojaxhiu), Roman Catholic nun

Emmeline Blanche Woodward Wells, Mormon community leader and suffragist

BELVA Feminine form of **Belveder.** Italian, "handsome." **Belvia**

BENA Feminine form of **Ben.** Hebrew, "son." **Bina, Buna, Bunie**

BENEDICTA Feminine form of **Benedict.** Latin, "blessed." **Benedetta, Benedicte, Benedikta, Benetta, Benita, Benni, Bennie, Benny, Benoite, Bianie, Binny, Dixie**

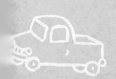

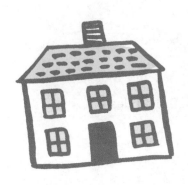

BENIGNA Latin. "Benevolent."

BENJAMINA Feminine form of **Benjamin.** Hebrew, "son of the right hand." **Benay, Jamina**

BENITA Spanish variant of **Benedicta.** Latin, "blessed."

BENTLEY Old English. "Meadow with coarse grass." **Bentlea, Bentlee, Bentleigh, Bently**

BERA Teutonic. "Bear."

BERDINE Old German. "Bright maiden."

BERENGARIA Old English. "Maiden of the bear-spear."

BERIT Scandinavian. "Gorgeous," "splendid," or "magnificent." **Beret, Berett**

BERNADETTE Feminine form of **Bernard.** Old German, "courageous." **Berna, Bernadett, Bernadetta, Bernee, Berneta, Bernetta, Bernette, Bernie, Bernita, Berny, Detta, Dette**

BERNADINE Feminine form of **Bernard.** French, "courageous." **Berna, Bernadeena, Bernadina, Bernadyna, Bernardyne, Bernee, Bernie, Berny**

BERNICE Greek. "She who brings victory." **Barri, Barrie, Barry, Beranice, Beraniece, Beranyce, Berenice, Bereniece, Berenyce, Bern, Bernee, Berneece, Bernelle, Berni, Bernie, Berniece, Berny, Bernyce, Berry** et al., **Bunni, Bunnie, Bunny**

BERRY English. "Berry." Also diminutive of **Alberta, Bernice, Beryl. Berie, Berrie**

BERTA Short form of **Alberta, Gilberta, Roberta;** variant of **Bertha.**

BERTHA Old German. "Bright." **Barta, Bartha, Berrta, Berrte, Berrti, Berrtina, Berrty, Berta, Berte, Berthe, Bertie, Bertina, Bertine, Bertuska, Berty, Bird** et al.

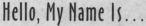

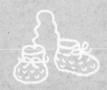

BERTILDE Old German. "Shining battle-maiden." **Bertilda, Berthilda, Berthilde**

BERTINA Variant of **Bertha**. Old German, "bright."

BERTRADE Old English. "Bright adviser."

BERURA Hebrew. "Pure."

BERURIA Hebrew. "Selected by God."

BERYL Greek. A pale green gemstone. **Berry** et al., **Beryle**

BESS Short form of **Elizabeth**. Hebrew, "pledged to God." **Bessie, Bessy**

BETA Greek. Second letter of the Greek alphabet.

BETH Hebrew. "House." Also short form of **Elizabeth, Bethany**.

BETHANY Hebrew. "House of poverty." **Bethanie, Bethanne, Bethannie, Bethanny**

BETHEL Hebrew. "House of God." **Bethell, Bethuel, Bethuna, Bethune**

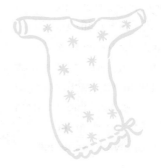

BETHESDA Hebrew. "House of mercy." Also a city in Maryland.

BETHIA Hebrew. "Daughter of Jehovah." **Betia, Bithia**

BETSY Short form of **Elizabeth**. Hebrew, "pledged to God."

BETTINA Diminutive of **Elizabeth**. Hebrew, "pledged to God." **Betina, Bettine**

BETTULA Persian. "Young women."

BETTY Diminutive of **Elizabeth**. Hebrew, "pledged to God." **Bet, Bett, Betta, Bette, Betti, Bettie, Bettina, Bettine, Bettye**

BEULAH Hebrew. "Married." **Beula**

BEVERLY Old English. "Beaver stream." **Bev, Beverle, Beverlee, Beverley, Beverlie, Beverlye, Bevlyn, Bevverlie, Bevverly, Bevvy, Buffy, Verlee, Verlie, Verly, Verlye**

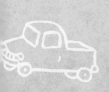

Head majorettes at the University of Tennessee

If, as someone once said, America's greatest contribution to art is the halftime show, majorettes are the Jackson Pollocks of our time. They prance, they wear glittery outfits, they throw batons in the air, and they catch them—most of the time. Here are some names of the finest practitioners of this most feminine art, from 1957 forward, at the University of Tennessee.

Ann-Dale Guinn
Claudette Riley
Helen Newport
DeAnna Smith
Judy Barton
Brenda Flowers
Connie Phillips
Rosemary Payne
Kathy McCarrell
Susan Huntington
Nancyjean Dolfi
Debra McCarrell
Eileen Keeler

Angela Floyd
Dawn James
Julie Watson
Monica Rahimzadeh
Sarah East
Kristi Ward
Pamela Beason
Heather Norman
Jennifer Whitehead
Carrie Delozier
Jessica Adams
Lanie Blankenship

BEVIN Irish. "Singer." **Bevan**

BIANCA Italian. "White." **Biancha**

BEYONCÉ Contemporary American. A currently popular singer.

BIBI French. "Toy." **Bebe, Beebee**

BIBIANA Spanish variant of **Vivian**. Latin, "full of life." **Bibiane, Bibianna, Bibianne, Bibyana**

BIENVENIDA Spanish. "Welcome."

BIJOU French. "Jewel."

BILHAH Hebrew. "Weak." **Baila**

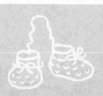

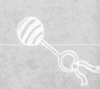

BILLIE Old English diminutive of **Wilhelmina;** variant of **Bella.** **Billee, Billey, Billi, Billy, Willa**

BINA Hebrew. "Knowledge" or "perception." **Binah, Buna**

BIRD English. "Bird." Also nickname for **Bertha. Birdey, Birdie, Birdy, Byrd, Byrdie**

BIRGIT Norse. "Splendid." **Birget, Birgett, Birgitt, Birgitta, Birgitte**

BITA Persian. "Unique."

BITHRON Hebrew. "Daughter of song."

BLAINE Irish. "Slender." **Blane, Blayne**

BLAIR Scottish. "Wicker basket." **Blaire**

BLAISE Latin. "One who stutters." **Blaize, Blase, Blasia, Blaze**

BLAKE Old English. "Bright meadow." **Blakelee, Blakeleigh, Blakeley, Blakely, Blakenee, Blakeney, Blakeny**

BLANCA Spanish. "White." **Bellanca, Blancha, Blanka**

BLANCHE French. "White." **Balaniki, Blanch, Blinni, Blinnie, Blinny**

BLANCHEFLEUR French. "White flower."

BLANDA Latin. "Smooth." **Blandina, Blandine**

BLASIA Variant of **Blaise.** Latin, "one who stutters."

BLESSING Old English. "Consecration."

BLIMA Hebrew. "Blossom." **Blimah, Blime**

BLISS Old English. "Happiness." **Blisse, Blyss**

BLODWEN Welsh. "White flower." **Blodwyn**

BLONDELLE French. "Little pale one." **Blondell, Blondie, Blondy**

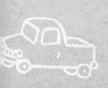

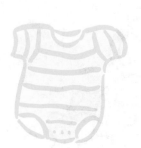

BLOSSOM Old English. "Flower."

BLYTHE Old English. "Happy, carefree." **Bliss, Blisse, Blithe**

BO Chinese. "Precious."

BOBBIE Diminutive of **Barbara. Bobbe, Bobbe, Bobby, Bobbye**

BOENN Irish. Unknown meaning.

BOGDANA Polish. "Gift from God." **Bogna, Bohdana**

BOLADE Nigerian. "The coming of honor."

BOLANILE Nigerian. "This house's riches."

BONA Arabic, "builder." Latin, "good."

BONFILLA Italian. "Good daughter."

BONITA Spanish. "Pretty." **Bo, Bonie, Bonnie, Bonny, Nita**

BONNIE Scottish. "Good looking." Also diminutive of **Barbara, Bonita. Bonne, Bonnee, Bonni, Bonny, Bunny** et al.

BONNIEBELLE Combination of **Bonnie** and **Belle. Bonnebell, Bonnibel, Bonnibell**

BORBALA Hungarian. "Foreigner." **Bora, Boriska, Borka, Borsala, Borsca**

BRACHA Hebrew. "Blessing."

BRADLEY Old English. "Broad field." **Bradlea, Bradlee, Bradleigh, Bradly**

BRANDY English. A liqueur. **Brandais, Brande, Brandea, Brandde, Branddie, Brandee, Brandi, Brandice, Brandie, Brandye, Branndais, Branndea, Branndi**

BRENDA Feminine form of **Brendan.** Old English, "burning." **Bren, Brenn, Brennda, Brenndah**

BRENNA Irish. "Black-haired." **Bren, Brenn, Brennah, Brenne**

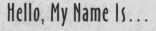

BRETT Latin. "From Britain." **Brette, Britt**

BRIA City in the Central African Republic.

BRIANA Feminine form of **Brian.** Irish, "strong one." **Brana, Breana, Breanne, Breeann, Breeanna, Breeanne, Breena, Bria, Brianna, Brianne, Brina** et al., **Briney, Briny, Bryana, Bryann, Bryanna, Bryanne**

BRICE Welsh. "Prize." **Bryce**

BRIDGET Celtic. "Strength" or "power." In myth, goddess of fire and poetry. St. Bridget, Scandinavian founder of the Bridgettine order. **Bedelia** et al., **Berget, Bergett, Bergette, Biddie, Biddy, Birkita, Birkitta, Birkitte, Birte, Bitta, Breeda, Bride, Bridee, Bridey, Bridgett, Bridgette, Bridgit, Bridgitt, Bridgitta, Bridgitte, Bridie, Bridy, Brietta, Briget, Brigett, Brighid, Brigid, Brigida, Brígida, Brigit, Brigitt, Brigitte, Brijet, Brijette, Brijit, Brijitte, Brita, Britt, Britta, Britte, Brydie, Brydget, Brydgit, Brydgitta, Brydgitte, Brydjette, Brydjitt, Bryget, Brygette, Brygit, Brygitte, Bryjet, Bryjit, Gitta** et al.

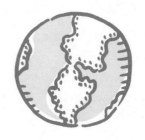

BRIE French. "Strong." Also a soft, rich French cheese. **Bree, Brielle, Briette**

BRIER French. "Heather." **Briar**

BRILLIANTE French. "Shining." **Brilliana**

BRINA Feminine form of **Brian.** Irish and Scottish, "defender." **Brinn, Brinna, Bryn, Bryna, Brynn, Brynna, Brynne**

BRIT Celtic. "Freckled." Also short form of **Brittania.**

BRITANNIA Latin. "Britain." **Brit, Brita, Britta**

BRITES Portuguese. "Power."

BRITTA Variant of **Bridget**; short form of **Brittania, Brittany.**

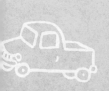

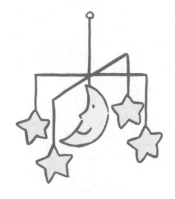

BRITTANY Latin. "Britain." Also the province of France settled by Gaels. **Brett** et al., **Brit, Briteny, Britney, Britni, Britny, Britta, Brittan, Brittaney, Brittani, Britteny, Brittnee, Brittney, Brittni, Brittny**

BRONWYN Welsh. "Fair breast." **Bronnie, Bronny, Bronwen, Bronya**

BROOKE Old English. "Small stream." **Brook, Brookie, Brooks, Brooky**

BRUCIE Feminine form of **Bruce.** Old French, "brushwood thicket." **Brucina, Brucine**

BRUNA Feminine form of **Bruno.** Italian, "brown-skinned" or "brown-haired."

BRUNELLA Old French. "Little one with brown hair." **Brunelle, Brunetta, Brunette**

BRUNHILDA Old German. "Armor-wearing fighting maid." **Brinhild, Brinhilda, Brinhilde, Brunhild, Brunhilde, Brunnhilda, Brunnhilde, Brynhild, Brynhilda, Brynhilde, Hilda** et al.

BUNNY English. "Bunny." Nickname for **Bernice,** variant of **Bonnie. Bunni, Bunnie**

BUNTY English. "Bunny.

CADENCE Latin. "With rhythm." **Cadena, Cadenza, Cadina, Kadenza** et al.

CADY Old English. **Cade, Cadee, Cadey, Cadi, Cadie, Cadye, Kade, Kadee, Kadi, Kadie, Kady, Kadye**

 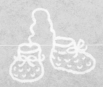

CAL Vietnamese. "Feminine."

CAITLIN Irish variant of **Catherine.** Greek, "pure." **Cait, Caitilin, Caitlan, Caitlann, Caitlinn, Caitlyn, Caitlynn, Caity, Catlin, Catlinn, Kaitlin** et al.

CALA Arabic. "Castle, fortress."

CALANDRA Greek. "Lark." **Cal, Calandre, Calandria, Calendre, Callee, Calley, Calli, Callie, Cally, Kalandra**

CALANTHA Greek. "Lovely flower." **Cal, Calanthe, Callee, Calley, Calli, Callie, Cally, Kalantha**

CALEDONIA Latin. "Scotland."

CALIDA Spanish. "Heated." **Cali, Calla, Calli, Callida**

CALLA Greek. "Beautiful." Also a type of lily.

CALLAN Old Norse. "To call loudly."

CALLIDORA Greek. "Gift of beauty."

CALLIGENIA Greek. "Daughter of beauty."

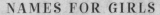

CALLIOPE Greek. In myth, the Muse of epic poetry. **Callia, Callyope, Kalliope, Kallyope**

CALLISTA Greek. "Most beautiful." **Cala, Calesta, Calista, Calla, Callesta, Calli, Callie, Cally, Callysta, Calysta, Kallista** et al.

CALLISTO Greek. In myth, a princess whom Zeus turned into first a bear, and then into the Great Bear constellation.

CALLULA Latin. "Small beauty."

CALPURNIA Greek. "Beauty."

CALTHA Latin. "Golden flower."

CALVINA Feminine form of **Calvin.** Latin, "hairless." **Calvine, Kalvina**

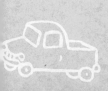

MOSLEM NAMES

oslem parents almost always give their children names that are from the Koran or related to Mohammed, his family, or early leaders of the faith. The most popular name in the world may be *Mohammad,* if its variants are included in the count.

According to the Koran, Allah has 99 good qualities: The Beneficent, The Just, The Pardoner, The Most High, The Protector, The Giver of Life, and so on. Each of these qualities is a possible name. Here are some examples:

Ar-Rehman	"The Compassionate"
Al-Malik	"The Holy"
As-Salam	"The Peace"
Al-Muhaymin	"The Protector"
Al-Jabber	"The Compeller"
Al-Aleem	"The Knower"

The rise of the Nation of Islam brought many Moslem names into the United States, as African-Americans changed their names to Arabic ones. The most famous change was made by the heavyweight boxer Cassius Clay, who became Muhammad Ali. Lew Alcindor, a basketball player, changed his name to Kareem-Abdul Jabbar, and Louis Eugene Wolcott, a calypso singer, became Louis Farrakhan, who heads the Nation of Islam.

Following are some popular Moslem boys' names and their meanings.

Ayaan	"God's gift"
Aadil	"just, upright"
Rayn	one of the gates of heaven
Zain	"friend" or "beloved"
Aahil	"prince"
Aalee	"high"
Aamir	"civilized"
Aariz	"respectable man"
Ali	"noble, sublime"
Daanish	"wisdom," "learning," or "science"
Deen	"religious"
Eshan	"in God's grace, worthy"
Keyaan	"crown" or "king"
Rayyan	"full" or "pretty"
Shayaan	"intelligent"

Here are some Moslem girls' names and their meanings.

Aaliyah	"tall, towering"
A'idah	"guest" or "the one who is returning"
Aishah	wife of the Prophet Mohammed

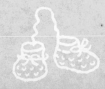

Aleena	"silk of heaven"	**Eshal**	a flower in Heaven
Alesha	"protected by God"	**Maira**	"moon"
Alina	"beautiful"	**Maya**	"princess"
Alisha	"honest, truthful"	**Nadia**	"hope"
Aliza	daughter of Prophet Ali	**Sabrina**	"white rose"
Amelia	"trustworthy" or "beautiful"	**Sarah**	"pure" or "happy"
Ariana	"full of life"	**Selina**	"moon" or "salty"
Eliza	"unique" or "precious"	**Sofia**	"beautiful"

CALYPSO Greek. "She who hides." In myth, the nymph who cared for Odysseus for over a year.

CAMELIA New Latin. A flowering evergreen shrub, named for Georg Josef Kamel. **Camellia**

CAMILLA Latin. In the *Aeneid*, the fleet-footed queen of the Volscians. **Cam, Cama, Camala, Cami, Camila, Camile, Camilla, Camille, Cammi, Cammie, Cammilla, Cammille, Cammy, Cammylle, Camyla, Camylla, Camylle, Kamilla** et al., **Milla, Mille, Milly** et al.

CAMEO Italian. A semi-precious stone. **Cammeo**

CANACE Greek. "Daughter of the wind." **Canice**

CANDACE Latin. "Brilliantly white." **Candee, Candi, Candie, Candies, Candis, Candy, Dacey** et al., **Kandace** et al.

CANDIDE Latin. "White." **Candi, Candida, Candie, Candy**

CANDRA Latin. "Glowing." **Candi, Candie, Candy, Kandra** et al.

CANTARA Arabic. "Little bridge."

CAPRICE French, from Italian. "Whim." **Caprisse**

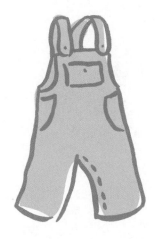

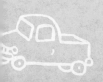

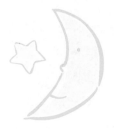

CAPUCINE French. "Cowl."

CARA Latin. "Darling." **Caralie, Carrie, Carry, Kara, Karina, Karine, Karrah, Karrie, Karry**

CAREY Welsh. "Near the castle."

CARI Latin. "Keel." **Cairenn, Carin, Carine, Caryn, Karin, Karine, Karyn**

CARINA Italian. "Dear little one." **Careena, Caren, Carena, Carin, Carine, Karena, Karina, Karine**

CARINTHIA A region in Austria.

CARISSA Greek. "Grace." **Caresa, Caressa, Carisa, Chareese, Charis, Charissa, Charisse, Karisa, Karissa**

CARITA Latin. "Kindness." **Caritta, Carrita, Carritta, Karita** et al.

CARLA Feminine form of **Carl.** Old German, "man." **Carlla, Karla, Karlla**

CARLIE Feminine form of **Carl.** Old German, "man." **Carl, Carlee, Carley, Carlita, Carly, Carlye, Carlyta, Karlee, Karli, Karlicka, Karlie, Karlika, Karlita, Karly, Karlyta**

CARLENE Feminine form of **Carl.** Old German, "man." **Carleen, Carlina, Carline, Carlyne, Karleen, Karlena, Karlene, Karline, Karling, Karlinka**

CARLIN Irish and Scottish. "Little champion." **Carlen, Carling, Carlinn, Carlyn, Carlynn, Carlynne, Karlin, Karling, Karlinn**

CARLOTTA Italian variant of **Charlotte;** feminine form of **Charles.** Old German, "man." **Carlota**

CARMA Arabic. "Vineyard." **Carmania, Carmia, Carmie, Carmine, Carmit, Carmita, Carmiya, Carmy, Kaarmia, Karma, Karmit**

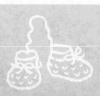

CARMEL Hebrew. "Garden." **Carma, Carmela, Carmelina, Carmeline, Carmelita, Carmina, Carmy, Karmel, Karmela, Karmelit, Lina, Lita, Melina, Meline, Melita, Mina**

CARMEN Latin. "Song." **Carmencita, Carmie, Carmina, Carmine, Carmita, Carmyna, Carmyta, Charmaine, Karmen** et al., **Mina**

CARNA Arabic. "Horn." **Carniela, Carniella, Carnit, Carnyella, Karniela** et al.

CARNATION Latin. "Becoming flesh." Also a flower, *Dianthus Caryophyllus.*

CARNELIAN English. Semi-precious red stone.

CAROL Feminine form of **Carl, Charles.** Old German, "man." **Carel, Carey, Cari, Caro, Carola, Carole, Caroll, Carri, Carrie, Carroll, Carry, Cary, Caryl, Caryll, Karel, Kari, Karole, Karryl, Karryll, Karyl, Karyll, Kerril, Kerryl, Keryl**

CAROLINDA Combination of **Carol** and **Linda.**

CAROLINE Feminine form of **Carl, Charles.** Old German, "man." **Caraleen, Caraleena, Caraline, Caralyn, Caralyne, Caralynn, Carlyn, Carlyna, Carlyne, Carlynn, Carlynne, Carol** et al., **Carolena, Carolin, Carolina, Carollyn, Carolyn, Carolyne, Carolynn, Carolynne, Ina, Karaleen, Karaleena, Karlen, Karolina** et al., **Lena** et al., **Roline** et al.

CARPATHIA Greek. "Fruit."

CARYS Welsh. "Love."

CASEY Irish. "Watchful." **Cacey, Cacie, Caisee, Caisey, Caisi, Caisie, Casee, Casi, Casie, Caycee, Caycey, Cayci, Caycie, Caysee, Caysey, Caysi, Caysie, Kacey** et al.

CASILDA Latin. "Dwelling place."

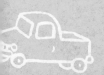

CASS Short form of **Cassandra, Catherine. Cassey, Cassi, Cassie, Cassy**

CASSANDRA Greek. In myth, a Trojan princess and prophet whom no one believed. **Casandera, Casandra, Cass** et al., **Cassandre, Cassandry, Cassaundra, Cassi, Cassie, Cassondra, Cassy, Kassandra** et al., **Sandra** et al.

CASSIA Greek. "Cinnamon."

CASSIDY Irish. "Clever."

CASTA Latin. "Modest."

CATHERINE Greek. "Pure." **Caitlin** et al., **Caitrin, Caitrine, Caitrinn, Cass** et al., **Cat, Catarina, Catarine, Caterina, Catha, Catharin, Catharina, Catharine, Catharyna, Catharyne, Cathelin, Cathelina, Cathelle, Catherin, Catherina, Catherinn, Cateryn, Cathirin, Cathiryn, Cathleen** et al., **Cathrine, Cathrinn, Cathryn, Cathrynn, Cathy** et al., **Catia, Catina, Catlaina, Ekaterina, Kaki, Karen** et al., **Kasja, Kaska, Kaslenka, Kass** et al., **Kasya, Kat, Kata, Katalina, Katarina, Katchen, Kate** et al., **Katenka, Kateri, Katerina, Katerinka, Katha, Katherine** et al., **Kathleen** et al., **Kathrina, Kathrine, Kathryn, Kathy** et al., **Kathyrine, Katica, Katina, Katinka, Katlaina, Katoushka, Katrina** et al., **Katty, Katushka, Katya, Kay** et al., **Kayla** et al., **Kitty** et al., **Thrine, Yekaterin, Yekaterina**

CATHLEEN Irish variant of **Catherine**. Greek, "pure." **Cataleen, Cataleena, Catalin, Catalina, Catelina, Cathaleen, Cathaline, Cathlene, Cathyleen.**

CECILIA Feminine form of **Cecil**. Latin, "blind one." **Cacilia, Cacilie, Cacily, Ceceley, Cecely, Cecil, Cecile, Ceciley, Ceciliane, Cecilija, Cecilla, Cecily, Cecilyann, Cecyl, Cecyle, Cecylia, Ceil, Cele, Celia, Celie, Cesia, Cesya,**

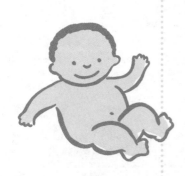

Cicely, Cici, Cicily, Cile, Cilia, Cilka, Cilly, Cycalye, Cycly, Kikelia, Kikylia, Sasilia, Sasilie, Saelia, Saelie, Saely, Sasilia, Sela, Sessaley, Sesseelya, Sessile, Sessilly, Sessily, Sheila et al., **Sile, Sileas, Siseel, Sisely, Sisile, Sisiliya, Sisslya, Sissela, Sissy** et al.

CELANDINE Greek. "Swallow." Also a perennial plant with yellow blossoms. **Celanda, Celandia, Celenda, Celendia, Celendine, Celinda, Celindia, Celindine, Lindi, Lindie, Lindy**

CELENA Variant of **Selena.** Greek goddess of the moon. **Cela, Celeena, Celene, Celie, Celina, Celinda** et al., **Celine, Celinka, Cellina, Celyna**

CELESTE Latin. "Heavenly." **Cela, Celesta, Celestena, Celestene, Celestia, Celestijna, Celestina, Celestine, Celestyne, Celie, Saleste, Salestia, Seleste, Selestia, Selestina, Selestine, Selestyna, Selestyne, Silesta, Silestia, Silestijna, Silestina, Silestyna, Silestyne, Tina** et al., **Tinka**

CELINDA Variant of **Selena.** Greek goddess of the moon. **Celinde, Salinda, Salinde, Selinda, Selinde**

CELOSIA Greek. "Flame." Also a flowering plant with flame-like blossoms.

CENA Variant of **Xenia.** Greek, "hospitable host."

CENOBIA Greek. "Power of Zeus."

CERES Latin. "Springtime." **Cerelia, Cerella**

CERIDWEN Welsh. "Sweet poetry." **Ceridwin, Ceridwyn**

CERISE French. "Cherry." **Cherice, Cherise, Sherise**

CESARINA Feminine form of **Caesar.** Latin clan name. **Cesarea, Cesarie, Cesarine, Kesare**

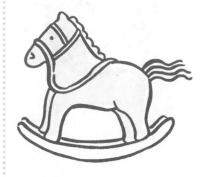

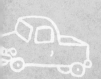

NAMES FOR GIRLS

53

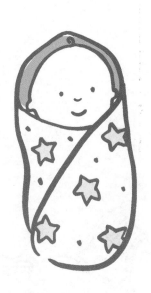

CHANAH Hebrew. "Grace." **Chana, Chani, Channa, Channah, Hannah** et al.

CHANDELLE French. "Candle." **Chanda, Chandel, Chendel, Chendelle**

CHANDRA Sanskrit. "Moon." **Candra, Chanta, Chantha, Kandra, Kanthra, Shandra**

CHANEL French. A famous perfume. **Chanelle, Channelle, Shanel, Shanell, Shanelle, Shannel, Shannelle**

CHANTAL Feminine form of **Chanticleer.** Middle English, from Old French, "to sing clearly." **Chantalle, Chantel, Chantele, Chantelle, Chantial, Chantialle, Shantal** et al.

CHARILL Contemporary American. Feminine form of **Charles.** Old German, "man." **Charille**

CHARIS Greek. "Grace."

CHARITY Latin. "Brotherly love." **Charita, Charitee, Charitey, Charitye, Cherry** et al., **Sharitee, Sharitey, Sharity, Sharitye**

CHARLOTTE French. Feminine form of **Charles.** Old German, "man." **Carlota, Carlotta, Char, Chara, Charla, Charlotta, Charly, Charo, Karlotta, Karlotte, Lolotte, Lottchen, Lottie** et al., **Sharea, Sharla, Totti, Tottie, Totty**

CHARMAINE Latin. Clan name. **Charmain, Charmane, Charmayne, Charmion, Charmyn, Charmyne, Sharmain, Sharman, Sharmane, Sharmayne, Sharmian, Sharmion, Sharmyn**

CHARMIAN Greek. "Joy." **Charmeyen, Charmiane, Charmien, Charmion, Charmyan**

CHASIDAH Hebrew. "Devout woman."

CHASTITY Latin. "Purity."

CHAVA Hebrew. "Life." **Chabah, Chaya, Chayka, Eva, Hava, Haya, Kaija**

CHAVIVA Hebrew. "Beloved."

CHAVONNE American variant of **Sioban**, Irish variant of **Joan. Chevonne, Chivon, Shavonne** et al.

CHAYA Feminine form of **Chaim.** Hebrew, "life."

CHEERA Greek. "Pleasing features." **Cheara, Cheare, Cheere, Shera**

CHELSEA Old English. "Port." **Chellsea, Chellsee, Chellsey, Chelsee, Chelsey, Chelsie, Chelsy**

CHENETTA French. "Oak tree." **Chanet, Chanetta, Chanette, Chenet, Chenette, Janet, Janeta**

CHENOA Native American. "Dove."

CHEPHZIBAH Hebrew. "My delight is in her."

CHER Variant of **Chère**; short form of **Cheryl.** Cher, contemporary popular entertainer.

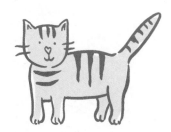

CHÈRE French. "Beloved." **Cher, Chere, Cheree, Cherey, Cheri, Cherida, Chérie, Cherie, Cherita, Cherry** et al., **Chery, Cherye, Sher, Shere, Sherry** et al.

CHERAMIE Combination of **Chère** and **Amie** (French, "friend"). **Cherami**

CHERISH English. "Cherish."

CHERRY English, from Old French. "Cherry." Also short form of **Charity**; variant of **Chère, Sherry. Cherrey, Cherri, Cherrie, Chery**

CHERYL Feminine form of **Charles.** Old German, "man." **Charil, Charyl, Cher, Cheri, Cherie, Cherryl, Cheryll, Cherylle, Sheryl** et al.

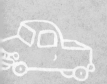

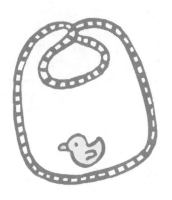

CHERIANN Combination of **Cheryl or Cherry** and **Ann. Cherianne, Sherianne**

CHERILYN Combination of **Cheryl** and **Lynn. Charalin, Charalyn, Charalynn, Charalynne, Charelin, Charelyn, Charelynn, Charelynne, Charilyn, Charilynn, Cheralin, Cheralyn, Cheralynn, Cheralynne, Cherilin, Cherilynn, Cherilynne, Cherlyn, Cherralyn, Cherrilyn, Cherrylene, Cherrylin, Cherryline, Cherrylyn, Cherylin, Cheryline, Cheryllyn, Cherylyn, Sherilyn** et al.

CHERYLEE Combination of **Cheryl** and **Lee. Cherylie**

CHESNA Slavic. "Peaceful." **Chessa, Chesse, Chessey, Chessi, Chessie, Chessy, Chezna**

CHEYENNE Sioux. "People of different speech."

CHIARA Italian. "Bright." **Chiarra, Ciara**

CHILALI Native American. "Bird of the snow."

CHIQUITA Spanish. "Little girl." **Chica, Chickie, Chicky, Chiquin, Chiquina**

CHITA Hindi "Spotted one."

CHIZU Japanese. "A thousand storks."

CHLOE Greek. "Young green shoot." **Clo, Cloe**

CHLORIS Greek. "Pale." **Chlori, Chlorie, Chlorin, Chlorine, Chlorise, Chlorisse, Chlorit, Chlory, Clori, Clorie, Clorin, Clorine, Cloris, Clorise, Clorisse, Clorit, Clory, Lois, Lori, Lorice** et al.

CHO Japanese. "Butterfly."

CHOLENA Delaware tribe. "Bird."

CHOOMIA Romanian. "Kiss."

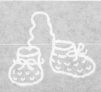

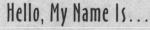

Wild women

These lively souls are remembered for their misdeeds as well as their rebellious spirits.

Lizzie Andrew Borden, who gave her mother 40 whacks

Lucrezia Borgia, poisoner and woman about Rome

Calamity Jane, frontier character

Charlotte Corday, who stabbed French revolutionary Jean-Paul Marat

Emma Goldman, anarchist

Emma Hamilton, recipient of Lord Nelson's Column

Tonya Harding, figure skater, hard competitor, and boxer

Monica Lewinsky, most famous White House intern

Mata Hari, spy

Messalina, Roman empress and woman about Rome

Lola Montez, dancer famous for "Whatever Lola wants, Lola gets"

Bonnie Parker, who died with Clyde

Belle Starr, big-time outlaw in the West

CHRISTA Varian of **Krista.** Greek, "Christian." St. Cristeta of Avila. **Cristeta**

CHRISTABEL Latin. "Beautiful Christian." **Christa, Christabel, Christabell, Christabella, Christabelle, Christey, Christie, Christobel, Christobella, Christy, Chrystabel, Chrystabelle, Chrystebel, Chrystebelle, Chrystobel, Cristabel, Cristabella, Cristabelle, Cristie, Cristy, Crystabel, Crystabella, Crystabelle**

CHRISTINE Feminine form of **Christian.** Greek, "Christian." **Cairistina, Cairistine, Cairistiona, Chris, Chrissie, Chrissy, Chrisstan, Chrissten, Chrissti, Chrisstie, Chrissty, Christan,**

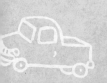

Christeen, Christeena, Christen, Christi, Christian, Christiana, Christiane, Christiania, Christianna, Christie, Christin, Christina, Christinn, Christy, Christyna, Chrystee, Crete, Cris, Crissey, Crissie, Crissy, Cristen, Cristena, Cristi, Cristin, Cristina, Cristine, Cristiona, Cristy, Crystena, Crystene, Crysti, Crystina, Crystine, Crystyna, Karstin, Kersti, Khristna, Khristya, Kina, Kirsten et al., Kirsto, Kit, Kris, Kriss, Krissie, Krissy, Krista et al., Kristen et al., Kristi, Kristine et al., Krystka, Kristy, Krystyan, Stina, Stine, Tina et al., Xena, Xina

CHRISTMAS Old English. "Christ's mass," mid-winter holiday.

CHRYSEIS Latin. "Golden daughter." **Chrysilla, Chrysis**

CHRYSANTHEMUM Latin, from Greek. "Golden flower." Also any plant of the genus *Chrysanthemum.*

CHRYSOGON Greek. "Born of gold." **Chrisogone, Chrisogonia, Grisigon** et al.

CHUMANI Sioux. "Drops of dew."

CIA Contemporary American.

CIMA Greek. "Symbol." **Cyma, Seema** et al.

CINDERELLA French. "Little ash-girl." **Cindy** et al., **Ella, Elle**

CINDY Diminutive of **Cinderella, Cynthia, Lucinda. Cindee, Cindi, Cindie, Cyndee, Cyndie, Cyndy, Sindee, Sindi, Sindie, Sindy, Syndi, Syndie, Syndy**

CIPRIANA Italian. "From Cyprus." **Cipriane, Ciprianna, Ciprianne, Cypriana, Cyprianne, Cyprienne**

CLAIRE Latin. "Clear." **Cheeara, Chiara, Chiarra, Ciara, Clair, Claira, Claireen, Clairene, Claireta, Clairetta, Clairette, Clairey, Clairinda, Clairy, Clara, Clarabella** et al., **Clare,**

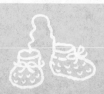

Clareen, Clarene, Clares, Claresta, Clareta, Claretha, Claretta, Clarette, Clarey, Clari, Clarice et al., Clarina, Clarinda, Clarine, Clariscia, Clarissa et al., Clarita, Clarrie, Clarry, Clarus, Clary, Clatie, Clayre, Clayrette, Clayrinda, Cliara, Klaire, Klara et al., Klaretta, Klaricka, Klayre, Kliara, Klyara

CLARAMAE English. Combination of **Clara** and **Mae. Claramay**

CLARABELLE Combination of **Clara** and **Belle. Clarabel, Clarabella, Claribel, Claribella, Claribelle**

CLARICE Variant of **Claire.** Latin, "clear." **Clairice, Claris, Clarise, Clarissa** et al., **Clarisse, Claryce, Clerisse, Cleruce, Clerysse, Klarice, Klaryce**

CLARIMOND Latin, German. "Shining defender." **Clarimonde**

CLARISSA Variant of **Claire. Clairissa, Claricia, Clarisa, Clayrissa, Clerissa, Clyrissa, Klarissa, Klarisza, Klaryssa**

CLAUDIA Feminine form of **Claude.** Latin, "clear." **Claudella, Claudelle, Claudetta, Claudette, Claudey, Claudie, Claudina, Claudine, Claudy, Clodia, Klaudia, Klaudya**

CLEANTHA Greek. "Glory." **Cleanthe, Cliantha, Clianthe**

CLELIA Latin. "Glorious."

CLEMATIS Greek. "Brushwood." Also a flowering vine.

CLEMENTIA Latin. "Granting mercy." **Clem, Clemence, Clemency, Clemense, Clementina, Clementine, Clementya, Clementyn, Clementyna, Clemmie, Clemmy, Klementina** et al., **Tina**

CLEOPATRA Greek. "Her father's glory." **Clea, Cleo, Cleothe, Cleta**

CLEVA Feminine form of **Cleve, Clive.** Old English, "cliff."

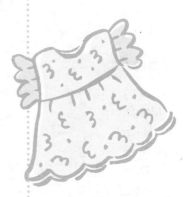

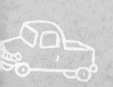

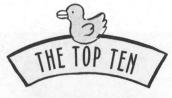

THE TOP TEN

NAMES OF 1903

The Year of the Wright
Brothers' First Flight

BOYS

John
William
James
George
Joseph
Charles
Robert
Frank
Walter
Henry

GIRLS

Mary
Margaret
Helen
Anna
Ruth
Marie
Elizabeth
Florence
Dorothy
Lillian

CLIANTHA Greek. "Glory flower." **Cleantha, Cleanthe, Clianthe, Kliantha, Klianthe**

CLIO Greek. "To praise." In myth, the Muse of history. **Cleo, Cleon, Cleona, Cleone, Cleora, Cleoria**

CLOELIA Latin. In Roman legend, Cloelia was given as hostage to an Estruscan invader, and escaped by swimming across the Tiber River. **Clelia, Cloela, Cloeli, Clola, Cloli, Clolia**

CLORINDA Latin. "Renowned beauty."

CLOTILDA German. "Renowned battle." **Clothilda, Clothilde, Clotilde, Klotild** et al.

CLOVE Latin. "Nail." The dried bud of a tropical tree, used as a spice. **Clova, Clovah, Clovi, Clovie, Clovy**

CLOVER Old English. "To cling." Also a low-growing leguminous plant.

CLYMENE Greek. "Famous one." **Climena, Climene, Climenia, Clymena, Clymenia**

CLYTIE Greek. "Lovely one." **Clita, Cliti, Clitia, Clitie, Clity, Clyta, Clyti, Clytia, Clytie**

COCHAVA Hebrew. "Star."

CODY Old English. "Pillow." **Codee, Codey, Codi, Codie, Kodey, Kodi, Kodie, Kody**

COLETTE Diminutive of **Nicole**. French, from Greek, "people of victory." **Coleta, Colete, Coletta, Collet, Collete, Collette, Nicholette, Nicoletta, Nicolette, Nikoleta, Nikoletta**

COLLEEN Irish. "Girl." **Coleen, Colena, Colene, Colina, Coline, Collie, Colline, Colly, Kolleen**

COLUMBA Latin. "Dove." **Collie, Colly, Colombe, Colombia, Columbia, Columbine** et al.

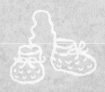

COLUMBINE Latin. "Dove." Also a perennial flowering plant. **Columba** et al., **Columbina, Columbinia**

COMFORT French. "To strengthen."

CONCEPCIÓN Spanish. "Conception." **Cetta, Chiquin, Chita, Conception, Concetta**

CONCHA Greek. "Shell." **Conchata, Concheta, Conchita**

CONCORDIA Latin. "Harmony." **Concorda, Concordi, Concordie, Concordya**

CONRADINE Feminine form of **Conrad.** Old German, "wise counselor." **Connee, Connie, Conny, Conrada, Conradeen**

CONSTANCE Latin. "Steadfastness." **Con, Coneta, Conetta, Connee, Conney, Conni, Connie, Conny, Constancia, Constancy, Constanta, Constantia, Constantija, Constantina, Constantine, Constantinia, Constantya, Constanz, Conte, Costanza, Custance, Custancia, Custans, Custins, Konstanze** et al., **Tina**

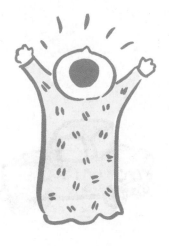

CONSUELO Spanish. "Consolation." **Chela, Chelo, Consolata, Consuela, Consuelia**

CONTENT Latin. "Fulfilled." **Contenca, Contencha, Contenchia, Contencia, Contenta, Contentia**

CORA Greek. "Maiden." **Coree, Corela, Corella, Coreta, Coretta, Corette, Corey, Cori, Corie, Corilla, Corillia, Corinne** et al., **Corita, Corrella, Correlle, Correnda, Correndia, Correnza, Corretta, Corrette, Correy, Corri, Corrie, Corry, Cory, Coryssa, Kora** et al.

CORABELLE Combination of **Cora** and **Belle. Corabel, Corabela, Corabella, Corabellita, Korabel, Korabell, Korabella, Korabelle**

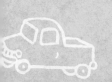

CORAL Latin. "Pebble." **Coralee, Coraleen, Coralena, Coralie, Coraline, Coraly, Coralyn, Coralyne, Coreli, Cori, Corie, Corry, Kora, Koralie** et al.

CORAZÓN Spanish. "Heart." **Corazona, Corazone, Corazonia, Corrazon, Corrazona, Corrazone, Corrazonia**

CORDELIA Feminine form of **Cordell**. Old French, "rope maker." **Cordeilia, Cordelie, Cordell, Cordella, Cordelle, Cordey, Cordi, Cordie, Cordula, Cordulia, Cordulla, Cordullia, Cordy, Della** et al., **Kordelia** et al.

COREY Irish. "A hollow." **Cori, Corrie, Corry, Cory, Korey, Korie, Korry, Kory**

CORINNE French variant of **Cora**. **Carine, Carinna, Carinne, Carynna, Carynne, Corena, Corene, Corenna, Corenne, Corina, Corine, Corinn, Corinna, Correen, Correna, Correne, Corrianne, Corrienne, Corrina, Corrine, Corrinn, Coryna, Corynna, Corynne, Karinne, Karynna, Korinne** et al.

CORLISS Old English. "Benevolent, cheery." **Corlee, Corley, Corlie, Corly**

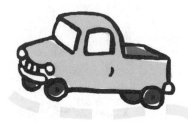

CORNELIA Feminine form of **Cornelius**. Latin, "like a horn." **Cornalia, Corneeliya, Cornela, Corneli, Cornelie, Cornelija, Cornella, Cornelle, Cornelya, Cornie, Korneelia, Korneelya, Kornelia, Kornelija, Kornelya, Neel, Neely, Nela, Nelia, Nell** et al.

CORONA Spanish. "Crown." **Coronetta**

CORVINA Latin. "Like a raven."

COSETTE Variant of **Nicole**, feminine form of **Nicholas**. Greek. "People of victory." **Cosetta**

COSIMA Feminine form of **Cosmo**. Greek, "organization." **Cosimè, Cosimo, Cosma, Cosmè, Cosmina, Kosima, Kosma, Kosmo**

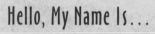

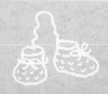

COURTLAND Old English. "Land owned by the court." **Cortland**

COURTNEY Old English. "Court-dweller." **Cortnee, Cortney, Cortnie, Cortny, Courtenay, Courtnay, Courtnee, Courtnie, Courtny, Kourtney** et al.

CREOLA French. "Home-raised." **Creoli, Creolia, Creolie**

CRESCENT Old French. "Increasing." **Crescence, Crescentia, Cressant, Cressent, Cressentia, Cressentya**

CRISELDA Variant of **Griselda.** Old German, "gray fighting maid." **Chriselda**

CRISPINA Feminine form of **Crispin.** Latin, "curly-haired." **Crispa, Crispine**

CRISTINA Variant of **Christine.** Latin. "Christian."

CRYSTAL Greek. "Ice." **Christal, Christalle, Chrystal, Chrystalle, Chrystel, Chrystelle, Chrystle, Cristal, Cristall, Cristel, Cristelle, Cristle, Crysta, Crystel, Crystelle, Crystle, Krystal** et al.

CSILLA Hungarian. "Defenses."

CUTHBERGA Feminine form of **Cuthbert.** Old English, "famous" or "brilliant."

CYANEA Greek. "Sky blue."

CYBELE Greek. A Phrygian goddess. **Cybebe, Cybela, Cybil, Cybill, Cybilla, Cybillia, Cyble**

CYMRY Welsh. "From Wales." **Cymri, Cymria, Kymry** et al.

CYNARA Greek. "Thistle." **Cynaria, Synara, Synaria**

CYNTHIA Greek. "From Cynthos." **Cinda, Cindy** et al., **Cinnie, Cinny, Cinthia, Cintia, Cyn, Cynda, Cyndia, Cynnie, Cynth,**

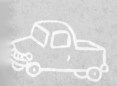

Cynthea, Cynthiana, Cynthie, Cynthya, Kynthia, Kynthija, Synthia et al.

CYPRIS Greek. "Cyprus." Ciprian, Cipriana, Cyprian, Cyprien, Cyprienne, Cyprus

CYRA Feminine form of Cyrus. Persian, "sun." Cira, Ciri, Cyr, Cyri

CYRILLA Feminine form of Cyril. Latin, "lordly." Cira, Ciri, Cirilla, Cirillia, Cyrillia, Syrilla et al.

CYTHEREA Greek. "From the island of Cythera." Cithera, Citherea, Cythera, Sytherea et al.

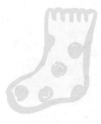

DACEY Irish. "From the south." Also diminutive of Candace. Dace, Dacee, Dacia, Dacie, Dacy, Daicee, Daicey, Daicy, Daisey, Daisy

DACIA Latin. A Roman province.

DADA Nigerian. "Curly-haired."

DAFFODIL Old French. Spring-flowering bulb in the genus *Narcissus.* Daffy, Dilly, Lill, Lilly

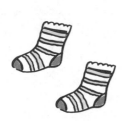

DAGANIA Hebrew. "Grain." Daganya, Degania, Deganya

DAGMAR Danish. "Joy."

DAHLIA Tuberous-rooted flowering plant from Mexico and Central America, named for Swedish botanist Anders Dahl. Dahlya, Dalya

DAI Japanese. "Great."

DAISY Old English. "Eye of the day." Also variant of **Dacey.**
   Daisee, Daisey, Daisie, Dasi, Dasie

DALE Old English. "Valley." **Dael, Daile, Dayle**

DALIA Hebrew. "Branch." **Dalya**

DALILA Swahili. "Delicate." **Lila, Dahlila, Dahlilah**

DALLAS Scottish. "Skilled." A village in Scotland, and a city in
   Texas.

DALMACE French, from Latin. Dalmatia, a region of Croatia.
   Dalma, Dalmacie, Dalmassa, Dalmatia

DAMA Latin. "Noblewoman." **Dame, Damita**

DAMALIS Greek. "Conqueror."

DAMARIS Greek. "Calf." **Damara, Damaress, Dameris,**
   Dameryss, Damiris, Damris, Demaras, Demaris, Demarys,
   Mara, Mari, Maris

DAMIA Greek. "Fate." **Damian, Damiana, Damiane,**
   Damienne, Damya, Damyan, Damyana, Damyen,
   Damyenne

DAMITA Spanish. "Little noblewoman."

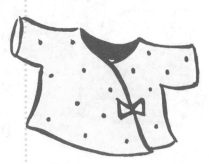

DANA Old English. "From Denmark." **Dane, Dania, Danna,**
   Danni, Danny, Dannye, Dayna

DANAË Greek. In myth, the mother of Perseus. **Danae, Danay,**
   Dee, Denae, Dene

DANICA Old Slavic. "Dawn." **Danicka, Danika**

DANIELLE Feminine form of **Daniel.** Hebrew, "God is my
   judge." **Danee, Danele, Danella, Danelle, Danet, Danette,**
   Daney, Dani, Danica, Danice, Danie, Daniela, Daniella,
   Danila, Danit, Danita, Danitza, Danna, Danney, Danni,
   Danny, Dannyce, Dany, Danya, Danyelle

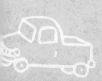

DANTEL Feminine form of **Dante.** Italian, "lasting." **Dantal, Dantelle, Dantia**

DAPHNE Greek. "Laurel tree." In a story told by Ovid, Daphne was a hunter with whom Apollo fell in love. In escaping him, she turned into a laurel tree. **Daff, Daffi, Daffie, Daffy, Dafna, Dafne, Dafnee, Dafnit, Dafny, Daph, Daphna, Daphney, Daphnit, Daphny**

DARA Hebrew. "Courage and compassion." **Darda, Dare, Darelle, Dareth, Darra**

DARALIS Old English. "Beloved." **Daralice**

DARALYN Combination of **Darrel** and **Lynn. Darrelyn, Darrilyn, Darryleen, Darrylene, Darryline, Darrylyn, Darylene, Darylin, Daryline, Darylyne**

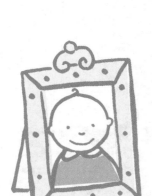

DARBY Old English. "Park with deer." **Darb, Darbee, Darbey, Darbi, Darbie, Darrbey, Darrbi, Darrbie, Darrby**

DARCIE Irish. "Dark." **D'Arcy, Darcee, Darcey, Darci, Darcy, Darsee, Darsey, Darsi, Darsie, Darsy**

DARIA Feminine form of **Darius.** Greek, "great." **Dari, Darian, Darice, Darien, Dariya, Darya, Dorian, Doriane**

DARLENE Old English. "Highly valued." **Dareen, Darelle, Darla, Darleen, Darline, Darlyne**

DARON Feminine form of **Darren.** Contemporary American.

DAVIDA Feminine form of **David.** Hebrew, "loved one." **Davita, Veda** et al., **Vida,** et al., **Vita** et al.

DAVINA Feminine form of **David.** Hebrew, "loved one." **Daveen, Davene, Davi, Daviana, Daviane, Davida, Davina, Davine, Davinia, Devina**

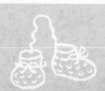

DAWN Contemporary American, from Old English. "Dawn." **Daun, Dauna, Daunna, Daunne, Dawna, Dawnita, Dawnyelle, Dawnysia**

DAY Old English. "Day."

DAYA Hebrew. "Bird."

DEA Latin. "Goddess." **Dia**

DEANNA Old English. "Valley." Also variant of **Diane. Deana, Deann, Deanne, DeeAnn, DeeAnna, DeeAnne, Dena** et al.

DEBORAH Hebrew. "Bee." **Deb, Debb, Debbe, Debbee, Debbera, Debbey, Debbi, Debbie, Debbra, Debby, Debee, Debera, Deberah, Debi, Debir, Debo, Debor, Debora, Debra, Debrah, Debs, Deva, Devora, Devorah, Devorit, Devra, Dobra, Dovra, Dvora, Dvorit**

DECIMA Latin. "Tenth." **Decia, Declan, Deka**

DEE Welsh. "Dark." Also short form of **Deirdre, Delicia, Diana. Dei, Dede, Dedie, DeeDee, Di, Didi**

DEEDAR Persian. "Awake."

DEGULA Hebrew. "Excellent."

DEIFILIA Latin. "God's daughter."

DEIRDRE Irish. "Sorrow." In Irish legend, a beautiful woman whose elopement from the court of King Conchobar led to sorrow and disaster. **Dedra, Dee** et al., **Deedre, Deerdre, Deidra, Deidre, Deidrie, Derdre, Derdriu, Diedra, Diedre, Dierdra, Dierdre**

DEL short form of **Adelaide, Adel, Delia**

DELANEY Irish. "Offspring of the challenger." **Delaine, Delainey, Delainy, Delane, Delani, Delanie, Delany**

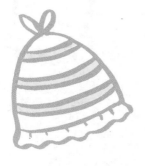

DELIA Greek. "From Delos." **Dehlia, Del, Delinda, Della**

DELICIA Latin. "Delight." **Dee** et al., **Dela, Delice, Delise, Delisha, Delizia, Della, Delyse, Delysia**

DELIGHT English. "Delight."

DELILAH Hebrew. "Delicate." In the Bible, a Philistine woman who outwitted Samson. **Dalila, Delila, Lila, Lilah**

DELLA Short form of **Adelle, Cordelia. Del, Delia, Delie, Delle, Delli**

DELMAR Spanish. "Of the sea." **Delma, Delmara**

DELPHINE Greek. "Dolphin." **Delfin, Delfina, Delfine, Delfyne, Delpha, Delphina, Delphine, Delphinea, Delphinia, Delphinie, Delphinium**

DELTA Fourth letter of the Greek alphabet. **Deltha**

DEMELDA Greek. "To utter aloud."

DEMELZA Cornish. "Fort on the hill."

DEMETRIA Greek. Goddess of fertility. **Demeter, Demetra, Demetris, Demi** et al., **Dimitra, Dimity**

DEMI Short form of **Demetria. Demie, Demmi, Demmie**

DENA Old English. "Valley." Also variant of **Diane. Deana, Deane, Deanna** et al., **Deena, Denah, Dene, Denna, Denni, Dina**

DENISE Feminine form of **Dennis.** French, from Greek, "follower of Dionysus." **Denese, Deney, Deni, Denice, Deniece, Deniese, Denis, Denize, Dennet, Denni, Dennie, Dennise, Denny, Denyce, Denys, Denyse, Deonysia, Dinnie, Dinny, Dionysia**

DEOLINDA Portuguese. "Beautiful God." **Linda**

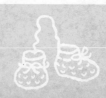

DERINDA Contemporary American. **Dorinda**

DERORA Hebrew. "Flowing stream." **Derorit**

DERYN Welsh. "Bird." **Deren, Derin, Deron, Derrine, Derron**

DESDEMONA Greek. "Wretchedness." The wife of Shakespeare's Othello, who kills her. **Desdemone, Desmona, Desmone**

DESIRÉE French. "Desired." **Desideria, Desir, Desirae, Desirat, Desire, Desiri, Deziree** et al.

DESMA Greek. "Oath."

DESTINÉE Old French. "Fate." **Destiny**

DETTA Short form of **Benedetta**. Latin, "blessed." **Dette**

DEVA Hindi. "God-like." **Devaki, Devi**

DEVIN Irish. "Poet." **Devan, Devinne**

DEVON Old English. A county in southern England. **Devona, Devondra, Devonne**

DEXTRA Feminine form of **Dexter.** Old English, "dyer." Latin, "right-handed."

DEZIREE Contemporary American variant of **Desirée**. French, "desired." **Dezira, Deziray, Dezyrae**

DIAMANTE French. "Diamond." **Diamanta**

DIAMOND English, from French. "Diamond."

DIANA Latin. "Divine." Roman goddess of the hunt. **Danne, Dayann, Dayanna, Dayanne, Deanna** et al., **Deannis, Dee** et al., **Dena** et al., **Di, Diahann, Diahanna, Diahanne, Dian, Diandra, Diane, Diann, Dianna, Dianne, Didi, Dyan, Dyana, Dyane, Dyann, Dyanna, Dyanne**

Names of the Staples Singers

The Staples Singers, a black family that began in gospel and crossed over into the pop charts, had very distinctive names. The founder was the father, the late Roebuck "Pop" Staples. His children include daughters Cleotha, Yvonne, and Mavis, and son Pervis. The group is most famous for their songs "Respect Yourself," "I'll Take You There," and "Let's Do It Again."

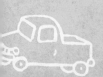

Famous female artists with interesting names

Berenice Abbott, American photographer of New York City

Cecilia Beaux, American figure and portrait painter of the 1890s

Rosalba Carriera, eighteenth-century Italian portrait painter

Malvina Hoffman, twentieth-century American sculptor

Frida Kahlo, twentieth-century Mexican painter known for self-portraits

Dorothea Lange, American Depression-era photographer

Edmonia Lewis, Chippewa/African-American sculptor famed for "Death of Cleopatra"

Nampeyo, Hopi potter

Louise Nevelson, Russian-born sculptor and print maker

Georgia O'Keeffe, American painter of flowers and skulls

Beatrix Potter, creator and illustrator of Peter Rabbit and friends

Patience Lovell Wright, eighteenth-century American sculptor

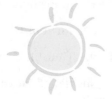

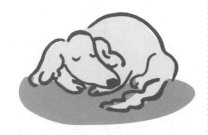

DIANTHE Greek. "Flower of the gods." **Diandre, Diantha**

DIARA African. "Gift." **Diera, Dierra, Dyara**

DICKLA Hebrew. "Palm tree." **Dicey, Dicia**

DIDESSA A river in Ethiopia.

DIDI Diminutive of **Diana, Deirdre.**

DIDIA French. "Desired one." **Didiane, Didiere**

DIDO Greek. In the *Aeneid,* the founding queen of Carthage.

DIDRIKA Feminine form of **Dietrich.** Old German, "people's ruler."

DIELA Greek. "Worships God." **Diella**

DIGNA Latin. "Worthy." **Dinya**

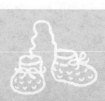

DILLIAN Latin. "Object of worship." **Dilli, Dilliana, Dillien, Dilliena, Dillo**

DILYS Welsh. "True." **Dillis, Dylis, Dyllis, Dylys**

DIMITRA Variant of **Demetria.**

DINAH Hebrew. "Justified." **Dina, Dyna, Dynah**

DIONNE Greek. In the *Iliad,* the mother of Aphrodite. **Deonne, Dion, Diona, Dione, Dionée, Dionetta, Dionis, Dionna**

DIONYSIA Greek. "Follower of Dionysus." **Denise** et al. **Deonysia**

DITA Variant of **Edith.** Old English, "prosperity."

DITZA Hebrew. "Joy." **Ditzah, Diza**

DIVINA Italian. "Divine." **Divinia**

DIXIE French, "tenth." American, "southern United States," i.e., south of the Mason-Dixon line. **Disa, Dix, Dixee**

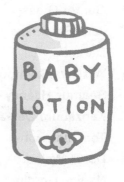

DODIE Hebrew. "Well loved." Also nickname for **Dora, Dorothy. Doda, Dodee, Dodey, Dodi, Dody**

DOLCILA Latin. "Gentle." **Docila, Docilla**

DOLLY Diminutive of **Dorothy. Doll, Dollee, Dolley, Dolli, Dollie**

DOLORES Spanish. "Sorrows (of Christ)." **Dalores, Delora, Delores, Deloria, Deloris, Delorita, Dolorcita, Dolorcitas, Dolorita, Doloritas, Dolours, Lola, Lolita**

DOMINA Latin. "Lady."

DOMINIQUE French feminine form of **Dominic.** Latin, "lord." **Domenica, Domeniga, Dominga, Domini, Dominica, Dominika, Dominizia, Domitia, Mika**

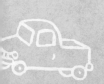

Winners of the Nobel Prize in Literature

These men and women, who together have named thousands of fictional characters, have a great array of names.

2004 **Elfriede Jelinek**—Austria

2003 **J. M. (John Maxwell) Coetzee**—South Africa

2002 **Imre Kertész**—Hungary

2001 **V. S. (Vidiadhar Surajprasad) Naipaul**—Trinidad & Tobago

2000 **Gao Xingjian**—China

1999 **Günter Grass**—Germany

1998 **José Saramago**—Portugal

1997 **Dario Fo**—Italy

1996 **Wislawa Szymborska**—Poland

1995 **Seamus Heaney**—Ireland

1994 **Kenzaburo Oe**—Japan

1993 **Toni Morrison**—United States

1992 **Derek Walcott**—St. Lucia

1991 **Nadine Gordimer**—South Africa

1990 **Octavio Paz**—Mexico

1989 **Camilo José Cela**—Spain

1988 **Naguib Mahfouz**—Egypt

1987 **Joseph Brodsky**—Russia/UnitedStates

1986 **Wole Soyinka**—Nigeria

1985 **Claude Simon**—France

1984 **Jaroslav Seifert**—Czechoslovakia

1983 **William Golding**—United Kingdom

1982 **Gabriel García Márquez**—Colombia

1981 **Elias Canetti**—United Kingdom

1980 **Czeslaw Milosz**—Poland/United States

1979 **Odysseus Elytis**—Greece

1978 **Isaac Bashevis Singer**—United States

1977 **Vicente Aleixandre**—Spain

1976 **Saul Bellow**—Canada/United States

1975 **Eugenio Montale**—Italy

1974 **Eyvind Johnson, Harry Martinson**—Sweden, Sweden

1973 **Patrick White**—Australia

1972 **Heinrich Böll**—Germany

1971 **Pablo Neruda**—Chile

1970 **Alexander Solzhenitsyn**—Russia

1969 **Samuel Beckett**—Ireland

1968 **Yasunari Kawabata**—Japan

1967 **Miguel Angel Asturias**—Guatemala

1966 **Samuel Agnon, Nelly Sachs**—Israel, Germany

1965 **Michail Sholokhov**—Russia

1964 **Jean-Paul Sartre** (declined)—France

1963 **Giorgos Seferis**—Greece

1962 **John Steinbeck**—United States

1961 **Ivo Andric**—Yugoslavia

1960 **Saint-John Perse**—France

1959 **Salvatore Quasimodo**—Italy

1958 **Boris Pasternak**—Russia

1957 **Albert Camus**—France

1956 **Juan Ramón Jiménez**—Spain

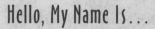
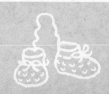

1955	Halldór Laxness—Iceland	1922	Jacinto Benavente—Spain
1954	Ernest Hemingway—United States	1921	Anatole France—France
1953	Winston Churchill—United Kingdom	1920	Knut Hamsun—Norway
1952	François Mauriac—France	1919	Carl Spitteler—Switzerland
1951	Pär Lagerkvist—Sweden	1917	Karl Gjellerup, Henrik Pontoppidan—Denmark, Denmark
1950	Bertrand Russell—United Kingdom		
1949	William Faulkner—United States	1916	Verner von Heidenstam—Sweden
1948	T. S. (Thomas Stearns) Eliot—United States	1915	Romain Rolland—France
1947	André Gide—France	1913	Rabindranath Tagore—India
1946	Hermann Hesse—Germany	1912	Gerhart Hauptmann—Germany
1945	Gabriela Mistral—Chile	1911	Maurice Maeterlinck—Belgium
1944	Johannes V. Jensen—Denmark	1910	Paul Heyse—Germany
1939	Frans Eemil Sillanpää—Finland	1909	Selma Lagerlöf—Sweden
1938	Pearl Buck—United States	1908	Rudolf Eucken—Germany
1937	Roger Martin du Gard—France	1907	Rudyard Kipling—United Kingdom
1936	Eugene O'Neill—United States	1906	Giosuè Carducci—Italy
1934	Luigi Pirandello—Italy	1905	Henryk Sienkiewicz—Poland
1933	Ivan Bunin—Russia	1904	Frédéric Mistral, José Echegaray—France, Spain
1932	John Galsworthy—United Kingdom		
1931	Erik Axel Karlfeldt—Sweden	1903	Bjørnstjerne Bjørnson—Norway
1930	Sinclair Lewis—United States	1902	Theodor Mommsen—Germany
1929	Thomas Mann—Germany	1901	Sully Prudhomme—France
1928	Sigrid Undset—Norway		
1927	Henri Bergson—France		
1926	Grazia Deledda—Italy		
1925	George Bernard Shaw—Ireland		
1924	Wladyslaw Reymont—Poland		
1923	William Butler Yeats—Ireland		

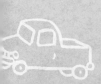

DONALDA Scottish. "World-mighty." **Dona, Donaldina, Donaline, Donelda**

DONATA Latin. "Given."

DONNA Italian. "Lady." **Domella, Dona, Donella, Donelle, Donetta, Donia, Donica, Donielle, Donita, Donnelle, Donni, Donnie, Donnis, Donny, Ladonna** et al.

DORA Greek. "Gift." Also short form of **Adora, Eldora, Eudora, Isadora, Theodora. Dodie** et al., **Doralia, Doralice, Doralie, Dorelia, Dorelle, Dorellia, Doretta, Dorette, Dori, Dorie, Dorika, Dorina, Dorinda, Dorita, Dorra, Dorrie, Dory**

DORCAS Greek. "Gazelle." **Dorca, Doricia**

DORÉ French. "Gilded." **Dorée, Dory**

DOREEN Irish. "Brooding." **Dorena, Dorene, Doreyn, Doryne**

DORINDA Spanish variant of **Dora**. Greek, "gift."

DORIS Greek. "From the ocean." **Dori, Dorice, Dorie, Dorisa, Dorise, Dorith, Doritt, Dorrie, Dorris, Dorry, Dorrys, Dory, Dorys, Doryse**

DORMA Latin. "To sleep."

DORONIT Aramaic. "Gift."

DOROTHY Greek. "Gift of God." **Dee** et al., **Dodie** et al., **Dodo, Doe, Doortje, Dori, Dorlisa, Doro, Dorota, Dorotea, Doroteya, Dorothea, Dorothée, Dorrit, Dorthea, Dorthy, Dory, Dottie, Tea, Thea**

DORY Variant of **Doré**; diminutive of **Dorothy, Isadora.**

DOUCE French. "Sweet."

DREAMA Old English. "Make joyful noise."

DRUELLA Old German. "Clever."

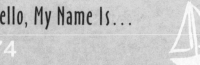

DRUSILLA Latin. "Soft-eyed one." **Drewsila, Dru, Drucella, Druci, Drucie, Drucilla, Drucy, Druscilla, Drusie, Drusus, Drusylla, Drusy**

DUANA Feminine form of **Duane.** Irish, "swarthy." **Duan, Duna, Dwana, Swana**

DUDEE Old English. "Star."

DUEÑA Spanish. "Owner."

DULCIE Latin. "Sweet." **Delcina, Delcine, Delsine, Dulce, Dulcea, Dulcee, Dulci, Dulcia, Dulciana, Dulcibelle** et al., **Dulcina, Dulcine, Dulcinea, Dulcy, Dulsea, Dulsia, Dulsiana, Dulsine**

DULCIBELLE Combination of **Dulcie** and **Belle. Dulcibel, Dulcibella**

DUNA Variant of **Iduna.** Old Norse, "loving one." **Dunia**

DUSHA Russian. "Soul."

DUSTY Feminine form of **Dustin.** Old German, "brave warrior."

DYLANA Feminine form of **Dylan.** Welsh, "from waves." **Dylane**

DYMPNA Irish. "Fawn." **Dymphna** St. Dympna

DYSIS Greek. "Sunset." **Disis, Disys, Dysys**

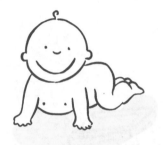

EARLA Feminine form of **Earl.** Old English, "nobleman." **Earleen, Earlene, Earley, Earlie, Earline, Earlla, Erleen, Erlene, Erlina, Erline, Erlla, Urla**

EARTHA Old English. "Earth." **Erda, Erde, Ertha, Herta** et al.

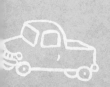

EASTER Spring holiday, originally held in honor of the goddess Eastre.

EBERTA Teutonic. "Bright."

EBONY Name of the wood, known for its black color. **Ebboney, Ebbony, Ebonee, Eboney, Eboni, Ebonie, Ebonney, Ebonni, Ebonnie, Ebonny**

EBIERE Nigerian. Unknown meaning.

ECHO Greek. In myth, a beautiful nymph whom Hera condemned never to speak except to repeat what was said to her.

EDA Old English. "Wealthy." **Edda, Ede**

EDANA Feminine form of **Aidan.** Irish and Scottish, "fire." **Aidana, Aydana, Edanna**

EDELINE Variant of **Adeline.** Old German, "noble."

EDEN Hebrew. "Pleasure, delight." **Eaden, Eadin, Edin, Edna** et al.

EDGA Feminine form of **Edgar.** Old English, "wealthy spearman."

EDINA Old English. "From Edinburgh." **Edeena, Edine, Edyna, Idina**

EDITH Old English. "Prosperity." **Ardith, Dita, Eade, Eadie, Eadita, Eadith, Eady, Eda, Ede, Edi, Edie, Edita, Editha, Edithe, Edy, Edyth, Edytha, Edythe, Eidith, Eidyth, Eidytha, Eyde, Eydie**

EDLYN Old English. "Small noble one."

EDMONDA Feminine form of **Edmund.** Old English. "Wealthy protector." **Edma, Edmée, Edmonde, Edmunda, Edmunde**

EDNA Variant of **Eden.** Hebrew, "pleasure, delight." **Adna, Eddi, Eddie, Eddna, Eddnah, Eddy, Ednah**

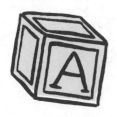

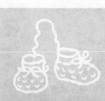

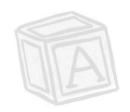

EDREA Old English. "Wealthy, powerful." **Adria, Aydrah, Edra, Eidra, Eydra**

EDRIS Feminine form of **Edric.** Old English, "wealthy ruler." **Edrice, Edriss, Edryce, Edrys, Eidris, Eidriss, Eydris, Idrice, Idris, Idrys**

EDWARDINE Feminine form of **Edward.** Old English, "wealthy defender." **Edwarda, Edwardeen, Edwardene, Edwardyne**

EDWIGE French, from Old German. "Happy battle." **Edvig, Edwidge, Edwig, Edwigge**

EDWINA Feminine form of **Edwin.** Old English, "wealth." **Edweena, Edwena, Edwiena, Edwyna, Edwynna**

EFFAM Variant of **Euphemia.** Greek, "pleasant speech." **Effie** et al, **Effim, Effum, Epham**

EFFIE Diminutive of **Euphemia, Effam.** Greek, "pleasant speech." **Effi, Effy, Ephie, Ephy, Eppie**

EFRATA Hebrew. "Respected." **Efratta**

EFRONA Feminine form of **Efron.** Hebrew, "singing bird."

EGBERTA Feminine form of **Egbert.** Old English, "shining sword." **Egbertha, Egbertina, Egbertine, Egbertyne**

EGIDIA Feminine form of **Giles.** Greek, "young goat." **Giddy**

EGLANTINE Old French. "Sweetbrier." **Eglanti, Eglanty, Eglantyne**

EIBHLIN Irish. "Shining, brilliant."

EILEEN Irish variant of **Helen.** Greek, "bright one." **Ayleen, Eila, Eilean, Eilene, Eiley, Eilidh, Eily, Lena** et al., **Lianna, Lina**

EILUNED Welsh. "Idol." **Eilunet, Eluned** et al., **Linnet** et al., **Luned, Lunet, Lunette**

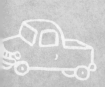

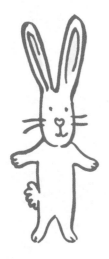

EIR Old Norse. "Peacefulness."

EIRA Welsh. "Snow."

EIREEN Variant of **Irene.** Greek, "peace." **Eiren, Eirena, Eirene**

EIRIAN Welsh. "Silver." **Eeryan**

EITHNE Variant of **Aithne.** Irish, "fire." **Ethnah, Ethnea, Ethnee**

EKATERINA Slavic variant of **Catherine.** Greek, "pure." **Katerina**

ELAINE Old French variant of **Helen.** Greek, "bright one." **Alaina** et al., **Elaina, Elana, Elane, Elanna, Elayne, Ellaina, Ellaine, Ellane, Ellayne, Helaine, Helayne, Lainey** et al.

ELANA Variant of **Elaine, Ilana.**

ELATA Latin. "Elevated." **Lata**

ELBERTA Feminine form of **Elbert.** Old English, "noble," "shining." **Elbertha, Elberthina, Elberthine, Elbertina, Elbertine**

ELDORA Spanish. "The guilded one." **Eldorée, Eldoria, Eldoris, Dora, Dory, L'Dora**

ELEANOR Greek. "Mercy." **Aleanor, Alenor, Aleonore, Alianora, Alienor, Alienora, Eleanora, Eleanore, Elenor, Elenora, Elenore, Eleonora, Eleonore, Elianora, Elianore, Elie, Elien, Elinor, Elinore, Elinorr, Ella** et al., **Elleanor, Elleanora, Ellenor, Ellenora, Ellenore, Elleonor, Ellette, Ellinor, Ellinore, Elly, Elna, Elnora, Elnore, Elyenora, Enora, Heleanor, Heleonor, Helenora, Leanora, Lena, Lenny, Lina, Nelda, Nell** et al., **Nonnie, Nora, Norah, Noreen**

ELECTRA Greek. "Brilliant." **Elektra, Lektra**

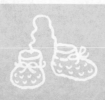

ELENA Spanish variant of **Helen.** Greek, "bright one."

ELFRIDA Old English. "Elf-power." **Elfie, Elfre, Elfredah, Elfredda, Elfreeda, Elfrida, Elfrieda, Elfryda, Elfrydah, Ellfreda, Ellfrida, Elva, Elvah, Freda** et al.

ELGA Slavic variant of **Helga.** Old German, "sacred." **Elgiva, Olga** et al.

ELIANE Feminine form of **Elias.** French, from Hebrew, "Jehovah is God." **Elia, Eliette, Eline, Elyann, Elyanne, Elyette**

ELIDA Variant of **Alida.** Latin, "winged one." **Lida**

ELIDI Greek. "Gift of the sun." **Lidi, Lidy, Liti**

ELIORA Hebrew. "The Lord is my light." **Eleora, Eleorah, Elleora, Leora** et al.

ELISE French variant of **Elizabeth.** Hebrew, "pledged to God." **Eliese, Elisa, Elisée, Elize, Elyse, Liese, Liesel, Lison, Lize**

ELISHEVA Hebrew. "The Lord is my pledge." **Eliseva, Elisheba**

ELISSA Variant of **Alice, Elizabeth. Alisa, Alissa, Allissa, Allyssa, Alyssa, Elissia, Ellissa, Elysa, Elyssa, Elyssia, Ilissa, Ilysa, Ilyssa, Lissa, Lissy, Lyssa**

ELITA Latin. "The chosen." Also variant of **Alida. Lita**

ELIZA Short form of **Elizabeth.** Hebrew, "pledged to God." Arabic, "unique" or "precious." **Elisa**

ELIZABETH Hebrew. "Pledged to God." **Bess** et al., **Beth, Betsy** et al., **Betty** et al., **Buffy, Eilsa, Elisa, Elisabet, Elisabeth, Elisabetta, Elise** et al., **Elisheba, Elissa, Eliza, Elizabet, Elizabetta, Elizabette, Elize, Elle, Elliza, Ellsee, Ellsey, Ellsi, Ellyse, Ellyssa, Ellyza, Elsa** et al., **Elsabet, Elsebin, Elsie** et al., **Elspeth** et al., **Elsy, Elyse, Elyssa, Elyza,**

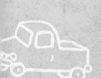

PERSIAN NAMES

The country now known as Iran was once the fabled land of Persia, where people spoke an Indo-European language called Farsi. When Arabs invaded Persia in the sixth century A.D., they introduced many Arabic names and words into the language. Iranians still speak Farsi, but because the country has been invaded by a variety of peoples, Persian names have origins that are hard to determine.

Here are some Persian boys' names and their meanings:

Ali	"elevated"
Amir	"prince"
Anoosh	"joyful"
Arash	a legendary hero
Arman	"ideal"
Bamdad	"morning"
Danesh	"knowledge"
Fateh	"victorious"
Hadi	"leader"
Navid	"good news"
Parsa	"pious"
Perooz	"victorious"
Shaheen	"royal falcon"
Shayan	"suitable"
Zhian	"strong"

And here are some Persian girls' names and their meanings:

Aram	"calm"
Arezou	"desire"
Azadeh	"liberated"
Bita	"unique"
Deedar	"awake"
Ghazalleh	"graceful youth"
Halleh	"halo"
Mahtab	"moonlight"
Negar	"image"
Neheed	goddess of water
Pari	"fairy"
Parvaneh	"butterfly"
Setareh	"star"
Sousan	"flower"
Zalleh	"dew"

Elzbieta, Erzabet, Helsa, Ila, Isabel et al., Letha, Lety, Lilibet et al., Lilla, Lillah, Lisa, Lisbet, Lisbeth, Lisbett, Lisbetta, Lisbette, Lise, Lisel, Liselotte, Lisenka, Lisette, Lisi, Liza, Lizabeth, Lizbeth, Lusa, Lusabet, Lusabeth,

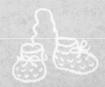

Lusabette, Lysa, Lysbet, Lysbeth, Lysbette, Lyzbet, Lyzbeth, Lyzbette, Orszebet, Tet, Tetsy, Tetty, Ylisabet, Ylisabette

ELKANA Hebrew. "Made by God." **Elkanah**

ELKE Variant of **Alice.** Old German, "noble." **Elka, Ilka, Ilke**

ELLA Old German. "All, completely." Also short form of **Eleanor.** **Ala, Alla, Ela, Elladine, Elle, Ellee, Elletta, Ellette, Elley, Elli, Ellie, Ellina, Elly, Hela, Hele**

ELLAMAE English. Combination of **Ella** and **May. Ellamay, Elliemae, Ellymae, Ellymay**

ELLEN Variant of **Helen, Eleanor. Elan, Elen, Elena, Elene, Eleni, Elenita, Elenyi, Elin, Ellan, Ellene, Ellie, Ellin, Ellon, Elly, Ellyn, Elon, Elyn, Elynn**

ELLICE Feminine form of **Elias.** Greek, "the Lord is God." **Elice, Elise**

ELMA Turkish. "Apple." Also variant of **Alma, Elmina. Ellma, Elm**

ELMINA Short form of **Wilhelmina.** Old German, "will-helmet." **Almina** et al., **Elma, Elmeena, Elmena, Elmine**

ELMIRA Arabic. "Aristocratic lady." **Almera** et al., **Elmeera, Ellmeera, Ellmera, Ellmeria, Elmeera, Elmera, Elmeria, Elmerya, Elmyra, Elmyrah, Mera** et al., **Mira** et al.

ELOISE French form of **Louise.** Old German, "renowned in battle." **Eloisa, Elouise, Eloize, Heloisa, Heloise**

ELRICA Old German. "Ruler over all." **Elricka**

ELSA Short form of **Elizabeth.** Also variant of **Ailsa. Ellsa, Else, Elsha, Elshe, Ilsa, Ilse**

ELSIE Diminutive of **Elizabeth, Alcina. Ellsee, Ellsey, Ellsi, Ellsie, Ellsy, Elsea, Elsee, Elsey, Elsi**

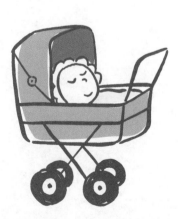

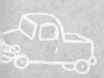

ELSPETH Scottish variant of **Elizabeth. Ellspet, Ellspeth, Elsbet, Elsbeth, Elsbethe, Elspet, Elspie**

ELUNED Welsh. "Idol" or "image." **Eiluned, Elined, Lanet, Lanette, Linet, Linette** et al, **Luned, Lunet, Lynette** et al.

ELVA Irish. Unknown meaning. **Elfie, Elvia, Elvie, Elvra**

ELVINA Feminine form of **Elvin.** Old English, "of the elves." **Alvina** et al., **Elveena, Elvena, Elvene, Elvenia, Elvine, Elvinia, Vina** et al.

ELVIRA Latin, "fair one." Teutonic, "stranger." **Ellvira, Elveera, Elvera, Elvire, Elvyra, Elwira, Lira, Vira**

ELYSIA Greek. "Utopia." In myth, the Elysian Fields were the peaceful, beautiful home of the spirits of good people after death. **Eleese, Elisia, Elyse, Ilysia** et al.

EMANUELA Spanish feminine form of **Emanuel.** Hebrew, "God is with us." **Emanuelita, Manuela, Manuelita**

EMELINE Variant of **Amelia.** Old German, "hard-working." **Ema, Emaleen, Emalene, Emaline, Emalyn, Embline, Emblyn, Eme, Emelen, Emelyn, Emiline, Emlyn, Emm, Emma, Emmalee, Emmalene, Emmaline, Emmalyn, Emmalynne, Emmeline, Emmiline, Emylin, Emylinn, Emylynn**

EMERALD English. "Emerald." **Emeralda, Emeraldina, Emeraldine, Emerant, Emeraude, Emerlin, Emerline, Emmie, Esmeralda** et al.

EMILY Teutonic. "Hard-working." **Aimil, Amalea, Amalia, Amalie, Amelia, Amelie, Ameline, Amelita, Eimile, Em, Emalee, Emalia, Eme, Emelda, Emele, Emelea, Emelia, Emelita, Emely, Emelyne, Emila, Emilea, Emilee, Emiley, Emili, Emilia, Emilie, Emilla, Emillea, Emilley, Emillie, Emilly, Emma** et al., **Emmalee, Emmalie, Emmelee,**

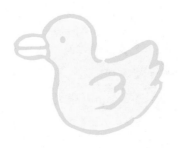

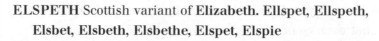

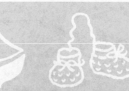

Emmeleia, Emmely, Emmey, Emmi, Emmie, Emmile, Emmilee, Emmily, Emmlee, Emmy, Emmye, Emyle, Emylee, Milly et al.

EMINA Latin. "Eminent."

EMMA Old German. "Universal." Also a variant of **Amelia, Emeline, Emily. Em, Ema, Emm, Emme, Emmet** et al., **Emmi, Emmie, Emmy, Emmye, Ima, Imma, Irma** et al., **Ymma**

EMMANUELLE French feminine form of **Emmanuel.** Hebrew, "God is among us."

EMMETT Old German. "Universal." **Emmet, Emmete, Emmette, Emmot, Emmota, Emmote, Emmott**

EMOGEN Variant of **Imogen.** Latin, "imitation."

EMUNA Arabic. "Faith." **Emunah, Emunda, Emundah, Iman, Imana, Imani**

ENA Variant of **Aithne.** Irish, "fire." **Eithne** et al., **Enah, Enna, Ina**

ENID Welsh. "Life, spirit." **Eanid, Enidd, Enyd, Enydd**

ENRICA Feminine form of **Enrico,** variant of **Henry.** Old German, "estate ruler." **Enrichetee, Enrichetta, Enrika, Enriqueta**

EOLANDE Greek. "Dawn."

ERENE Variant of **Irene.** Greek, "peace." **Erena**

ERICA Feminine form of **Eric.** Scandinavian, "all-ruler." **Airica, Airika, Eraca, Ericka, Erika, Erricka, Errika, Eyrica, Rica** et al., **Ricky** et al.

ERIN Irish. "Of the island to the west," that is, Ireland. **Eire, Eirin, Eirinn, Eiryn, Eirynn, Erina, Erinn, Eryn, Erynn**

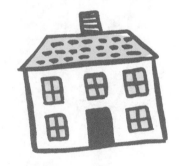

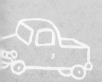

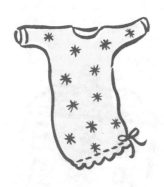

ERLINDA Hebrew. "Spirited." **Erlin, Erlynda**

ERMA Old German. "Universal." **Irma** et al.

ERMINE Old French. "Weasel." **Ermin, Ermina, Erminia, Erminie, Erminn, Ermyne**

ERNESTINE Feminine form of **Ernest.** Old English, "sincere." **Erna, Ernaline, Ernalynn, Ernesta, Ernestina, Ernestyne**

ERWINA Feminine form of **Erwin.** Old English, "boar-friend." **Irwina**

ESHAL Arabic. A flower in heaven.

ESMÉ French. "Esteemed." **Esme, Esmée, Esma**

ESMERALDA Spanish. "Emerald." **Esma, Esmaralda, Esmarelda, Esmaria, Esmie, Esmiralda, Esmiralde, Esmirelda, Ezmeralda**

ESPERANZA Spanish. "Hope." **Esperance, Esperansa, Esperanta, Esperantia**

ESTELLE Old French. "Star." **Essie, Estée, Estel, Estele, Stella, Stelle**

ESTHER Persian. "Star." In the Bible, the Jewish queen of Persia who saved her people from slaughter. **Eister, Essa, Essie, Essy, Esta, Ester, Eszter, Ettey, Etti, Ettie, Etty, Hester** et al.

ESTRELLA Spanish. "Star." **Estrellita, Trella**

ETANA Feminine form of **Ethan.** Hebrew, "steadfastness."

ETHEL Old English. "Noble." **Edel, Ethelda, Ethill, Ethille, Ethyl, Ethyll**

ETHELDREDA Old English. "Noble power."

ETHELINDA Old German. "Noble serpent." **Athelina, Ethelind, Ethelinde, Etholinda, Ethylind**

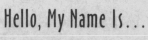

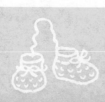

ETHELINE Old English. "Noble." **Ethelene, Ethelin, Ethelyn, Ethelynn, Ethelynne, Ethylyn, Ethylynn, Ethylynne**

ETSU Japanese. "Delight."

ETTIE Diminutive of Harriet, Henrietta. Old German, "estate ruler." **Etta, Etti, Etty**

EUCLEA Greek. "Glory." **Euclaya**

EUDOCIA Greek. "Well regarded." **Docie, Doxie, Doxy, Eudosia, Eudoxia**

EUDORA Greek. "Gifted." **Dora, Eudore**

EUGENIA Feminine form of **Eugene.** Greek, "well-born." **Eugenie, Gene** et al., **Genia, Gina** et al., **Ina, Janie, Jean** et al., **Jenna, Jennie**

EULA Variant of **Ula.** Celtic, "gem of the sea."

EULALIA Greek. "Sweet-speaking." **Eula, Eulalee, Eulaliah, Eulalie, Eulaylia, Eulaylie, Lalie, Lally**

EUNICE Greek. "Victorious." **Euniss, Unice, Uniss, Younice**

EUPHEMIA Greek. "Pleasant speech." **Effam, Effie** et al., **Effim, Effum, Epham, Eufemia, Eupham, Eupheme, Euphemie, Euphie, Phamie, Phemie, Fanny** et al.

EURYDICE Greek. Bride of Orpheus, who followed her to Hades when she died. **Euridice**

EUSTACIA Feminine form of **Eustace.** Greek, "fertile." **Stacie, Stacy** et al., **Stasia**

EVA Spanish, Portuguese variant of **Eve;** short form of **Evangeline.**

EVADNE Greek. "Fortunate." **Evadney, Evadnie, Evanne**

EVANGELINE Greek. "Good news." **Angela, Engie, Eva,**

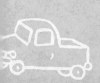

Latin entertainers

Christina Aguilera, singer

Desi Arnaz, Cuban band leader, husband of Lucille Ball, and TV producer

Rubén Blades, Panamanian actor, singer, and political figure

Lynda Carter, actress and wonder woman

Dolores Del Rio, sultry actress from the 1920s through the 1970s

Cameron Diaz, actress whose first big role was in *The Mask*

Gloria Estefan, singer from Miami

Emilio Estevez, actor and director

Salma Hayek, actress whose breakout role was *Frida*

Rita Hayworth, actress whose career soared in the 1930s

Trinidad (Trini) Lopez, singer whose first big hit was "If I Had a Hammer"

Ricardo Montalban, actor and godfather of suave sophistication

Carlos Santana, guitar virtuoso

Selena, singer who died too soon

Lupe Velez, Mexican film actress from 1927 to 1943

Raquel Welch, actress and poster girl in a million dorm rooms

Evangelia, Evangelina, Evangelista, Evangeliste, Eve, Vangie, Vangy

EVANIA Greek. "Peaceful." **Evanne, Evannie, Evanny, Evanya, Vanya**

EVE Hebrew. "Life." In the Bible, Adam and Eve were the first humans on Earth. Also variant of **Evelyn;** short form of **Evangeline. Eba, Ebba, Eeve, Ev, Eva, Evetta, Evette, Evey, Evie, Evienne, Evota, Evvie, Evvy, Evy**

EVELYN Old German. "Hazelnut." **Avelina, Aveline, Avelyn, Avi, Eva, Evaleen, Evalina, Evaline, Eve, Eveleen, Evelene,**

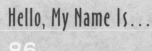

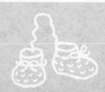

Evelina, Eveline, Evelyne, Evelynn, Evelynne, Evie, Evleen, Evlin, Evline, Evlyn, Evlynn, Evlynne, Evy

EVETTE Variant of **Yvette.** French, "little archer."

EVONNE French variant of **Yvonne. Eevonn, Evon, Evona, Eyvonne**

EYOTA Sioux. "Greatest." Pronounced "EE-yo-tah."

FABIA Feminine form of **Fabian.** Latin, "bean." **Fabian, Fabiana, Fabiane, Fabianna, Fabianne, Fabienne, Fabiola**

FABRIZIA Italian. "Works with the hands." **Fabrice, Fabricia, Fabrienne, Fabritzia, Fabriza**

FAIDA Arabic. "Plentiful." **Fayda, Faidah**

FAITH English, from Old French. "Faith." **Fae, Faithe, Fay, Faye, Fayth, Faythe**

FALASHINA A language spoken in Ethiopia.

FALINE Latin. "Cat-like." **Falene, Fayleen, Faylene, Fayline, Felina, Feyline**

FALLON Irish. "Descended from a ruler."

FANCY English, from French. "Imagine." **Fancee, Fancie**

FANNY Short form of **Euphemia, Frances. Fan, Fannee, Fanney, Fannie**

FAREN Middle English. "Traveler." **Faron, Farren**

FARICA Short form of **Frederica.** Old German, "peaceful ruler." **Faricia, Farisha**

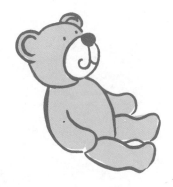

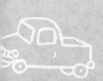

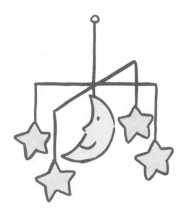

FARRAH Middle English. "Lovely, pleasant." **Fara, Farah, Farra**

FATIMA Arabic. A daughter of the prophet Mohammed. **Fatimah, Fatma**

FAUSTINE Feminine form of **Faust.** Latin, "of good fortune." **Fausta, Fauste, Faustina**

FAWN Old French. "Offspring." **Faina, Fanya, Faun, Fauna, Faunia, Faunita, Fawna, Fawne, Fawnia, Fawnya**

FAY Old French. "Fairy." Also variant of **Faith. Fae, Faye, Fayette, Fayina, Fée**

FAYME Latin. "Acclaim." **Faim, Faym**

FEDORA Variant of **Theodora.** Greek, "gift of God." **Fadora, Fedorla, Fedorn, Fedorna, Fieodora, Fyodora**

FELDA Old German. "Field." **Feldah**

FELICIA Feminine form of **Felix.** Latin, "happy." St. Feliciana. St. Felicísima. **Falecia, Falice, Falicia, Falisha, Falishia, Felcia, Felecia, Felice, Feliciana, Felicidad, Félicie, Felicienne, Felicísima, Felicit, Felicite, Felicity, Felis, Felisa, Felise, Felisha, Felisia, Feliss, Felisse, Felita, Feliz, Feliza, Felysse, Filisia**

FELICIDAD Spanish. "Happiness."

FELIPA Spanish variant of **Philippa.** Greek, "lover of horses."

FEN Chinese. "Fragrant."

FENELLA Irish. "White shoulder." **Fenel, Fenell, Finella, Fynella**

FERN Old English. "Fern." Also short form of **Fernanda. Ferne**

FERNANDA Spanish feminine form of **Ferdinand.** Old German, "explorer." **Anda, Ferdinanda, Ferdinande, Fern, Fernande, Fernandina, Fernandine, Nan, Nanda, Nandie, Nandy**

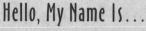

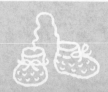

FERNLEY Old English. "Fern meadow." **Fernlee, Fernleigh, Fernly**

FIALL Irish. Unknown meaning.

FIDELITY English, from Latin. "Loyalty." **Fidela, Fidele, Fidelia, Fidella**

FIFI French diminutive of **Josephine.** Hebrew, "the Lord provides." **Fifine, Fifita**

FILIA Greek. "Friendship."

FILIPPA Italian variant of **Philippa.** Greek, "lover of horses." **Fillipa**

FILOMELA Italian variant of **Philomela.** Greek, "lover of song."

FILOMENA Italian variation of **Philomena.** Greek, "beloved."

FINA Spanish. Short form of **Josefina.** Hebrew, "the Lord provides."

FIONA Irish. "Fair, pale." **Fee, Fione, Fionna, Nona**

FIONNULA Irish. "White shoulder." **Fenella, Finella, Finnuala, Finola, Fionnuala, Nuala** et al.

FIORA Italian. "Flower." **Fiore, Fiorella, Fiorentine**

FLAMINIA Latin. "Priestess." **Flamina, Flaminya**

FLANNA Irish. "Russet hair." **Flana, Flannah**

FLAVIA Latin. "Blonde hair." **Flava, Flavah, Flavie, Flaviere, Flavya, Flavyere**

FLETA Old English. "Immaculate."

FLEUR French. "Flower." **Fleurette, Fleurina, Fleurine**

FLORA Latin. "Flower." **Fiora** et al., **Flo, Flor, Flore, Florella, Florelle, Flori, Floria, Florie, Florissa, Florita, Florrie, Florry, Flossie** et al.

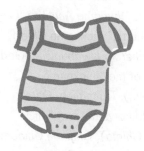

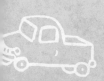

Choosing eight names at once

In December 1998, a Nigerian-born mother gave birth in Houston, Texas, to octuplets—six girls and two boys. The couple gave the children traditional Ibo names from Nigeria. The daughters were named *Chukwuebuka Nkemjika* ("God is great," nickname *Ebuka*), *Chidinma Anulika* ("God is beautiful," nickname *Chidi*), *Chinecherem Nwabugwu* ("God thinks of me," nickname *Echerem*), *Chimaijem Otito* ("God knows my way," nickname *Chima*), *Chijindu Chidera* ("God has my life," nickname *Odera*), and *Chinagorom Chidiebere* ("God is merciful," nickname *Gorom*). The sons were named *Chukwubuikem Maduabuchi* ("God is my strength," nickname *Ikem*) and *Chijoke Chinedum* ("God is my leader," nicknamed *Jioke*).

FLORENCE Latin. "Flowering." **Fiorenza, Flonda, Flora** et al., **Florance, Floreen, Floren, Florense, Florencia, Florentia, Florentina, Florentyna, Florenz, Florenza, Floriana, Floriane, Florice, Florida, Florina, Florinda, Florine, Florise, Florissa, Floryn, Florynce**

FLOSSIE Diminutive of **Flora, Florence. Floss, Flossi, Flossy**

FLOWER Middle English. "Flower."

FONDA French. "Melting." **Fon, Fondea, Fonta**

FORTUNA Latin. "Good fate." **Fortunata, Fortunate, Fortune, Fortunella**

FRAN Short form of **Frances.** Latin, "from France." **Fanny** et al., **Frannee, Franni, Frannie, Franny**

FRANCES Feminine form of **Francis.** Latin, "from France." **Fancey, Fanchette, Fanchon, Fancie, Fancy, Fanechka, Fanny** et al., **Fannya, Fannye, Fanya, Fran, France, Franceline, Francene, Francesca, Francetta, Francette, Francey, Franchesca, Franci, Francie, Francina, Francine, Francisca, Franciska, Françoise, Franconia, Francyne, Frania, Franika, Franja, Frank, Frankie, Franky, Franni, Frannie, Franny, Franzetta, Franzi, Franziska, Franziske, Fronia**

FRANCESCA Italian feminine form of **Francis.** Latin, "from France." **Franchesca**

FRANCISCA Spanish feminine form of **Francis.** Latin, "from France." **Franciska**

FRANÇOISE French feminine form of **Francis.** Latin, "from France."

FRAYDA Hebrew. "Joy." **Frayde, Fraydyne**

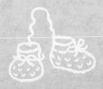

FREDA Old German. "Peaceful." Also short form of **Alfreda, Elfreda, Winnifred. Freada, Fredda, Freddi, Freddie, Freddy, Fredi, Fredy, Fredyne, Freeda, Freedah, Freida, Freide, Frida, Fridha, Frieda, Friedah, Fryda, Frydda**

FREDELLA Combination of **Fred** and **Ella. Fredelle**

FREDERICA Feminine form of Frederick. Old German. "Peaceful ruler." **Farica** et al., **Federica, Feriga, Fred, Fredalena, Fredda, Freddee, Freddey, Freddi, Freddie, Freddy, Fredericka, Frederickina, Frederine, Frederique, Fredi, Fredia, Fredie, Fredricia, Fredrika, Frerika, Friederike, Fyrdryka, Rica, Rickie** et al.

FREYA Scandinavian. "Highborn lady." Norse warrior goddess of love and beauty. **Fraya, Freja**

FRITZI Feminine form of **Fritz.** Old German, "peaceful ruler." **Fritsey, Fritze, Fritzey, Fritzy**

FULVIA Latin. "Blonde one."

GABRIELLE French, from Hebrew. "Heroine of God." **Gabay, Gabbe, Gabbi, Gabbie, Gabby, Gabel, Gabell, Gabey, Gabi, Gabie, Gabriel, Gabriela, Gabriele, Gabriell, Gabriella, Gabrila, Gabryel, Gabryell, Gabryella, Gabryelle, Gaby, Gavrielle, Gavrila** et al.

GADA Hebrew. "Fortunate." **Gayda**

GAEA Greek. "The Earth." **Gaia, Gaiea, Gala, Kaia**

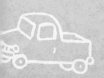

GAETANA Italian. "From Gaeta," a city in southern Italy. **Gaetane, Gaetanya**

GAIL Short form of **Abigail.** Hebrew, "my father rejoices." **Gael, Gahl, Gaila, Gaile, Gaill, Gale, Gayel, Gayelle, Gayle, Gayleen** et al., **Gayll, Gaylle**

GAL Hebrew. "Spring." **Gali, Galit, Galy**

GALATEA Greek. "White as milk." **Galatée**

GALIENA Old German. "High one." **Galiana, Galianna, Galya, Galyena**

GALINA Russian variant of **Helen.** Greek, "bright one." **Galena, Galita**

GALLIA Latin. "Gaul." Also variant of **Galya. Gala, Galla**

GALYA Hebrew. "The Lord has redeemed." **Galia, Gallia, Gallya**

GANA Hebrew. "Garden." **Ganah, Ganit, Ganna, Gannah, Ganya**

GARDENIA A shrub with fragrant white flowers, named for the Scottish naturalist Alexander Garden.

GARLAND Old French. "Garland." **Garlande, Garlend**

GARNET Old French. "Garnet. "**Garnette, Garnia, Garniata**

GAVRILA Hebrew. "Heroine of God." **Gabrielle** et al., **Gavi, Gavra, Gavrilla, Gavryla, Gavrylla**

GAY Old French. "Lighthearted." **Gae, Gai, Gaye**

GAYLENE American variant of **Gail,** short form of **Abigail.** Hebrew, "my father rejoices." **Gaylene, Gayline**

GAYNOR Irish. "Daughter of the fair-skinned one." **Gaenor, Gayna, Gayner, Gaynora, Gaynore**

GAYORA Hebrew. "Valley of light." **Gayorla, Gayorna, Gayorra**

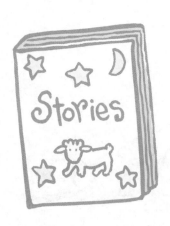

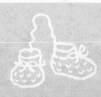

GAZELLA Latin. "Delicate." **Gazelle, Gazellya**

GEDUAL Hebrew. "Big one." **Gedua, Gedula, Gedulah**

GEMINI Greek. "Twin." **Gemella, Gemelle, Gemina, Geminay, Gemine**

GEMMA Latin. "Fullness." **Jema, Jemma**

GENE Greek. "Well-born." Also variant of **Jean**; short form of **Eugenia, Geneva, Genevieve, Virginia. Geena, Geenia, Geenya, Gena, Genie**

GENEVA Old French. "Juniper." Also a city in Switzerland. **Gene** et al., **Genever, Genevia, Genevra, Genevre, Genna, Genovera, Ginebra, Ginevra, Ginevre, Janeva, Janevra**

GENEVIEVE Old German. "Of woman." **Genavieve, Gene** et al., **Geneveeve, Genivieve, Gennie, Genny, Genovefa, Genovera, Genoveva, Gina** et al., **Jenevieve, Jennie** et al.

GENNIE Variant of **Jennie. Genna, Genni, Genny**

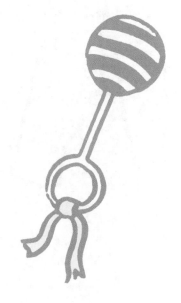

GEORGETTE French feminine form of **George**. Latin, "farmer." **Georgetta**

GEORGIA Feminine form of **George**. Latin, "farmer." **George, Georgea, Georgess, Georgie, Georgina** et al., **Giorgia**

GEORGINA Feminine form of **George**. Latin, "farmer." **Georgeann, Georgeanna, Georgeanne, Georgeen, Georgeina, Georgena, Georgene, Georgiana, Georgiann, Georgianna, Georgianne, Georgienne, Georgine, Georgyana, Georgyann, Georgyanne, Giorgina, Giorgyna, Jorgi**

GERALDINE Feminine form of **Gerald**. Old German, "spear ruler." **Deena, Dina, Dyna, Geralda, Geraldeen, Geraldene, Geraldina, Gereldina, Gereldine, Gerildine, Gerrie** et al., **Gerroldine, Jeraldine** et al., **Jerilene, Jerrie** et al.

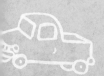

GERALYN Combination of **Gerald** and **Lynn. Geralynn, Geralynne, Gerilyn, Gerilynn, Gerrilyn, Jeralleen, Jerilene**

GERANIUM Latin, from Greek. "Geranium" or "little crane."

GERDA Old Norse. "Shelter." **Garda**

GERHARDINE Old German. "Spear ruler." **Gerhardina**

GERMAINE French. "From Germany." **Germain, Germana, Germane, Germayn, Germayne, Jermaine** et al.

GERRIE Diminutive of **Geraldine. Geri, Gerri, Gerry, Jerrie** et al.

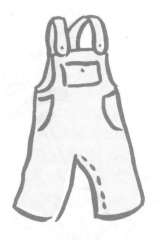

GERTRUDE Old German. "Spear." **Gatt, Gatty, Gerda, Gert, Gerta, Gerte, Gerti, Gertie, Gertina, Gertraud, Gertrud, Gertruda, Gertrudis, Gerty, Traudi, Trudel, Trudy** et al.

GHALIYA Arabic. "Sweet-smelling." **Ghalya**

GHAZALLEH Persian. "Graceful youth."

GHISLAINE French. "A pledge."

GHITA Italian. Short form of **Margherita**. Greek, "pearl." **Chita, Gita**

GIACINTA Italian variant of **Hyacinth**. Greek, "hyacinth." **Giacinda, Giacintha, Giacinthia**

GIANA Italian feminine form of **John**. Hebrew, "the Lord is gracious." **Gianetta, Gianina, Giannine, Ginetta, Ginette, Ginnette, Jeanine** et al., **Nina**

GIANETTA Italian variant of **Jeanette**, feminine form of **John**. Hebrew, "the Lord is gracious."

GIDGET Contemporary American. From a 1957 book by Frederick Kohner and movies based on it.

GIGI Diminutive of **Gilberte, Ginger.**

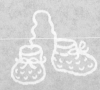

GILA Hebrew. "Joy." **Chila, Geela, Geelan, Ghila, Gilah, Gilana, Gili, Gilla, Gillia, Gilliah**

GILBERTE Feminine form of **Gilbert.** Old German, "shining pledge." **Berta, Berte, Bertie, Berty, Gigi, Gilberta, Gilbertina, Gilbertine, Gill, Gillie, Gilly**

GILDA Old English. "Gilded."

GILLIAN Feminine form of **Julius.** Latin clan name, "youthful." **Gilian, Gill, Gillan, Gillianne, Gillie, Gillot, Gilly, Gillyanne, Jill** et al., **Jillian** et al.

GINA Short form of **Regina, Eugenia, Virginia. Geina, Gene** et al., **Ginah, Gini, Ginie, Ginna, Jena, Jeena**

GINGER English, from Latin. "Ginger." Also variant of **Virginia. Gingie, Jinger, Jinjer**

GINNY Diminutive of **Virginia.** Latin, "virgin." **Ginnee, Ginni, Ginnie, Jinnie, Jinny**

GIOVANNA Italian feminine form of **John.** Hebrew, "the Lord is gracious."

GISELLE Old German. "Protector." **Ghisele, Ghisella, Ghislaine, Ghislane, Ghislayne, Gisela, Giselda, Gisele, Gisella, Giza, Gizela, Gizella**

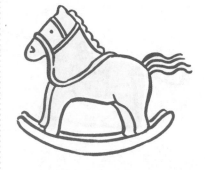

GITANA Spanish. "Gypsy." **Gitane, Gitanna, Kitana**

GITTA Short form of **Brigitta, Brigitte.** Irish, "strength." **Gita, Gitte**

GIULDITTA Italian variant of **Judith.** Hebrew, "Jewish."

GIULIA Feminine form of **Giulio.** Italian, from Latin, "youthful." **Giula, Giuliana, Giulietta, Julia** et al.

GIUSEPPA Feminine form of **Giuseppe.** Italian, from Hebrew, "the Lord provides." **Giuseppina**

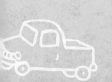

GIUSTINIA Feminine form of **Giustino.** Italian, from Latin, "just." **Giustina, Giustinana**

GLADYS Welsh. "Princess." **Glad, Gladdi, Gladdie, Gladdis, Gladdys, Gladi, Gladie, Glady, Gladyss, Gleda, Gwladys, Gwyladyss**

GLENDA Welsh. "Fair and good." **Glendi**

GLENNA Feminine form of **Glenn.** Irish, "glen." **Glen, Gleneen, Glenene, Glenine, Glenn, Glenne, Glennene, Glennie**

GLENYS Welsh. "Holy." **Glenice, Glenis, Glennice, Glennis, Glennys**

GLORIA Latin. "Glory." **Glora, Gloree, Glori, Gloriana, Gloriane, Glorianna, Glorianne, Glorie, Glorria, Glory**

GLYNIS Welsh. "Narrow glen." **Glinyce, Glinys, Glinyss, Glynnis**

GODIVA Old English. "God's gift." In legend, Lady Godiva rode naked through town so her husband would lower the people's taxes. Today, Godiva is the name of a large chocolate company.

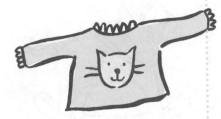

GOLDA Old English. "Gold." **Goldarina, Goldarine, Goldi, Goldia, Goldie, Goldina, Goldy, Goldya**

GOZALA Hebrew. "Young bird." **Gozalia, Gozalya**

GRACE Latin. "Pleasing, joyful." **Engracia, Gracee, Gracey, Gracia, Graciana, Gracie, Graciela, Grata, Gratia, Gratiana, Grayce, Grazia, Graziella, Grazina, Graziosa, Grazyna**

GRACILIA Latin. "Slender." **Gracilla, Grasilia, Grasilla**

GRAINNE Irish. "Love." **Grainnia, Grania**

GREER Scottish variant of **Gregory.** Latin, "alert." **Grier**

GREGORIA Feminine form of **Gregory**. Latin, "alert." **Gregorya**

GRETA German short form of **Margaret**. Greek, "pearl." **Greeta, Gretal, Grete, Gretel, Grethel, Gretl, Gretna, Gretta, Grette, Grietje, Grittie, Gritty, Gryta**

GRETCHEN German short form of **Margaret**. Greek, "pearl."

GRISELDA Old German. "Gray fighting maid." **Chriselda, Criselda, Griseldis, Grishelda, Grishilda, Grishilde, Grissel, Grizel, Grizelda, Grizzel, Gryselde, Gryzelde, Selda, Zelda**

GRISIGON Variant of **Chrysogon**. Greek, "born of gold." **Grisegod, Grisigion, Grisigonia, Grissecon, Grissecone**

GUADALUPE Mexican place name. The Virgin of Guadalupe is the patron saint of Mexico. **Lupe, Lupita**

GUCCI A contemporary fashion label.

GUDRÜN Scandinavian. "Battle." **Gudren, Gudrin, Gudrinn, Gudruna, Gudrune**

GUIDA Italian. "Guide."

GUILLERMA Spanish. Feminine form of **Willhelm**. Old German, "will-helmet."

GUINEVERE Welsh. "White and smooth, soft." **Gaenna, Guenever, Guenevere, Gueniveer, Guenna, Guennola, Guinna, Gwen et al., Gweniver, Gwennola, Gwynn et al., Jenifer et al., Wendy et al., Winnie et al.**

GUNHILDA Old Norse. "Battle-maid." **Gunhilde, Gunilda, Gunilla, Gunnhilda**

GUSTAVA Feminine form of **Gustav**. Scandinavian, "staff of the gods." **Gustaya, Gustha**

GWEN Short form of **Guinevere, Gwendolyn, Gwyneth**. **Gwenn, Gwenna, Gwenni, Gwennie, Gwenny, Gwynn et al.**

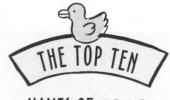

THE TOP TEN

NAMES OF 1912

The Year the *Titanic* Sank

BOYS

John
William
James
Robert
George
Joseph
Charles
Frank
Edward
Thomas, Walter (tie)

GIRLS

Mary
Helen
Dorothy
Ruth
Margaret
Anna
Mildred
Frances
Elizabeth
Marie

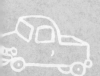

GWENDA Welsh. "Fair and good."

GWENDOLYN Welsh goddess of the moon. **Guendolen, Guenna, Gwen** et al., **Gwendaline, Gwendolen, Gwendolene, Gwendolin, Gwendoline, Gwendolynn, Gwendolynne, Gwenna, Gwenndolen, Gwynn** et al., **Wendy** et al., **Winnie** et al., **Wynelle, Wynette, Wynne** et al.

GWYNETH Welsh. "Happiness." **Gweneth, Gwenette, Gwenith, Gwenyth, Gwineth, Gwinyth, Gwynet, Gwynith, Gwynna, Gwynne, Gwynneth, Winnie** et al., **Wynne** et al.

GWYNN Welsh. "Fair, blessed." **Gwyn, Gwynne, Winne** et al.

GYPSY Old English. "Romany." **Gipsi, Gipsy, Gypsi**

HABIBAH Arabic. "Lover." **Habiba**

HADASSAH Hebrew. "Victory." **Dasi, Dassi, Hadassa, Hadasseh**

HADRIA Feminine form of **Hadrian.** Latin, "make beautiful." **Hadara, Hadrianna, Hadrien, Hadrienne, Hadrya, Haydria, Haydrya**

HAIDÉE Greek. "Modest."

HALCYONE Greek. "Kingfisher" (bird).

HALDANA Old Norse. "Half Danish." **Haldane, Haldanna**

HALEY Old Norse. "Hero." **Haile, Hailie, Halie, Hallie, Hally, Hayley**

HALFRIDA Old German. "Peaceful heroine."

HALIMAH Arabic. "Gentle, soft-spoken." **Halima**

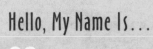

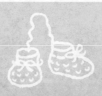

HALIMEDA Greek. "Thinking of the sea." **Halette, Hali, Hallie, Halymeda, Meda, Medie**

HALINA Hawaiian. "Resemblance."

HALLEH Persian. "Halo."

HANA Japanese. "Flower." Also variant of **Hannah. Hanae, Hanako**

HANNAH Hebrew. "Grace." **Ann** et al., **Chanah** et al., **Hana, Hanita, Hanna, Hanne, Hannele, Hannelore, Hanni, Hannie, Hanny, Honna, Nan** et al.

HAPPY English. "Cheerful." **Happi**

HARALDA Old Norse. "Army ruler." **Halley, Hallie, Hally, Haroldena, Haroldine**

HARLEY Old English. "Long meadow." **Arley** et al., **Harlea, Harlee, Harleigh, Harly**

HARMONY Latin. "Agreement." **Harmonia, Harmonie**

HAROLDINE Old Norse. "Army ruler." **Haralda** et al., **Haroldena**

HARRIET Feminine form of **Henry, Harry.** Old German, "estate ruler." **Ettie** et al., **Harrie, Harriett, Harrietta, Harriette, Harriot, Harriott, Hatsie, Hatsy, Hattie, Hatty, Henka, Hettie** et al., **Rita, Yetta, Yette**

HARUKO Japanese. "Spring child."

HASIA Hebrew. "Protected by God." **Haisa, Hasya, Haysa, Haysia**

HATTIE Diminutive of **Harriet, Henrietta.** Old German, "estate ruler." **Hatty**

HAWA Arabic. "Breath of life." **Hawah**

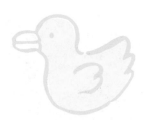

HAYAT Arabic. "Life."

HAYFA Arabic. "Slender, well-shaped." **Haifa**

HAYLEY Old English. "Hay meadow." **Hailea, Hailee, Haileigh, Haily, Haleigh, Halie, Hally, Haylea, Haylee, Hayleigh**

HAZEL Old English. "Hazelnut tree." **Hasse, Hazele, Hazell, Hazelle**

HEATHER Middle English. "Heather," a flowering shrub. **Hetter**

HEBE Greek. "Youth." In myth, the daughter of Hera and the wife of Hercules.

HEDDA Old German. "Warfare." **Heda, Heddi, Heddie, Hedi, Hedy, Hetta**

HEDWIG Old German. "Happy battle." **Hadvig, Hadwig, Hedvig, Hedviga, Hedvige, Hedwiga, Hedwige, Hedy**

HEDY Greek. "Delightful, sweet." **Heddy, Hedia, Hedyla**

HEIDI Short form of **Adelaide**. Old German, "noble." **Heida, Heidy**

HELAINE French variant of **Helen**. Greek, "bright one." **Helayne, Elaine** et al.

HELEN Greek. "Bright one." In the *Iliad*, the wife of Menelaus, king of the Spartans. **Aileen** et al., **Alena, Alene, Alina, Aline, Eileen** et al., **Elaine** et al., **Eleanor** et al., **Elena, Ella** et al., **Ellen** et al., **Galina** et al., **Halina, Helaine, Helayne, Helena, Hélène, Helina, Hella, Hellen, Hellena, Hellene, Ilene** et al., **Iliana** et al., **Ilona** et al., **Jelena** et al., **Leanora** et al., **Lena** et al., **Lina** et al., **Nelda, Nell** et al., **Nonnie, Olena** et al., **Yelena** et al.

HELGA Old German. "Sacred." **Elga, Elgiva, Olga** et al.

HELICE Greek. "Spiral." **Helike**

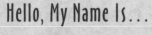

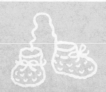

Rainbow names

The Rainbow Family of Living Light gathers every summer on public land, where they camp, have drum circles, and practice (temporarily, for some) the hippie lifestyle circa 1969. They have no official leaders, preferring to make decisions by consensus. Participants traditionally adopt "Rainbow names," such as the following:

Sunflower
Dan D
Papabear Rainbow
7 Song
Aspen Moon
Butterfly Bill
Vermin Supreme
Pie Man
Granola Jay
Guano
Jaydreaming
Sun Gypsy
Stardust

Trading Bill
Spaceman
Dovid
Shadow
Crystalhawk
Rich in Spirit
Piet
Mabl
Tommy Gunn
Spiritbik
Fraglthndr
Lady Saavedra
Starrchild

HELMA Old German. "Helmet." Also short form of **Wilhemina. Helmina, Helmine, Helminette**

HELOISE French variant of **Louise.** Old German, "renowned warrior." **Eloise** et al., **Heloisa**

HELSA Danish variant of **Elizabeth.** Hebrew, "consecrated to God."

HENRIETTA Feminine form of **Henry.** Old German, "estate ruler." **Enrica** et al., **Ettie** et al., **Harriet** et al., **Hatsie, Hatsy, Hattie, Hatty, Hendrika, Henia, Henie, Henka, Hennie, Henrie, Henrieta, Henriette, Henrika, Henryetta, Hettie** et al., **Yenta, Yente, Yetta** et al.

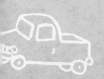

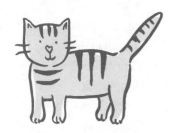

HEPZIBAH Hebrew. "My delight is in her." **Eppie, Hepsie, Hepsibah, Hephzibah**

HERA Greek. "Queen." In myth, the wife of Zeus and protector of marriage.

HERMA Latin. "Stone pillar."

HERMIONE Greek. "Earthly." In myth, the daughter of Helen and Menelaus, and the wife of Achilles's son Neoptolemus and also of Orestes. In contemporary fiction, a main character in the Harry Potter series. **Hermia, Hermina, Hermine, Herminia, Herminie**

HERMOSA Spanish. "Beautiful."

HERO Greek. "Hero." Priestess of Aphrodite who killed herself over the loss of her lover, Leander. Also a character in Shakespeare's *Much Ado About Nothing*.

HERTHA Old English. "Earth." **Eartha** et al., **Herta, Herti**

HESPER Greek. "Evening star." **Hespera**

HESPERIA Latin. "The western land," Italy.

HESTER Greek. "Star." **Hesther, Hestie, Hettie** et al., **Hittie**

HETTIE Diminutive of **Harriet, Henrietta, Hester. Hetta, Hetti, Hetty**

HIALEAH Creek. "Pretty prairie." Pronounced "HI-ah-lee-ah."

HIAWASSEE Cherokee. "Meadow."

HIBERNIA Latin. "Ireland."

HIBISCUS Latin. "Mallow." A large genus of flowering herbs, shrubs, and trees.

HILA Hebrew. "Praise."

HILARY Greek. "Cheerful." **Hilaria, Hilarie, Hillary, Hillery, Hilliary**

HILDA Old German. "Battle woman." **Hilde, Hildie, Hildy, Hylda**

HILDEGARDE Old German. "Battle stronghold." **Helle, Hilda** et al., **Hildagard, Hildagarde, Hildegaard, Hildegard, Hildegunn, Hille**

HILDEMAR Old German. "Battle-renowned."

HILDRETH Old German. "Battle counselor." **Hildred**

HILMA Short form of **Wilhelmina**. Old German, "will-helmet." **Halma, Helma**

HINDA Hebrew. "Female deer." **Hynda**

HIPPOLYTA Greek. "She who frees the horses." In myth, the queen of the Amazons; Hercules killed her for her girdle. **Hippolita**

HISA Japanese. "Longevity." **Hisae, Hisako, Hisaye, Hisayo**

HOLDA Old German. "Hidden." **Holde, Holle, Hulda**

HOLLAND English. "Netherlands." Holland Coors, doyenne of the Colorado beer company.

HOLLIS Old English. "Holly bushes." **Holis**

HOLLY Old English. "Holly." **Holley, Holli, Hollie, Hollye**

HONELLA Variant of **Onella**. Greek, "light."

HONEY Old English. "Honey."

HONORA Latin. "Honored one." **Honor, Honorah, Honorata, Honorée, Honoria, Honorine, Honorita, Honour, Nora** et al., **Onora** et al.

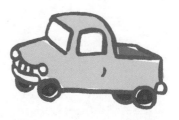

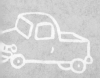

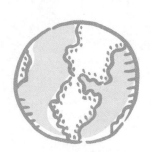

HOPE Old English. "Hope."

HORATIA Latin. Clan name. **Horacia**

HORTENSE Latin. Clan name. **Hortensia, Hortenspa, Ortensia**

HOSHA Japanese. "Star."

HUBERTA Feminine form of **Hubert.** Old German, "shining intellect."

HUETTE Feminine form of **Hugh.** Old German, "intellect." **Huetta, Hugette, Hughette, Hughina**

HULA Hebrew. "Make music."

HULDA Old German. "Loved one." **Huldah, Huldie**

HYACINTH Greek. "Hyacinth." **Cinthia, Cinthie, Cinthy, Giacinta, Giacintia, Hyacintha, Hyacinthe, Hyacinthia, Hyacinthie, Hyacintia, Jacinta** et al., **Jacinthe, Jackie** et al.

HYPATIA Greek. "Highest." **Hypacia**

IANA Variant of **Aya.** Hebrew. "Bird." **Ianna**

IANTHA Greek. "Purple flower." **Ianthe, Ianthia, Ianthina, Janthia**

IDA Unknown meaning. **Idaleen, Idalene, Idalia, Idalina, Idaline, Idalya, Idalyne, Idana, Idande, Iddes, Ide, Idel, Idell, Idella, Idelle, Idena, Ideny, Idetta, Idette, Idhuna, Idona, Idonia, Idony, Ita**

IDALEE Combination of **Ida** and **Lee.**

IDALOU Combination of **Ida** and **Lou.**

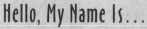

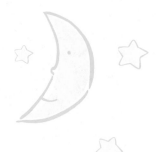

IDINA Variant of **Edina.** Old English, "from Edinburgh."

IDRA Aramaic. "Scholarly."

IDRIS Welsh. "Fiery champion."

IDUNA Old Norse. "Loving one." **Duna, Dunia, Idunia, Idunna**

IEESHA Variant of **Aisha.** Arabic, "woman;" Swahili, "life." **Ieasha, Ieashia, Ieashiah, Iesha, Ieshah**

IGNACIA Feminine form of **Ignatius.** Greek, "fire." **Ignatia, Ignazia, Iniga**

ILA Old French. "Island."

ILANA Hebrew. "Tree." **Elana, Ilanit, Lani**

ILENE Contemporary variant of **Aileen.** Greek, "light." **Ilean, Ileen, Ileene, Illene**

ILIANA Greek. "Trojan." **Ileana, Ileane, Ileanna, Ileanne, Illia, Illiana, Ilyana**

ILKA Slavic. "Flattering," "hardworking." **Ilke**

ILONA Hungarian variant of **Helen.** Greek, "light." **Illona, Ilone, Ilonka**

ILSA German variant of **Elizabeth.** Hebrew, "pledged to God." **Elsa** et al.

ILUMINADA Spanish. "Illuminated one."

ILYSIA Variant of **Elysia.** Greek. "Utopia." **Ileesia, Ilise, Ilysa, Ilyse**

ILYSSA Variant of **Alyssum.** Greek. "Sane."

IMA Variant of **Emma.** Old German. "Universal." **Imma**

IMANA Variant of **Emuna.** Arabic, "Faith." **Imani**

IMELDA Old German and Italian. "All-consuming fight." **Imalda**

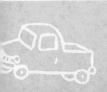

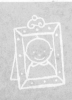

IMMACULADA Spanish. "Flawless." **Immaculata**

IMOGEN Latin. "Imitation." **Emogen, Emogene, Imagina, Imogene, Imogenia, Imogine, Imojean, Imojeen**

IMPERIA Latin. "Imperial." **Impericia, Imperiza, Imperizia**

INDIA Country name. In Latin America, "indigenous woman."

INEZ Spanish variant of **Agnes**. Greek, "pure" or "virginal." **Ines, Inesa, Inesita, Inessa, Ynez** et al.

INGA Scandinavian. "Guarded by Ing." **Ingaberg, Ingaborg, Inge, Ingeberg, Ingeborg, Ingerith, Ingune, Inka**

INGARET Variant of **Angahard**. Welsh, "greatly loved." **Ingaretta**

INGRID Scandinavian. "Beautiful." **Inger**

INOCENCIA Spanish. "Innocence." **Inocenta, Inocentia**

IOANNA Greek variant of **Hannah**. Hebrew, "grace."

IOLA Greek. "Cloud of dawn." **Iole, Iolia**

IOLANTHE Greek. "Violet flower."

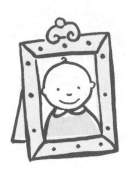

IONA Greek feminine form of **John**. Hebrew, "the Lord is gracious." Also an island off the coast of Scotland. **Ione, Ionia**

IONE Greek. "Violet." **Ionia, Ionie**

IPHIGENIA Greek. "Sacrifice." **Iphigenie, Genia**

IRENE Greek. "Peace." **Arina, Eireen** et al., **Erena, Erene, Ihrin, Ira, Ireen, Iren, Irena, Irenea, Irenee, Irenka, Irina, Irine, Iryna, Orina, Oryna, Rena, Rene** et al., **Renette, Rina, Yarina**

IRIS Greek. "Rainbow." A Greek and Roman goddess of the rainbow. **Irisa, Irita, Iryl, Irys**

IRIT Hebrew. "Daffodil."

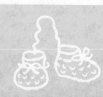

IRMA Old German. "Universal." **Erma** et al., **Irmalin, Irmaline, Irmina, Irmine, Irminia**

IRVETTE Feminine form of **Irving.** Old English, "sea friend."

ISABEL Spanish variant of **Elizabeth.** Hebrew, "pledged to God." **Bel, Bela, Belia, Belicia, Belita, Bell, Bella, Belle, Bellita, Ezabel, Ib, Ibbie, Ibbot, Ibby, Isa, Isabeau, Isabele, Isabelita, Isabell, Isabella, Isabelle, Isbel, Isobel, Isobell, Isobella, Isobelle, Isopel, Issabell, Issie, Issy, Izabel, Izabell, Izabella, Izabelle, Izzie, Izzy, Nib, Tibbi, Tibbie, Tibbs, Tibby, Ysabeau, Ysabel** et al.

ISADORA Feminine variant of **Isidore.** Latin, "gift of Isis." **Isadore, Isidora, Isidore**

ISIS Egyptian goddess of the moon. **Isys**

ISLA A river in Scotland. Also Spanish, "island."

ISMENIA Unknown origin. **Ismania, Ismena, Ismentia, Ismenya**

ISOLDE Celtic. In Arthurian legend, the lover of Tristram. **Isaut, Iseult, Iseut, Isola, Isold, Isolda, Isolt, Isolte, Yseult, Yseulte, Yseut, Ysolda, Ysolde**

ITA Irish. "Thirst."

IVANA Feminine form of **Ivan,** Slavic variant of **John.** Hebrew, "the Lord is gracious." **Iva, Ivancha, Ivanka, Ivanna**

IVETTE French variant of **Yvette,** feminine form of **Yves.** French, "little archer." **Evette**

IVORY Latin. "Ivory." **Ivoreen, Ivorine, Ivrie, Ivry**

IVY Old English. "Ivy." **Ivee, Ivey, Ivie**

Girls' names show more creativity

According to scholars, American parents are more likely to be creative in choosing names for girls than for boys. In the *Proceedings of the Royal Society* in 2003, Matthew Hahn and Alexander Bentley made some interesting observations about American names. First, for boys as well as girls, a relatively few names are given to the vast majority of babies. No surprise there. What is odd is that the number of newly invented names is higher for girls than boys. For each ten thousand girls named, there are an average of 2.3 new names, whereas for the same number of boys named there are only 1.6 new names. This means that girls are 40 percent more likely than boys to be given a new name.

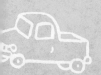

JACINTA Spanish variant of **Hyacinth**. Greek. "hyacinth." **Jacenda, Jacenta, Jacey, Jacie, Jacinda, Jacindia, Jacinna, Jacinth, Jacintha, Jacinthe, Jacinthia, Jacy, Jacynth, Jacyntha, Jacynthe, Jacynthia**

JACKIE Short form of **Jacqueline, Hyacinth. Jackee, Jackey, Jacki, Jacky, Jacquey, Jacqui, Jacquie**

JACOBINA Feminine form of **Jacob**. Hebrew, "he who supplants." **Jackie** et al., **Jacoba, Jacobetta, Jacobette, Jacobila, Jacobine**

JACQUELINE French. Feminine form of **Jacob**. Hebrew, "he who supplants." **Jacalin, Jacalyn, Jackalin, Jackalinne, Jackalyn, Jackalynn, Jackalynne, Jackelyn, Jackelynn, Jackelynne, Jacket, Jackett, Jacketta, Jackette, Jackie** et al., **Jacklin, Jacklyn, Jacklynn, Jacklynne, Jackqueline, Jacyn, Jaclyn, Jaclynn, Jaclynne, Jacolyn, Jacolynn, Jacolynne, Jacqualine, Jacqualyn, Jacquelean, Jacquelin, Jacquelyn, Jacquelynn, Jacquelynne, Jacquenetta, Jacquenette, Jacquetta, Jacquette, Jacquine, Jaculine, Jakolina, Jakoline, Jaqualine, Jaquelin, Jaqueline, Jaquelyn, Jaquelynn, Jaquelynne, Jaquetta, Jaquith**

JADA Spanish, "jade." Arabic, "goodness."

JADE English, from Spanish. "Jade." **Jayde**

JADWIGE Polish. "Safety in battle." **Jadwiga, Jadwigga**

JAEL Hebrew. "Mountain goat."

JAFIT Hebrew. "Beautiful." **Jaffa, Jafite, Yaffa** et al.

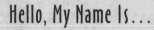
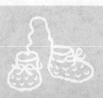

JAMIE Feminine form of **James.** Hebrew, "he who supplants." **Jaime, Jaimee, Jaimey, Jaimie, Jaimy, Jamee, Jamella, Jamesena, Jamesenya, Jamesina, Jamesine, Jami, Jayme, Jaymee, Jaymi, Jaymie, Jymie**

JAMILA Arabic. "Lovely." **Jamilah, Jamilla, Jamille, Jamillia**

JAN Feminine form of **John.** Hebrew, "the Lord is gracious." **Jann, Janna** et al.

JANE English feminine form of **John.** Hebrew, "the Lord is gracious." **Jaine, Jainee, Janaya, Janaye, Jandy, Janea, Janeczka, Janee, Janelle** et al., **Janerette, Janessa, Janet** et al., **Janey, Jani, Jania, Janica, Janice, Janie, Janique, Janita, Janith, Janka, Janna** et al., **Janney, Janny, Jantina, Jany, Jasisa, Jassisa, Jatney, Jayne, Jean** et al., **Jehane, Jenda, Jeni, Jenica, Jeniece, Jenie, Jensina, Jensine, Jinna, Joanna** et al., **Seonaid, Sheena** et al., **Sinead**

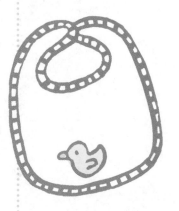

JANELLE Variant of **Jane,** feminine form of **John.** Hebrew, "the Lord is gracious." **Janel, Janela, Janella, Jannel, Jannelle, Jaynel, Jaynell, Jaynelle, Jeanelle, Jenella, Jenelle**

JANET Scottish variant of **Jane,** feminine form of **John.** Hebrew, "the Lord is gracious." **Gianetta, Jan, Janeta, Janetta, Janette, Janit, Jannet, Jannetta, Jenet, Jenett, Jenetta, Jenette, Jenit, Jennie** et al., **Nat, Nettie** et al.

JANICE Variant of **Jane,** feminine form of **John.** Hebrew, "the Lord is gracious." **Janiece, Janique, Janis, Janise, Janiss, Jannice, Janyce**

JANNA Variant of **Jan, Jane, Johanna,** feminine forms of **John.** Hebrew, "the Lord is gracious." **Jana, Janah, Janaya, Janne**

JANTHIA Variant of **Iantha.** Greek, "purple flower."

JAPONICA New Latin, from Japanese. "Japanese." **Japonicia**

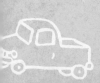

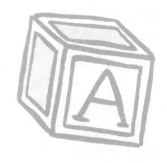

JASMINE Persian. "Jasmine." **Jasmin, Jasmina, Jassamayn, Jazan, Jazmin, Jesmond, Jess, Jessamina, Jessamine, Jessamy, Jessamyn, Jessie, Jessimine, Yasmin** et al.

JAY Middle English, from Middle French. "Jaybird." **Jae, Jaye, Jaylene**

JEAN Scottish variant of **Jane**. Also short form of **Eugenia**. **Gene** et al., **Genna, Jeana, Jeane, Jeanette** et al., **Jeanice, Jeanie, Jeanna, Jeanne, Jeannie, Jeany, Jeena, Jeenie, Jeeny, Jenat, Jenda, Jenica, Jennie** et al.

JEANETTE Variant of **Jane, Jean**, feminine forms of **John**. Hebrew, "the Lord is gracious." **Janetta, Janette, Jannetta, Jeannetta, Jeannette, Jenet, Jenett, Jenetta, Jenette, Jennet, Jennett, Jennetta, Jennette**

JEANNINE Feminine form of **John**. Hebrew, "the Lord is gracious." **Gianina, Janean, Janeen, Janene, Janina, Janine, Jannine, Jeaneen, Jeanene, Jeanine, Jeannean, Jenine, Jennine**

JELENA Russian variant of **Helen**. Greek, "light." **Jelina, Yelena**

JEMIMA Arabic. "Dove." **Jamima, Jem, Jemimah, Jemma, Jemmie, Jemmimah, Jemmy, Jona, Mima, Mimma, Yemima** et al.

JEMMA Variant of **Gemini, Jemima**.

JENA Arabic. "Little bird." **Jenna**

JENILEE Combination of **Jenny** and **Lee**. **Jennylee, Jennyleigh**

JENNIE Diminutive of **Genevieve, Janet, Jean, Jennifer. Jen, Jeni, Jennee, Jenney, Jenni, Jenny**

JENNIFER Welsh. "White, smooth, and soft." **Gennie** et al., **Gennifer, Genniver, Jena, Jenefer, Jenifer, Jeniffer, Jenn, Jenna, Jennica, Jennie** et al., **Jenniver, Jinny**

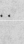

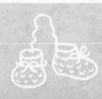

JERALDINE Variant of **Geraldine**. Old French, "spear ruler." **Jeraldeen, Jeraldene, Jerroldeen**

JEREMIA Feminine form of **Jeremiah**. Hebrew, "the Lord is exalted." **Jeree, Jeremina, Jeremiya, Jerrie**

JERRIE Diminutive of **Geraldine, Jeremia. Gerrie** et al., **Jere, Jeree, Jeri, Jerie, Jerree, Jerrey, Jerri, Jerry, Jery**

JERUSHA Hebrew. "Married." **Jarusha, Jeruscha**

JESSALYN Combination of **Jessica** and **Lynn. Jessalin, Jessalyne, Jessalynn, Jessalynne**

JESSICA Hebrew. "Rich gift." **Jess, Jessa, Jesse, Jesseca, Jessey, Jessicka, Jessie, Jessla, Jessy**

JESUSA Spanish feminine form of **Jesus**. Hebrew, "the Lord is salvation."

JETTE Danish. "Black." **Jet, Jeta, Jete, Jetta**

JEWEL English, from Old French. "Jewel." **Jewelia, Jewell, Jewelle, Jewelya**

JEZEBEL Hebrew. "Impure." **Jesabel, Jesabell, Jesabelle, Jessabel, Jessabell, Jessabella, Jessabelle, Jezabel, Jezabell, Jezabella, Jezebelle, Jezibel, Jezybell**

JIAO Chinese. "Beautiful."

JIA LI Chinese. "Good, beautiful."

JILL Diminutive of **Gillian, Jillian. Jilli, Jillie, Jilly**

JILLIAN English variant of **Gillian**. Latin, "youthful." **Jilan, Jilian, Jiliana, Jill** et al., **Jillana, Jillane, Jillayne, Jilleen, Jillene, Jilliana, Jillianne, Jillien, Jillyan, Jillyanna, Jilliyanne, Jillyen**

JIMENA Feminine form of **Jímen**, Spanish variant of **Simon**. Hebrew, "one who listened." **Jimenia, Jimenya, Ximenia** et al.

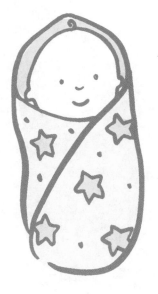

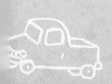

JING Chinese. "Sparkling."

JINNY Short form of **Virginia.** Latin, "virgin." **Ginnie, Ginny, Jinnie**

JINX Latin. "Spell." **Jynx**

JOAKIMA Feminine form of **Joachim.** Hebrew, "God will judge." **Joaka, Joakina, Joaquina, Joaquine, Joke**

JOAN Feminine form of **John.** Hebrew, "the Lord is gracious." **Ione, Jane** et al., **Joana, Joane, Joanie, Joanne** et al., **Joannie, Johan, Jone, Jonee, Jonet, Joni, Jonie, Siobhan**

JOANNE Variant of **Joan,** feminine form of **John.** Hebrew, "the Lord is gracious." **Jo, Joana, Joann, JoAnn, Jo Ann, Joanna, JoAnna, Jo Anna, Jo Anne, JoAnne, Joeann, Johanna, Johannah, Jojo, Jo Jo**

JOBETH Combination of **Jo** and **Beth.**

JOBY Feminine form of **Job.** Hebrew, "the afflicted." **Jobey, Jobi, Jobie, Jobina, Joby, Jobyna**

JOCASTA Greek. "Shining moon."

JOCELYN Latin. "The merry one." **Jocelin, Joceline, Jocelyne, Josalin, Josaline, Joscelin, Josceline, Joscelyn, Joselin, Joseline, Joselyn, Joselyne, Josilen, Josilin, Josiline, Josline, Josselyn, Jossline, Josslyn**

JOCOSA Latin. "Playful." **Giocosa, Giocossa, Jocossa**

JODY Hebrew. "Woman from Judea." Also diminutive of **Josephine,** variant of **Judy. Jodee, Jodene, Jodette, Jodey, Jodi, Jodia, Jodie**

JOELLE Feminine form of **Joel.** Hebrew, "God is willing." **Joel, Joela, Joelin, Joell, Joella, Joelliane, Joellin, Joelline, Joelly, Joely, Joelynn, Jowella, Jowelle, Jo Elle**

JOHANNA Feminine form of **Johann,** German variant of **John.** Hebrew, "the Lord is gracious." **Joanne** et al., **Johannah**

JOHNNA Feminine form of **John.** Hebrew, "the Lord is gracious." **Giana, Gianna, Johna, Jona**

JOLAN Greek. "Violet." **Jola, Jolanne, Jolanta, Jolantha**

JOLENE Contemporary American. **Joeleen, Joeline, Jolean, Joleen, Joleene, Jolina, Joline, Jolyn, Jolyna, Jolyne, Jolynn**

JOLIE French. "Pretty." **Jolee, Joley, Joli, Jolia, Jolie, Joly**

JONQUIL English, from French or Spanish. "Small, fragrant daffodil." **Jonquilla, Jonquille**

JORA Hebrew. "Summer rain shower." **Jorah**

JORDAN Hebrew. "Descend." **Jardena, Jordain, Jordana, Jordane, Jordanna, Jordena, Jorey, Jorie, Jorry, Jourdan**

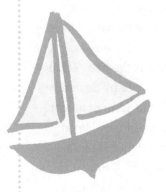

JOSEPHINA Feminine form of **Joseph.** Hebrew, "the Lord provides." **Fifi** et al., **Fina, Joe, Joette, Joey, Josee, Josefa** et al., **Josefena, Josefene, Josefina, Josefine, Josepha, Josephe, Josephene, Josephine, Josephyna, Josephyne, Josetta, Josette, Josey, Josie, Josy, Jozaa, Pepita, Peppie, Peppy, Pheenie, Pheeny, Phina, Yosepha** et al., **Yosephine**

JOVITA Latin. "Joyful." **Jovicia, Jovite, Jovitha**

JOY Middle English, from Old French. "Joy." **Gioia, Joi, Joia, Joie, Joya, Joyann, Joye**

JOYCE Middle English, from Middle French. "Merry." **Jocea, Jocey, Joice, Jossy, Joyous**

JOYCELYN Combination of **Joyce** and **Lynn. Joycelin, Joycelynn, Joycelynne**

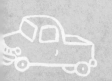

Names that make funny phrases

The following names look reasonably normal in print, but when you pronounce them they form unexpected—and often corny—phrases. Although jokes involving such names have been around a very long time (remember the book *Under the Bleachers* by Seymour Butt?), this form of humor has received new life on National Public Radio's *Car Talk* and *A Prairie Home Companion.* In naming a child, say prospective names aloud to make sure you don't add another bit of hilarity to the world of low humor.

Lisa Karr
Sara Bellum
Natalie Attired
Peter Abbott
Justin Time
Eileen Yourway
Pat McAnn
Ophelia Payne
Harry Butz
Yul Adenauer
Hyam Gone
Paige Turner
Sonny Day
Anita Bath
Dan Druff
Guy Wire
Heywood Jabuzzoff
Marge Inovera
Warren Peace

Walter Mellon
Tyrone Shoes
Biff Stew
Ivan Awfulich
Rose Busch
Pete Moss
Amanda B. Reckundwith
Xavier Onassis
Sandy Beach
Anne Chovy
Eileen Dover
Phil Harmonic
Al Fresco

JUANA Spanish feminine form of **John.** Hebrew, "the Lord provides." **Janita, Janitia, Juanita, Juniata, Junita, Nita**

JUBILEE Hebrew. "Ram's horn." **Jubilea, Jubilie**

JUDITH Hebrew. "Praised." **Eudice, Giuditta, Jehudit, Jehudith, Jody** et al., **Judee, Judi, Judie, Judit, Judita, Judite, Juditha, Judithe, Judy, Judye, Jutta, Yehudit, Yudith** et al.

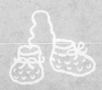

JUDY Short form of **Judith.** Hebrew, "praised." **Jody** et al., **Judee, Judey, Judi, Judie, Judye**

JULIA Feminine form of **Julius.** Latin, "youthful." **Giulia** et al., **Jiulia, Joleta, Joletta, Jolette, Juet, Juetta, Jules, Julie** et al., **Juliet** et al., **Julina, Julinka, Juliska, Julita, Julitta, Julyna, Yulenka, Yulia, Yuliya**

JULIANA Feminine form of **Julian.** Latin, "youthful." **Julian, Juliane, Juliann, Julianna, Julianne, Julieanna, Julieanne, Julienne, Julyan, Julyana, Julyane, Julyanna, Julyanne**

JULIE French feminine form of **Julius.** Latin, "youthful." **Jule, Julee, Juley, Juli, Julita, July**

JULIET Latin. Clan name. "Youthful." **Giulietta, Julieta, Juliett, Julietta, Juliette, Juiyet, Julette**

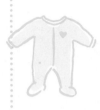

JUNE English, from Latin. "Youthful." Also the sixth month of the year. **Junella, Junelle, Junette, Junia, Juniata, Junieta, Junina, Junine, Une** et al.

JUNO Latin. In myth, the supreme goddess.

JUSTINE Latin. "Fair, righteous." **Giustina** et al., **Jussy, Justa, Justene, Justie, Justina, Justinn, Justy, Justyna, Justyne**

KACEY Variant of **Acacia, Casey. Kacie, Kacy, Kasey, Kasi, Kaycee, Kaycey, Kayci, Kaycie, Kaysee, Kaysey, Kaysi, Kaysy**

KADENZA Latin. "With rhythm." **Cadence** et al., **Kadena, Kadence, Kadensa, Kadenzia, Kadenzla**

KAGAMI Japanese. "Mirror." **Kagamee**

KAIA Variant of **Gaea**. Greek, "the Earth."

KAITLIN Variant of **Caitlin,** an Irish variant of **Catherine.** Greek, "pure." **Kaitlan, Kaitlann, Kaitlinn, Kaitlyn, Kaitlynn**

KALA Hindi. "Time." **Kalah**

KALANDRA Variant of **Calandra**. Greek, "lark."

KALANTHA Variant of **Calantha**. Greek, "lovely flower."

KALI Sanskrit. "Energy." Also the Hindu goddess of life and death. **Kalie, Kalli**

KALILA Arabic. "Beloved." **Kahlila, Kalilah**

KALLIOPE Variant of **Calliope**. In myth, the Muse of epic poetry. **Kallyope**

KALLISTA Variant of **Callista**. Greek, "most beautiful." **Kala, Kalesta, Kalista, Kalli, Kallie, Kally, Kallysta**

KALYCA Greek. "Rosebud." **Kalica, Kalicka, Kalika, Kaly**

KAMA Sanskrit. "Love." **Kamma**

KAMEKO Japanese. "Tortoise."

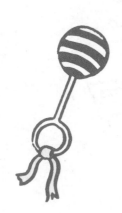

KAMILAH Arabic. "Perfect." **Kamila, Kamilla, Kamillah**

KAMILLA Variant of **Camille**. French, from Latin, "pure." **Kamila, Kamilka, Kamille, Kamyla, Milla, Millie**

KANANI Hawaiian. "A beauty."

KANDACE Variant of **Candace**. Latin, "brilliantly white." **Dacey** et al., **Kandi, Kandice, Kandie, Kandiss, Kandy**

KANDRA Variant of **Candra**. Latin, "glowing." **Kandi, Kandie, Kandy**

KARA Variant of **Cara**. Latin, "dear one." **Karrah, Karrie**

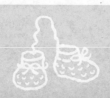

KAREN Danish variant of **Katherine**; variant of **Keren. Caren, Carin, Carine, Caron, Caronn, Caronne, Carren, Carri, Carrin, Carron, Caryn, Carynn, Carynne, Karena, Kari, Karin, Karon, Karri, Karrin, Karrina, Karryn, Karyn, Karynn, Kerran, Kerrin, Kerron, Kerynn, Kerynne**

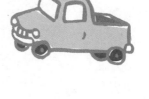

KARIMAH Arabic. "Giving." **Karima**

KARINA Variant of **Carina.** Italian, "dear little one." **Karena, Karine**

KARLA Variant of **Carla.** Old German, "man." **Karlla**

KARLOTTA German variant of **Charlotte.** French, from Old German, "man." **Karlota**

KARMA Hindi. "Destiny." **Carma, Carmah, Karmah, Kharma**

KARMITI Eskimo. "Trees."

KARNIELA Hebrew. "The Lord's horn." **Carniela, Carniella, Karna, Karniella, Karnit, Karnyella**

KAROLINA Slavic variant of **Caroline**; feminine form of **Carl, Charles.** Old German, "man." **Karalina, Karaline, Karalyn, Karalynn, Karalynna, Karalynne, Karlen, Karli, Karlie, Karlinka, Karoline, Karolinka, Karollina, Karolline, Karolyn, Karolyna, Karolyne, Karolynn, Karolynne, Leena, Lina, Lyna**

KASMIRA Feminine form of **Casimir.** Old Slavic, "bringing peace." **Kasmeera, Kasmirya**

KASSANDRA Variant of **Cassandra.** In the Odyssey, a Trojan princess and prophet whom no one believed. **Kass, Kassandera, Kassee, Kassey, Kassi, Kassie, Kassey, Kassy**

KASSIA Variant of **Cassia.** Greek, "cinnamon."

KATE Short form of **Katherine, Kathleen. Cait, Caitie, Cate, Catey, Cati, Catie, Caty, Cayt, Cayte, Cayti, Caytie, Cayty, Kaethe, Kait, Kaite, Kaitey, Kaitie, Katea, Katey, Kathe, Kati, Katie, Katy**

KATEESHA Contemporary American. **Kateeshia, Kateysha, Katisha**

KATHERINE Variant of **Catherine.** Greek, "pure."

KATHLEEN Irish variant of **Katherine.** Greek, "pure." **Cathleen** et al., **Katalina, Kathelina, Katheline, Kathileen, Kathleene, Kathlene, Kathlin, Kathline, Kathlyne, Kathyline, Katleen, Katlin, Katline, Katlyne**

KATHY Diminutive of **Katherine, Kathleen.** Greek, "pure." **Kathee, Kathey, Kathi, Kathie**

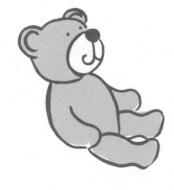

KATRINA Variant of **Katherine.** Greek, "pure." **Catreena, Catrin, Catrina, Catrine, Catrinn, Catriona, Catrionagh, Catrionaugh, Catrynn, Kaitreen, Kaitrin, Kaitrina, Kaitrine, Kaitrinna, Kaitrona, Katrena, Katreina, Katrine, Katriona, Katrionagh, Katrionaugh, Katryna, Trina** et al.

KAY Greek. "Rejoice." Also nickname for **Katherine, Kathleen** et al. **Caye, K, Kai, Kaye**

KAYA Hopi. "Older sister."

KAYLA Variant of **Katherine, Kelila.** Greek, "pure." **Cailya, Calya, Cayla, Caylia, Kaela, Kaila, Kalia, Kalya, Kaylah**

KAYLEY Irish. "Slender." **Cailey, Cailie, Caylie, Kailey, Kaily, Kaley, Kalie, Kaly, Kaylee, Kayley, Kaylie, Kayly**

KAYLYN Combination of **Kay** and **Lynn. Caylin, Kailyn, Kaylynn, Kaylynne**

KEDMA Hebrew. "Eastward." **Kedmah**

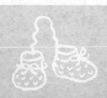

KEELY Irish. "Beauty" or "warrior maid." **Kealee, Kealey, Keali, Kealie, Kealy, Keeley, Keeli, Keelia, Keelie, Keighlee, Keighleigh, Keighley, Keighly**

KEFIRA Hebrew. "Young lioness." **Kefirah, Kefyra, Kefyrah**

KEISHA Contemporary American. **Keesha, Kesha, Kisha, LaKeisha, Lakisha**

KELDA Old Norse. "Deep mountain spring." **Keldah, Keldi, Keldine, Kellda, Kelldah**

KELILA Hebrew. "Crowned." **Kaile, Kayla** et al., **Kayle, Kaylee, Kelilah, Kelula, Kelulah, Kyla, Kyleen, Kylene, Kylila, Lila, Lyla**

KELLY Irish. "Warrior." **Keli, Kelie, Kellee, Kelley, Kellina, Kely**

KELSEY Middle English. "Keel." **Kelcey, Kelci, Kelcie, Kelcy, Kellsey, Kellsie, Kelsee, Kelseigh, Kelsie, Kelsy**

KEMBA Old English. "Lord." **Kem, Kembe**

KENDRA Old English. "Knowledgeable." **Ken, Kendis, Kenna, Kinna**

KENYA Country in East Africa.

KEREN Hebrew. "Animal horn." **Kaaren, Kareen, Karen, Karin, Karon, Karyn, Kerin, Keryn, Kyran**

KERENSA Cornish. "Love." **Karensa, Karenza, Kerenza**

KERRY Irish. "Dark one." Also a county in Ireland. **Keree, Keri, Kerrey, Kerri, Kerrie, Kery**

KESHET Hebrew. "Rainbow." **Kashet**

KESHISHA Aramaic. "Respected elder." **Keshishah**

KETIFA Arabic. "To pick a flower." **Ketifah**

KETURA Hebrew. "Incense." **Keturah**

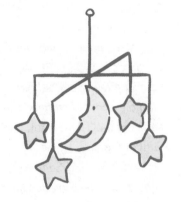

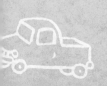

Gidget goes Chicago

Gidget—a name combining "girl" and "midget"— began as a 1957 book about a diminutive though spunky fifteen-year-old girl who took up the then all-male sport of surfing. The book spawned a series of movies: Gidget, Gidget Goes Hawaiian, Gidget Goes to Rome, *et cetera. In 1965, an eighteen-year-old Sally Field starred for one season on television as Gidget, and a year later a woman in Chicago was inspired to give her daughter this famous name. That little girl is now Gidget Ambuel.*

"My mother named me right out of the movies. She loved that show. I've had a great time with the name. I think it's fun. I say my name and people say, 'What?' or 'Did you really go to Rome? Did you really go to Hawaii?' I've always liked my name. It's a great conversation piece, and people always remember me—always.

"My mother wanted *Gidget* to be my first name, but the priest would not baptize me with the first name of *Gidget*. He said the first name must be a very Catholic name, so she had to name me *Christine Gidget*. Everybody thinks it's a nickname, but I have always gone by *Gidget*.

"My kids? I named my daughter *Ellie* and my son *Ian*. I always joked that I would like to name my daughter *Gidget,* but my friends said, 'There can't be two Gidgets in one family.'

"I'll always be Gidget. That name has made me."

KEVYN Feminine form of **Kevin**. Irish, "handsome." **Keveen, Kevina, Kevine**

KEZIA Hebrew. "Sweet-scented." **Kazia, Kerzia, Ketzia, Ketziah, Keziah, Kezze, Kezzie, Kissie, Kitzia, Kitzie, Kitzya, Kizzie, Kizzy**

KIA Contemporary American. **Keeya, Kiya, Kya**

KIANA Contemporary American. **Kia, Quiana, Quianna**

KIBA Variant of **Akiva**. Hebrew, "protect" or "shelter." **Kibah**

KICHI Japanese. "Lucky." **Kichy, Kitchi, Kitchie**

KIKU Japanese. "Chrysanthemum branch." **Kikuko, Kikuyo**

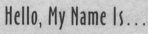 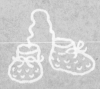

KIM Short form of **Kimberly. Kym**

KIMBERLY Old English. "Chief." **Kim, Kimba, Kimber, Kimberlee, Kimberleigh, Kimberley, Kimberlie, Kimberlyn, Kimbli, Kimbly, Kimblyn, Kimmie, Kimmy, Kym, Kymberlee, Kymberley, Kymberly**

KIMI Japanese, "the greatest." Algonquin, "secret." **Kimie, Kimiko, Kimiyo**

KIMINELA Sioux. "Butterfly." Pronounced "kih-mee-neh-la."

KIN Old English. "Family member." **Kinchen, Kinsey, Kinsy, Kyn, Kyne**

KINETA Greek. "Active one."

KINNERET Hebrew. "Harp." **Kineret, Kinnerett**

KINU Japanese. "Silk."

KIRBY Old Norse. "Church village."

KIRSTEN Scandinavian. "Christian." **Keerstin, Keirstin, Kersten, Kerstin, Kiersten, Kierstin, Kierstynn, Kirsteen, Kirsti, Kirstie, Kirstin, Kirsty, Kirstynn**

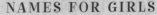

KISMET Persian. "Destiny." **Kissie, Kizmet, Kizzie, Kizzy**

KITANA Variant of **Gitana.** Spanish, "gypsy."

KITRA Hebrew. "Crown." **Kitrah, Kitrya**

KITTY Diminutive of **Katherine.** Greek, "pure." **Kit, Kittee, Kittey, Kitti, Kittie**

KIVA Variant of **Akiva.** Hebrew, "protect," "shelter." **Kivah, Kivi**

KIZZY Diminutive of **Kezia, Kismet. Kissie, Kizzie**

KLARA German, Hungarian variant of **Clara.** Latin, "bright." **Klarah, Klari, Klarika, Klarissa, Klarisza, Klaryssa**

KLAUDIA Polish variant of **Claudia.** Latin, "lame." **Klaudya**

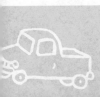

KLEMENTINA Variant of **Clementine.** Latin, "granting mercy." **Klementijna, Klementine, Klementyna**

KLOTILD Hungarian variant of **Clothilde.** German, "renowned battle." **Klothild, Klothilda, Klothilde, Klotilda, Klotilde**

KOKO Japanese. "Stork." **Koku**

KONEKO Japanese. "Kitten." Pronounced "ko-neh-ko."

KONSTANZE German variant of **Constance.** Latin, "steadfastness." **Konna, Konni, Konnie, Konny, Konstance, Konstantia, Konstantija, Konstantina, Kosta, Kostatina, Kostya, Stanze, Tina**

KORA Variant of **Cora.** Greek, "maiden." **Korella, Koren, Korena, Korenda, Korenza, Koretta, Korette, Korey, Kori, Korilla, Korissa, Korrie, Kory, Koryssa**

KORALIE Variant of **Coral.** Latin, "pebble." **Korali, Koraly**

KORDELIA Variant of **Cordelia.** Irish, "jewel of the sea." **Kordella, Kordula, Kordulia, Kordulla, Kordullia**

KORENET Hebrew. "To shine forth." **Koreneth**

KORINNE Variant of **Corrine.** French, from Greek, "maiden." **Koreen, Korina, Korinna, Korrina, Korrine, Koryne, Korynna**

KOURTNEY Variant of **Courtney.** Old English, "court dweller." **Kortnee, Kortney, Kortnie, Kourtnee, Kourtney, Kourtnie, Kourtny**

KORNELIA Variant of **Cornelia.** Latin, "like a horn." **Korneely, Korneelya, Kornelija, Kornellia, Kornelya**

KRISTA Variant of **Christine.** Greek, "Christian." **Chrissta, Christa, Crista, Crysta, Krysta**

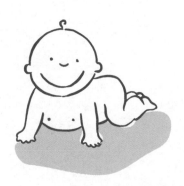

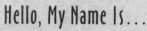

KRISTEN Combination of **Kirsten** and **Kristina**, both variants of **Christine**. Greek, "Christian." **Krissa, Krissie, Krissy, Kristan, Kristi, Kristin, Kristna, Kristyn, Krysten, Krystin**

KRISTINE Variant of **Christine**. Greek, "Christian." **Khristeen, Khristiana, Khristina, Khristine, Kirsteen, Kristeen, Kristian, Kristijna, Kristina, Krystyan, Krystyna**

KRYSTAL Variant of **Crystal**. Greek, "ice." **Khristalle, Khristel, Khrystalle, Khrystelle, Khrystle, Kristle, Krystalle, Krystelle, Krystle**

KUME Hawaiian. "Teacher."

KYLE Scottish. "Narrow spit of land." **Kylie**

KYNA Irish. "Wisdom."

KYNTHIA Variant of **Cynthia**. Greek, "from Mount Cynthos."

KYRA Greek. "Lady." **Keera, Keira, Kira, Kyria**

KYRENE Greek. "Lord." **Cyrene, Cyrine, Kyrina, Kyrine**

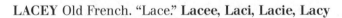

LACEY Old French. "Lace." **Lacee, Laci, Lacie, Lacy**

LADONNA Variant of **Donna**. Italian, "lady." **Ladona, Ladonia, Ledona, Ledonia, Ledonna**

LADY Short form of **Adelaide**. Old German, "noble." **Laidey**

LAILA Persian. "Dark." Also variant of **Layla. Laili, Lailia, Lailie, Laily, Laleh, Layla, Laylia, Laylie, Leila, Leilah, Lela, Lelah, Lelia, Leyla, Leylah**

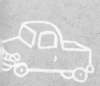

JEWISH NAMES

Jewish names permeate America. Virtually all of the names in the Bible, from *Adam* to *Zachariah,* are Jewish. Interestingly enough, given the political conditions in the Middle East, Jews and Arabs share many names—some spelled in the same way, such as *Sarah*—or slightly differently, as in *Abraham* or *Ibrahim.*

Naming customs among American Jews spring from two traditions, both of which began in Europe. Ashkenazic Jews lived in Germany and, later, in Poland and Lithuania, and spoke Yiddish. They would never give a baby the same name as a living relative, for they believed that when Death came for the older person it might take the baby instead. Because most American Jews come from the Ashkenazic tradition, you rarely find a Jewish man here with *Junior* appended to his name.

Sephardic Jews lived in Spain until 1492, when they were infamously expelled by King Ferdinand and Queen Isabella. They then dispersed into other southern European countries and along the Mediterranean coast of Africa. Among these people, the firstborn son was named after his paternal-grandfather, the second male child after his maternal grandfather,

the first daughter named after her paternal grandmother, the second female child after her maternal grandmother, the next child after a paternal uncle or aunt, the next after a maternal uncle or aunt, and so on. Although Sephardic parents had little choice in naming their children, at least they didn't have to listen to relatives complaining about the choices they made.

Two more factors have influenced Jewish names. Like other immigrants to America, Jewish families tried to help their children succeed in the new country by giving them popular American names. When the children grew up, they did the same for their offspring. American Jews of the third generation, however, sometimes embraced their ethnic roots by giving their children "ethnic" or "old country" names that would have been familiar to the children's great-grandparents.

The second factor influencing Jewish names was the decision by the founders of Israel to revive the Hebrew language and use it in the new country. Many Jews, in the United States as well as Israel, began to use Hebrew names, some old and some new. These took their place with *Adam* and *Aaron* and other biblical names.

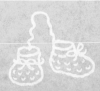

Here are some popular Jewish boys' names and their meanings:

Alon	"oak tree"
Amir	"strong"
Chaim	"life"
Dov	"bear"
Gil	"joy"
Hillel	"praised"
Isaac, Itzak, Yitzhak	"laugher"
Lev	"lion"
Navad	"giver"
Noam	"sweetness"
Ravid	"ornament"
Shamir	"strong"
Yakir	"precious"
Yotam	"God is perfect"
Zalman	"peace"

And these are some popular Jewish girls' names with their meanings:

Ariella	"lioness of God"
Bracha	"blessing"
Dalia	"branch"
Hila	"praise"
Irit	"daffodil"
Levana	"white"
Maayan	"spring, oasis"
Maya	"water"
Nirit, Nurit	"flower"
Ofira	"gold"
Raz	"secret"
Shir, Shira	"song"
Tamar	"palm tree"
Yona, Yonina	"dove"

LAINEY Short form of **Elaine.** Old French, from Greek, "bright one." **Lainee, Lainy, Laynee, Layney, Laynie**

LAKEISHA Contemporary American. **Lakeecia, Lakeesha, Laketia, Lakeysha, Lakicia, Lakisha, Lakitia, Lekeesha, Lekeisha, Lekisha**

LALA Slavic. "Tulip." **Lalah, Lalla, Lallah**

LALAGE Greek. "Babbler." **Lalaj, Lalash, Lallie** et al.

LALITA Sanskrit. "Honest." **Lalitah, Lallita, Lallitah**

LALLIE Diminutive of **Lalage.** Greek, "babbler." **Lali, Lalli, Lally**

LAMORNA Middle English. "The morning." **Lamorne, Lamurna**

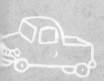

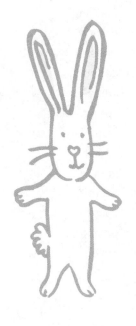

LANA Variant of **Alanna**, feminine form of **Alan**. Irish, "rock." **Lanae, Lanah, Lanette, Lanna, Lannah, Lanne, Lanny**

LANE Middle English. "Narrow road." **Laine, Layne**

LANI Hawaiian. "Sky." Also a variant of **Ilana**.

LAQUITA Contemporary American variant of **Poquita**. Spanish, "very little." **La Quita**

LARA Russian. "Lighthearted." Also a variant of **Laura**. **Larina**

LARAINE Variant of **Lorraine**. A province on the French-German border. **Laraene, Larayne, Lareine, Larina, Larine**

LAREINA Spanish. "The queen." **Larena, Lareyna**

LARISSA Russian, from Greek. "Lighthearted." **Larice, Larise, Laryssa, Lissa, Lyssa**

LARK Middle English. "Lark." **Larke**

LASSIE Middle English. "Little girl." **Lass**

LATA Variant of **Elata**. Latin, "elevated."

LATANYA Contemporary American. **Latania, Latanja, Latonia, Latonya, Tanya** et al.

LATISHA Variant of **Letitia**. Latin, "boundless joy."

LATOYA Contemporary American. **Latoia, LaToya, Latoyia**

LATRICE Contemporary American. "Noble." **Latrecia, Latreece, Latreese, Latreshia, Latricia, Letreece, Letrice, Letrisha**

LAUDOMIA Italian. "Praise to the house." **Laudomeya**

LAULANI Hawaiian. "Heavenly child."

LAURA Latin. "Laurel." **Lara, Lari, Laure, Lauren** et al., **Lauri, Laurice, Lauricia, Laurie, Lawrie, Lawry, Lollie, Lolly, Lora, Loreen** et al., **Lorelle** et al., **Loretta** et al., **Lori** et al., **Lorinda** et al., **Lorine, Lorita, Loura**

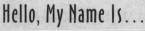
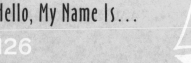

LAURALEE Combination of **Laura** and **Lee**. **Loralee**

LAUREL Latin. "Laurel tree." **Laural, Lauralle, Laurell, Loral, Lorelle** et al.

LAUREN Variant of **Laura**. **Lauran, Laurin, Lauryn, Laurynn, Laurynne, Loren, Lorin, Lorren, Lorrin**

LAURENCIA Feminine form of **Laurence**. Latin, "from Laurentium." **Laurena, Laurentia, Laurentine, Laurestine**

LAURIANNE Combination of **Lauri** and **Anne**. **Lauriane, Lauriann, Lorann, Loriann, Lori Ann, LoriAnn, Lorianne, Lori Anne, LoriAnne, Lourana, Louriann, Lourianne**

LAUVE Old English. "One of power." **Love**

LAVEDA Latin. "Cleansed." **Lavetta**

LAVENDER Latin. "Lavender."

LAVERNE English, from French. "Of spring." **Laverine, Lavern, Laverna, LaVerne, La Verne, Verne**

LAVINIA Latin. In myth, the mother of the Roman race. **Lavena, Lavenia, Lavina, Lavinie, Lavinya, Levene, Levenia, Levenya, Levinia, Levinya, Livinia, Lovina, Lovinia, Lovinya, Vinnie**

LAVONNE Contemporary American. **Lavon, Lavonna, Lavaughn, Lavonya, Levon, Levonne, Levonya**

LAYLA Arabic. "Wine." **Laila, Laya**

LEAH Hebrew. "Weary." **Lea, Lee, Leia, Leigha**

LEALA Old French. "Loyal." **Leale, Lealia, Lealie, Lela, Lelah**

LEANDRA Greek. "Lion woman." **Leanda, Leodora**

LEANNE Combination of **Lee** and **Anne**. **Leeann, Leeanna, LeeAnn, Lee Ann, Leeanne, LeeAnne, Lee Anne, LeighAnn, Leigh Ann, LeighAnne, Leigh Anne**

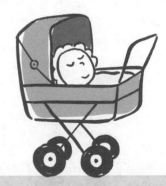

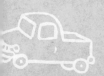

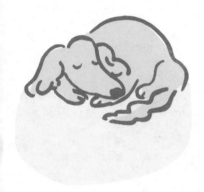

LEATRICE Combination of **Lee** and **Beatrice**. **Leatricia, Leetrice, Leetricia**

LEDA Variant of **Letitia**. Latin, "joy." In Greek mythology, the queen of Sparta. Impregnated by Zeus in the form of a swan, she gave birth to Helen of Troy. **Leta, Leyda, Lida**

LEE Old English. "Meadow." Also short form of **Leah**. **Lea, Leigh**

LEEBA Yiddish. "Loved one." **Leebah, Liba, Libah**

LEI Chinese. "Flower bud."

LEILA Arabic. "Night." **Layla, Laylah, Leela, Leelah, Leilah, Leilia, Lela, Lelah, Leyla, Lila, Lilah, Lyla**

LEILANI Hawaiian. "Flower from heaven." **Lei, Lelani**

LELIA Latin. Clan name. **Lelie, Lilia, Lilie**

LEMUELA Hebrew. "Devoted to God." **Lemuelah, Lemuelina, Lemueline, Lemuelita**

LENA Hebrew. "To sleep." Also variant of **Arlene, Caroline, Eileen, Helen, Madeline**, etc. **Leena, Leenah, Lenah, Lenea, Lenetta, Lenette, Lennete, Lennetta, Lina, Linah, Lyna, Lynah**

LENIS Latin. "Mild," "soft," "gentle." **Lene, Leneta, Lenice, Lenita, Lenos**

LENNA Old German. "Lion's strength." **Lenda, Lendie, Lendy**

LENORE Varian of **Helen**. Greek, "light." **Lenor, Lenora, Lenorah, Lienor**

LENUTA Romanian. "Mild." **Leunta**

LEODA Old German. "Of the people." **Leota, Leotha**

LEOMA Old English. "Brilliance."

LEONA Feminine form of **Leon.** Latin, "lion." **Leeota, Leoine, Leola, Leone, Leonel, Leonelle, Leonia, Leonie, Leonina, Leonine, Leontine, Leontyne, Leota, Lona** et al.

LEONARDA Feminine form of **Leonard.** Old German, "lion strength." **Leonarde**

LEONIE Feminine form of **Leon.** Latin, "lion." **Leoline, Leone, Leoni, Leonine, Leontine, Leony**

LEONORA Variant of **Helen.** Greek, "light." **Leanor, Leanora, Leanore, Lenore** et al., **Leonorah, Leonore, Nora, Norah**

LEOPOLDINE Feminine form of **Leopold.** Old German, "bold people." **Leopolda, Leopoldina**

LEORA Variant of **Helen.** Greek, "light." **Leorah, Liora, Liorah**

LESLIE Scottish. "Meadowlands." **Lea, Leslea, Leslee, Lesley, Lesli, Lesly, Lezlee, Lezley, Lezlie, Lezly**

LETA Latin. "Glad, joyful."

LETHA Greek. In myth, the river of forgetfulness in Hades. **Leitha, Leithia, Lethe, Lethia, Lethilia**

LETIFA Arabic. "Gentle." **Latifa, Latifah, Latipha, Letifah, Letipha**

LETITIA Latin. "Boundless joy." **Laetitia, Laetizia, Latashia, Latia, Latisha, Lecia, Letice, Leticia, Letizia, Letta, Lettice, Lettie, Lettitia, Letty, Loutisha, Loutita, Loutitia, Tish, Tisha, Titia**

LETTY Diminutive of **Aleta, Letitia.**

LEVANA Latin, "rising." Hebrew, "white." **Levania, Levanna, Levona, Levonia**

LEVIA Hebrew. "To join." **Livia, Liviya, Livya**

LEVINA Latin. "Lightning bolt." **Leveena, Leveenah, Levinah**

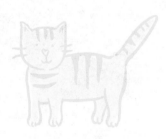

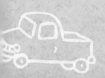

LEWANA Hebrew. "Shining white moon." **Levana, Levanna, Lewanah, Lewanna, Livana**

LEXIA Variant of **Alexandra.** Greek, "defender of humanity." **Lexa, Lexie, Lexina, Lexine, Lexy, Lexya**

LEXUS A luxury car.

LEYA Spanish. "Law." **Ley**

LI Chinese. "Beautiful."

LIANA French. "To bind." **Leana, Leanah, Leanna, Leannah, Liane, Lianna, Liannah, Lianne**

LIANE Variant of **Juliane, Liana, Lilliane. Lianna, Lianne**

LIBBY Diminutive of **Elizabeth.** Hebrew, "pledged to God." **Lib, Libbee, Libbey, Libbie, Liby**

LIBERTY Middle English, from Latin. "Freedom." **Berti, Bertie, Berty**

LIDA Slavic. "Loved by the people." Also a variant of **Alida. Lidah, Lyda**

LIESE German variant of **Elizabeth.** Hebrew, "pledged to God." **Liesa, Liesel, Lieselotte, Liesl, Lisel**

LIESELOTTE French variant of **Liese,** German variant of **Elizabeth.** Hebrew, "pledged to God." **Lieselotta, Liselotte**

LILA Variant of **Leila, Lily;** short form of **Delilah, Lillian.**

LILAC Persian, "indigo." English, "lilac."

LILIAS Scottish variant of **Lillian.** Latin, "lily." **Lillias**

LILIBET Variant of **Elizabeth.** Hebrew, "pledged to God." **Lilibette, Lillibet, Lillibette, Lilybet**

LILITH Arabic, Hebrew. "Woman from the night." **Lilis, Lilita, Lillith**

Country music singers

Any musical genre with song titles such as "You're the Reason Our Kids Are Ugly," "Did I Shave My Legs for This?," and "I Bought the Shoes that Just Walked Out on Me" has to have interesting names among its artists. Here are some of the most famous pickers and singers. All are members of the Country Music Hall of Fame.

Chet Atkins
Gene Autry
Owen Bradley
Boudleaux & Felice Bryant
Jethro Burns
Floyd Cramer
Lester Flatt
Red Foley
Lefty Frizzell
Homer Haynes
Harlan Howard
Waylon Jennings
Pee Wee King
Buck Owens

Dolly Parton
Minnie Pearl
Webb Pierce
Tex Ritter
Jimmie Rodgers
Earl Scruggs
Cliffie Stone
Merle Travis
Conway Twitty
Porter Wagoner
Kitty Wells
Hank Williams
Tammy Wynette
Faron Young

LILLIAN Latin. "Lily." **Lila, Lilia, Lilian, Liliana, Liliane, Lilias, Lilion, Lilione, Lillia, Lillianne, Lillias, Lillion, Lillione, Lillyan, Lillyanne, Lily** et al., **Lilyan, Lilyann, Lilyanne**

LILO Hawaiian. "Noble spirit." **Lylo**

LILY Latin. "Lily." Also short form of **Daffodil, Lillian.** Lil, Lila et al., **Lilas, Lili, Lilie, Lilla, Lilley, Lilli, Lillie, Lilly**

LIN Chinese. "Beautiful jade."

LINA Variant of **Lena;** short form of **Adina, Carolina, Helina, Karolina. Lena** et al, **Linah, Lino**

LINDA Spanish, Portuguese. "Pretty." Also short form of **Adelinda, Belinda, Deolinda, Lorinda, Melinda. Lin,**

Lindee, Lindey, Lindi, Lindie, Lindy, Linn, Lyn, Lyna, Lynda, Lynde, Lyndie, Lyndy, Lynn, Lynnda, Lynndie, Lynndy

LINDEN Old English. "Supple." Also a tree of the genus *Tilia.* **Linde, Lindenne, Lindi, Lindin**

LINDSAY Old English. "Island of linden trees." **Lind, Lindsea, Lindsee, Lindsey, Lindsi, Lindsie, Lindsy, Linzee, Linzi, Linzie, Linzy, Lyndsay, Lyndsey, Lynnsie, Lynnsey, Lynndsie, Lynnzey, Lynsey**

LINETTE Old French. "Linnet" (a small bird). Also variant of **Eiluned, Eluned. Lanette, Linet, Linnet, Linnetta, Linnette, Lyn, Lynet, Lynette, Lynnet, Lynnette**

LING Chinese. "Tinkling jade."

LINNEA Scandinavian. "Linden tree." **Linea, Lineya, Linnaea, Lynea, Lyneya, Lynnea, Lynneya**

LIOBA Old English. St. Lioba.

LIORA Short form of **Meliora.** Latin, "to better."

LIRION Hebrew. "My joyful song." **Lirione, Lyrion, Lyrione**

LIRIT Greek. "Pleasingly musical." **Lirith, Lyrit, Lyrith**

LISA Short form of **Elizabeth.** Hebrew, "pledged to God." **Leesa, Leeza, Liesa, Lise, Liseta, Lisetta, Lisette, Liszka, Lysa, Lyssa, Lyssie**

LISANDRA Variant of **Alexandra, Melisande. Lisandre, Lissandra, Lissandre**

LISSA Short form of **Elizabeth, Melissa, Millicent. Lisse**

LITA Diminutive of **Carmelita, Carmita** et al.

LIVIA Short form of **Olivia.** Latin, "olive." **Livya**

LI WEI Chinese. "Beautiful rose."

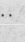

LIZ Short form of **Elizabeth.** Hebrew, "pledged to God." **Lizzi, Lizzie, Lizzy**

LIZA Short form of **Elizabeth.** Hebrew, "pledged to God." **Eliza, Lize, Lizette, Lizzie, Lyza, Lyzette**

LODEMAI Old English. "Guide." **Lodema, Lodemee, Lodemy**

LOELIA Arabic. "Night." **Loelya**

LOIS Old German. "Renowned in battle." **Lo**

LOLA Variant of **Dolores.** Spanish, "sorrows (of Christ)." **Lita, Loleta, Lolita**

LONA Variant of **Leona.** Latin, "lion." **Lonee, Lonie, Lonna, Lonnie**

LORA Variant of **Laura.** Latin, "laurel." **Lori** et al.

LOREEN Variant of **Laura.** Latin, "laurel." **Laureen, Laurene, Laurina, Laurine, Lorena, Lorene**

LORELEI German. In legend, a siren of the Rhein who lured men to destruction. **Loralee, Loralie, Loralyn, Lorely, Lorilee, Lorilyn, Lurleen** et al.

LORELLE Variant of **Laurel.** Latin, "laurel tree." **Laurella, Laurelle, Lorell**

LORENZA Feminine form of **Lorenzo.** Latin, "from Laurentium." **Lorensa**

LORETTA Variant of **Laura.** Latin, "laurel." **Larretta, Lauretta, Laurette, Lorettah, Lorette, Lorretta, Lorrette, Lurette**

LORI Diminutive of **Laura, Lorraine. Loree, Lorie, Lorri, Lorrie, Lorry, Lory**

LORICE Latin. "Slender." Also a variant of **Chloris. Loris, Lorrice, Lorris, Lorrise**

LORINDA Variant of **Laura.** Latin, "laurel." **Larinda, Laurinda**

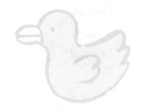

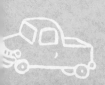

133

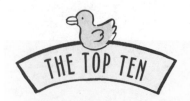

THE TOP TEN
NAMES OF 1925

The Year
The Great Gatsby
Was Published

BOYS

John
Robert
James
William
Charles
Joseph
George
Richard
Edward
Donald

GIRLS

Mary
Dorothy
Betty
Helen
Margaret
Ruth
Doris
Virginia
Elizabeth
Evelyn, Mildred (tie)

LORNA Scottish place name. *Lorna Doone*, a historical romance by R. D. Blackmore. **Lona, Lornah, Lornee, Lorrna, Lourna**

LORRAINE A province on the French-German border. **Laraine** et al., **Lauraine, Laurane, Laurraine, Lorain, Loraine, Lorayne, Lori, Lorine, Lorrain, Lorrayne**

LOTTIE Diminutive of **Charlotte, Carlotta. Lotie, Lotta, Lotte, Lottey, Lotti, Lotty**

LOTUS Greek. "Lotus."

LOU Short form of **Louise, Luella. Lu**

LOUANNE Combination of **Lou** and **Anne. Louann, LouAnn, Lou Ann, LouAnne, Lou Anne, Luann, LuAnn, Lu Ann, Luanne, LuAnne, Lu Anne**

LOUISE Feminine form of **Louis.** Old German, "renowned warrior." **Aloisia** et al., **Eloise** et al., **Heloisa, Heloise, Lewes, Lisette, Lois, Loise, Lou** et al., **Louie, Louisa, Louisetta, Louisette, Louisina, Louisiana, Louisiane, Louisine, Louiza, Lova, Lovisa, Lowise, Loyce, Loyise, Lu, Luisa, Luise, Luiza, Lujza, Lujzika, Lula, Lulita, Lulu**

LOURDES French place name, Catholic holy site. **Lordesse**

LOVE Old English. "Love." Also variant of **Lauve. Lovey**

LOVEDAY Old English. "A day appointed for a meeting with an amicable settlement of a dispute" or "the settlement of such a dispute." **Lovdie, Lowdy, Luveday**

LUANA Hawaiian. "Pleasure."

LUCANIA Italian. Place name. **Luca, Lucanya**

LUCERNE Latin, "lamp." English, "alfalfa." **Lucerna, Lucernia**

LUCETTA Italian variant of **Lucy.** Latin, "light." **Lucette**

LUCIA Latin. "Light." **Luciana, Lucida, Lucie, Lucienne, Luzia**

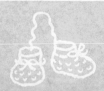

LUCILLE French variant of **Lucy.** Latin, "light." **Lucila, Lucile, Lucilia, Lucilla**

LUCINA Latin. Roman goddess of childbirth. **Lucine**

LUCINDA Variant of **Lucy.** Latin, "light." **Cindy, Lucinde**

LUCITA Diminutive of **Luz.** Spanish, "light."

LUCRETIA Latin. Clan name. **Lucrece, Lucrecia, Lucreecia, Lucretzia, Lucrezia**

LUCY Latin. "Light." **Lu, Luce, Lucetta, Lucette, Luci, Lucia** et al., **Lucie, Lucille** et al., **Lucinda** et al., **Lucyna, Lucza, Lus, Luse, Luz** et al., **Luze**

LUDELLA Old English. "Clever nymph." **Ludela, Ludelia, Ludie**

LUDMILLA Slavic. "Beloved of the people." **Ludmeela, Ludmelia, Ludmila, Lyudmila, Lyudmilia**

LUDOVICA Feminine form of **Ludovicus.** Latin, from Old German, "renowned warrior." **Ludova, Ludovika**

LUDWIGA Feminine form of **Ludwig.** Old German, "renowned warrior."

LUELLA Old English. "Renowned in battle." **Loella, Lou, Louella, Lu, Luelle, Lula**

LULA Variant of **Louise.** Old German, "renowned warrior." **Lulita**

LULIE Middle English. "To calm." **Luli, Lulli, Lullie, Luly**

LULU Variant of **Louise.** Old German, "renowned in battle." **Loulou, Lu**

LUMINOSA Spanish. "Bright."

LUNA Latin. "Moon." **Lunetta, Lunette, Lunneta, Lunya**

LUPE Spanish. Short form of **Guadalupe. Lupita**

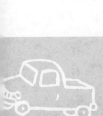

LURLEEN Variant of **Lorelei**. German. In legend, Lorelei was a siren of the Rhein who lured men to destruction. **Lura, Luralene, Luraline, Lurlene, Lurline**

LUZ Spanish. "Light." **Lucita, Luza**

LYDA Variant of **Alida, Lydia. Lydah**

LYDIA Greek. An ancient country in Asia Minor. **Lidia, Lidija, Lyda, Lydda, Lydie**

LYNETTE Welsh. "Idol." Also a variant of **Linette. Lynett, Lynetta, Lynnette**

LYNN Old English. "Bubbling brook." Also short form of **Linda, Madeline. Lin, Linn, Linne, Lyn, Lyndel, Lyndell, Lynelle et al., Lynna, Lynne**

LYNELLE Variant of **Lynn. Linnell, Lynell, Lynnelle**

LYUBOV Russian. "Love." **Luba, Lyuba**

MAAYA Hebrew. "Spring" or "oasis."

MAB Welsh, Irish. The queen of the fairies, according to Shakespeare and other poets. Probably a variant of **Maeve. Mabb**

MABEL Short form of **Amabel**. Latin, "lovable." **Amaybel, Amaybell, Amaybelle, Amayble, Mab, Mabe, Mabell, Mabelle, Mable, Maibel, Maible, Maybel, Maybell, Maybelle, Mayble**

MADELINE Variant of **Magdalene**. Greek, "from Magdala." **Dalanna, Dalenna, Lena, Line, Lynn, Mada, Madalena,**

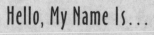

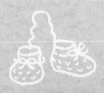

Madalyn, Madalynn, Maddalena, Maddie, Maddy, Madeena, Madel, Madelaine, Madelayne, Madeleina, Madeleine, Madelena, Madelene, Madelia, Madelina, Madella, Madelle, Madelon, Madge, Madlen, Madlin, Madlyn, Mady, Maidel, Maighdlin, Maj, Mala, Malena, Malin, Malina, Manda

MADGE Short form of **Madeline, Margaret. Maj**

MADONNA Latin. "My lady," the Virgin Mary. Madonna, contemporary pop singer, actress. **Medonna**

MADRE Spanish. "Mother." **Madra**

MAE Variant of **May**, short form of **Margaret. May**

MAEVE Irish. In legend, the queen of Connacht, who led a famous invasion of Ulster. **Maebe, Mave, Meave, Medb**

MAGDA Short form of **Magdalene.** Greek, "from Magdala." **Mada**

MAGDALENE Greek. "From Magdala." **Madeline** et al., **Magda, Magdala, Magdalen, Magdalena, Magdolna, Magli, Mala, Lena**

MAGGIE Diminutive of **Margaret, Magnolia. Maggey, Maggi, Maggy, Magi, Magie, Magy**

MAGNA Feminine form of **Magnus.** Latin, "great." **Magnah**

MAGNILDA Old German. "Strong in warfare." **Magnhilde**

MAGNOLIA Latin. A genus of trees and shrubs exhibiting large, showy flowers, named for the French botanist Pierre Magnol. **Maggie, Maggy, Nola**

MAHALA Hebrew. "Tender affection." Mahalia Jackson, American gospel singer, 1911–1972. **Mahalah, Mahalia, Mahaliah, Mahalla, Mahalya, Mahelia, Mehalia, Mehalya**

Would Fenway have sounded any better?

Shea Stadium, home to baseball's New York Mets, has provided a name for two children of ballplayers, a girl and a boy. Barry Larkin, shortstop for the Cincinnati Reds, named his daughter *Brielle D'Shea Larkin.* Chipper Jones, a third baseman for the Atlanta Braves who hit his first home run in the majors at Shea Stadium, named his son *Shea Logan Jones.*

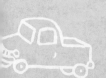

MAHINA Hawaiian. "Moon."

MAHIRA Hebrew. "Fast, energetic." **Mehira**

MAHOLA Hebrew. "Dance." **Maholah**

MAHTAB Persian. "Moonlight."

MAI Swedish variant of **Mary.**

MAIA Latin. "Star of the sea." In myth, the daughter of Atlas and mother of Hermes. Another Maia was the wife of Vulcan, sometimes called Bona Dea (Good Goddess). **Maaja, Maiah, Maila, Maj, Maja, Maya, Mya**

MAIDA Old English. "Maiden." **Maddi, Maddie, Maddy, Mady, Maidey, Maidi, Maidie, Maidy, Mayda, Maydena, Maydey**

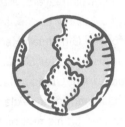

MAIRA Arabic. "Moon."

MAIREAD Irish. "To judge, officiate." **Maighread, Maired**

MAIRIN Irish variant of **Mary.** Hebrew, "bitter."

MAISIE Diminutive of **Margaret.** Greek, "pearl." **Maise, Maisey, Maisy, Maizie, Mazie**

MAJESTA Latin. "Majesty."

MAJIDAH Arabic. "Wonderful." **Majida**

MAKANI Hawaiian. "Wind."

MALA Short form of **Madeline, Magdalene.**

MALI Short form of **Amalia.** Also a West African country. **Malia, Malika**

MALKA Hebrew. "Queen." **Malca, Malcah, Malkah, Malkia, Malkie, Milcah**

MALLORY Old French. "Unhappy, unlucky." **Malloreigh, Mallorey, Mallorie, Malorey, Malorie, Malory**

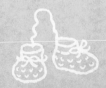

MALU Hawaiian. "Peace."

MALVA Greek, "slender, delicate." Latin, "mallow." **Malba**

MALVINA Irish. "Smooth-browed." Malvina Reynolds, twentieth-century American singer and songwriter. Malvina Hoffman, twentieth-century American sculptor. **Mal, Malvie, Malvinda**

MAMIE French. "My beloved." **Mame, Mayme, Maymie**

MANDA Short form of **Amanda**. Latin, "much loved." **Mandy** et al.

MANDISA South African. "Sweet." **Mandise, Mandissa, Mandisse**

MANDY Short form of **Amanda**. Latin, "much loved." **Mandee, Mandi, Mandie**

MANGENA Hebrew. "Song." **Mangina**

MANON French variant of **Mary**. Hebrew, "bitter."

MANSI Hopi. "Plucked flower."

MANUELA Spanish feminine form of **Emmanuel**. Hebrew, "God be with us." **Emanuela, Emanuelita, Manuelita**

MANYA Australian Aboriginal. "Small."

MARA Variant of **Amara, Demaris, Mary. Mahra, Marah, Maralina, Maraline, Mari, Marra, Marri**

MARCELLA Feminine form of **Marcellus**. Latin, "little warrior." **Marcela, Marcele, Marcelia, Marcelle, Marchella, Marchelle, Marcile, Marcille, Marcy** et al., **Maricel, Maricela, Maricella, Marisela, Mariselia, Marisella, Marsella, Marselle, Marshella, Marsiella**

MARCENE Feminine form of **Mark**. Latin, "warlike." **Marceen, Marcena, Marcenia, Marceyne, Marcina, Marcine, Mercena, Mercine**

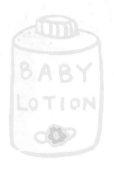

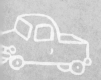

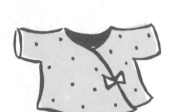

MARCIA Feminine form of **Mark.** Latin, "warlike." **Marchita, Marciane, Marcita, Marcy** et al., **Marquita, Marsha, Martia**

MARCILYN Feminine form of **Mark.** Latin, "warlike." **Marcelina, Marcelinda, Marceline, Marcellina, Marcellinda, Marcelline, Marcelyn, Marcelynn, Marcelynne, Marcilynn, Marcilynne**

MARCY Diminutive of **Marcella, Marcia.** Latin, "warlike." **Marcee, Marcey, Marci, Marcie**

MARDELL Disputed origin; possibly an inversion of the Spanish *del mar*, "of the sea." **Mardel, Mardelle**

MARE Latin. "Sea."

MARELDA Old German. "Renowned battle maid." **Mareldha, Mareldhe, Marilda**

MARGARET Greek. "Pearl." **Gita, Ghita, Greta** et al., **Gretchen, Madge, Mady, Maergrethe, Mag, Maggie** et al., **Mago, Maiga, Maisie, Maisy, Malgorzata, Marga, Margalit, Margalith, Margalo, Margareta, Margarete, Margaretha, Margarethe, Margaretta, Margarette, Margarida, Margarinda, Margarit, Margarita, Margarite, Margat, Marge** et al., **Margene, Margeret, Margeretta, Margerita, Margery** et al., **Marget, Margette, Margey, Marghania, Margharita, Margherita, Margiad, Margies, Margisia, Margit, Margita, Margo** et al., **Margret, Margreth, Margrett, Marguarette, Marguarita, Marguerite, Marguita, Margurite, Marketa, Markita, Marles, Megan** et al., **Mergret, Meta** et al., **Midge, Mittie, Peggy** et al., **Rita** et al.

MARGE Short form of **Margaret, Margery.** Greek, "pearl." **Margey, Margi, Margie, Margy, Marje, Marji, Marjie**

MARGERY French variant of **Margaret.** Greek, "pearl." **Marge** et al., **Margeree, Margerey, Margerie, Marjorie** et al.

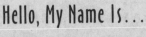
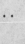

MARGO French variant of **Margaret.** Greek, "pearl." **Margaux, Margot**

MARGUERITE French variant of **Margaret.** Greek, "pearl."

MARIA Latin variant of **Mary.** Hebrew, "bitter." **Mariah, Mariya, Marja, Marya**

MARIAH Variant of **Maia, Maria, Moriah.**

MARIAN French. Combination of **Mary** and **Ann. Mariana, Mariane, Marianna, Marianne, Marion** et al., **Maryann, Mary Ann, Maryanne, Mary Anne**

MARIBEL Combination of **Mary** and **Belle. Marabel, Marabella, Marabelle, Mariabella, Maribell, Maribelle, Marybel, Marybell, Marybelle**

MARIE French, German variant of **Mary.** Hebrew, "bitter." **Maree**

MARIEL Dutch variant of **Mary. Marella, Marelle, Marial, Marialle, Mariela, Mariele, Mariella, Marielle, Marilla**

MARIETTA French variant of **Mary.** Hebrew, "bitter." Also a city in Georgia. **Maretta**

MARIGOLD English. Any of various plants with deep yellow flowers, usually of the genus *Tagetes.* **Marygold**

MARIKA Dutch variant of **Mary.** Hebrew, "bitter." **Marieke, Marijke, Marike, Mariska, Mariske, Maryk**

MARILEE Combination of **Mary** and **Lee. Marrilee, Marylea, Marylee**

MARILYN Variant of **Mary.** Hebrew, "bitter." **Maralin, Maralyn, Marelin, Marelyn, Marilen, Marilin, Marillyn, Marilynn, Marilynne, Marralyn, Marralynn, Marrilin, Marrilyn, Marrilynn, Marylin, Marylyn, Marylynn, Marylynne, Merilyn, Merilynn, Merilynne**

MARINA Latin. "From the sea." **Maren, Marena, Marin, Marine, Marinela, Marinna**

MARINI Swahili. "Vibrant, healthy."

MARION French variant of **Mary**. Originally a masculine form. **Maryon, Maryonn**

MARIS Latin. "Of the sea." **Marice, Marissa** et al., **Marris, Marys, Maryse, Meris**

MARISOL Spanish. Combination of **Maria** and *sol* ("sun").

MARISSA Latin. "Of the sea." **Maressa, Maricia, Marisa, Marise, Marisse, Marrisa, Marrise, Marysa, Maryse, Marysia, Merissa, Morissa**

MARJOLAINE French. "Marjoram," the herb. **Marjolain, Marjolaina, Marjolayne**

MARJORIE Variant of **Margery, Marge** et al. **Marjary, Marjery, Marjoree, Marjorey, Marjori, Marjorie, Marjory**

MARLA English. Variant of **Marlene**, combination of **Mary** and **Magdalene. Marlah, Marleah**

MARLENE Combination of **Mary** and **Magdalene. Marla** et al., **Marlaina, Marlane, Marlayne, Marlea, Marlee, Marleen, Marlen, Marlena, Marley, Marlie, Marlin, Marline, Marlyn, Marlyne, Marlynne**

MARLO Contemporary American. Marlo Thomas, actress and film producer. **Marloe, Marlon, Marlow, Marlowe**

MARMARA Greek. "Sparkling, shining." **Marmee**

MARNA Disputed origin. **Marne, Marney, Marni, Marnia, Marnie, Marnja, Marnya**

MARNINA Hebrew. "Celebrate." **Marninah, Marninya**

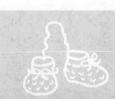

MARQUITA Diminutive of *marquise,* French for "marchioness," a noblewoman. **Markeesha, Marquitta, Marquisha**

MARSHA English variant of **Marcia.**

MARTA Spanish variant of **Martha.**

MARTHA Aramaic. "Lady." **Mart, Marta, Marth, Marthe, Marthena, Marti, Martie, Martita, Marty, Matti, Mattie, Merta, Mertha, Merthe**

MARTINA Feminine form of **Martin.** Latin, "warlike." **Marteena, Marti, Martie, Martine, Marty, Martyna, Martyne, Martynne, Tina, Tine**

MARVA Hebrew. "Sage," the herb.

MARVEL Old French. "Extraordinary." **Marva, Marvela, Marvele, Marvelina, Marvelita, Marvella, Marvelle**

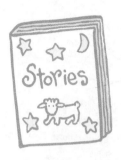

MARY Hebrew. "Bitter." **Mair, Maire, Mairin, Mal, Malia, Mallie, Manette, Manon, Manya, Mara, Mare, Maree, Mareea, Maren, Maretta, Marette, Mari, Maria, Marian** et al., **Marice, Maridel, Marie, Mariel** et al., **Marien, Mariesa, Mariessa, Marietta, Mariette, Marika** et al., **Marilyn** et al., **Mariquilla, Mariquita, Marita, Maritsa, Maritza, Marja, Marje, Marya, Maureen** et al., **Meridel, Mimi, Minette, Minnie, Miren, Miriam** et al., **Mirit, Maurya, Moira, Moire, Molly** et al., **Morag, Moya, Muire, Muriel** et al., **Polly** et al.

MASADA Hebrew. "Foundation." **Masadah, Massada, Massadah**

MATANA Hebrew. "Gift."

MATILDA Old German. "Battle-mighty." **Maltilde, Mat, Matelda, Mathilda, Mathilde, Matilde, Matti, Mattie, Matty, Maude** et al., **Metilda, Tilda, Tilde, Tildie, Tildy, Tilli, Tillie, Tilly**

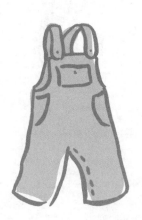

MATTEA Feminine form of **Matthew.** Hebrew, "gift of God." **Mathea, Mathia, Matthea, Matthia, Mattia**

MAUDE Variant of **Matilda.** Old German, "battle-mighty." **Maud, Maudene, Maudie, Maudine, Mawde**

MAURA Celtic. "Dark." **Maure, Moira, Mora**

MAUREEN Irish variant of **Mary, Maura. Mauren, Maurene, Maurine, Moreen, Morena, Morene, Morine**

MAURISE Feminine form of **Maurice.** Latin, "dark-skinned." **Maurita, Mauritia, Maurizia**

MAUVE French. "Mallow plant."

MAVIS French. "Thrush." **Mavise**

MAXINE Latin. "Greatest." **Massima, Max, Maxeem, Maxeen, Maxena, Maxene, Maxi, Maxie, Maxima, Maxime, Maxina, Maxy**

MAY English variant of **Maia.** Latin, "star of the sea." Also the fifth month of the year. **Mae, Maye, Mayella, Mayetta, Mayla**

MAYA Hindi, "creative force." Latin, "great one." Hebrew, "water." Maya Angelou, contemporary American writer.

MAZAL Hebrew. "Luck."

MEAD Middle English. "Meadow," "honey wine." **Meade**

MEADOW English. "Meadow."

MEARA Irish. "Gaiety."

MEATH Irish. A county in eastern Ireland. Pronounced "MEE-ath."

MEDEA Greek. "Ruling." In legend, a sorceress who helped Jason carry off the golden fleece and later, after he deserted her, murdered their two children. **Madora, Madorna, Medeia, Media, Medora, Medorah, Medorna**

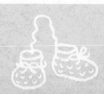

MEERA Short form of **Almera, Amira, Elmira. Meerah, Merah, Mere, Mira** et al.

MEG Short form of **Margaret.** Greek, "pearl."

MEGAN Welsh, Irish variant of **Margaret. Maegan, Meagan, Meaganne, Meaghan, Meg, Megen, Meggi, Meggie, Meggin, Meggy, Meghan, Meghann, Meghanne**

MEHITABEL Hebrew. "Benefited by God." **Mehetabel, Mehitabelle**

MEI Chinese. "Plum."

MEIRA Feminine form of **Meir.** Hebrew, "light."

MELANIE Greek. "Dark-skinned." **Malani, Malanie, Mel, Mela, Melanee, Melani, Melania, Melanney, Melannie, Melany, Mella, Mellanie, Melli, Mellie, Melloney, Melly, Meloni, Melonie, Melonnie, Melony**

MELANTHA Greek. "Dark flower."

MELBA Contemporary English. Dame Nellie Melba was the stage name of Helen Porter Mitchell (1859–1931), an Australian opera singer. Named for her are Melba toast and peach Melba (peach halves filled with ice cream and topped with raspberry-currant sauce).

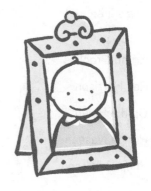

MELIA Greek. "Manna ash tree." **Malea, Malia, Maliah, Maliya, Meliah, Meliya**

MELINA Greek. "Honey." Also short form of **Carmelina** et al. **Meleana, Meline**

MELINDA Latin. "Honey." **Linda** et al., **Maillie, Malinda, Malinde, Mallie, Mally, Malynda, Melindah, Melinde, Melynda**

MELIORA Latin. "To better." **Liora, Meliorna, Melyorna**

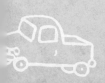

People with dogs' names

In Tennessee Williams's *Cat on a Hot Tin Roof*, Maggie scornfully asks her sister-in-law, Mae, why her children have dogs' names—*Buster, Trixie,* and *Dixie*. Now, a lot of dogs have people's names, but few people have dogs' names. These people haven't exactly led a dog's life:

Bruno Brookes

Rex Harrison

Goldie Hawn

Prince Naseem

Shep Pettibone

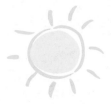

MELISANDE Combination of **Alessandra** and **Melissa**. **Lisandra** et al., **Malisande, Malissande, Malyssandre, Melesande, Melessande, Melisandra, Melisandre, Melisenda, Melissande, Melissandre, Mellisande, Melysande, Melyssandre, Sandra, Sandy** et al.

MELISSA Greek. "Honey bee." **Lissa, Lisse, Malissa, Mallissa, Mel, Melesa, Melessa, Meli, Melicia, Melisa, Melise, Melisse, Mellie, Mellisa, Melly, Melosa, Milli, Millie, Milly, Misha, Missy** et al.

MELITA Greek. "Honey." Also short form of **Carmelita**. **Mellita**

MELODY Greek. "Song." **Melodey, Melodi, Melodia, Melodie, Melodina, Melodyne**

MELORA Greek. "Golden apple."

MELOSA Spanish. "Honey-sweet." **Melosita**

MELVINA Feminine form of **Melvin**. Old French, "mill worker." **Mel, Melevine, Melva, Melveen, Melvena, Melvene, Melvine**

MERCEDES Spanish. "Mercies." **Merced, Mercede, Mercedez**

MERCIA Old English. Place name.

MERCY Latin. "Mercy." **Merci, Mercie, Mersey, Mersie, Mersy**

MEREDITH Old Welsh. "Great ruler." **Meredithe, Meridith, Merridie, Merry** et al.

MERI Hebrew. "Defiant." Also variant of **Merry**.

MERIEL Variant of **Muriel**. Irish, "sea-bright." **Merial, Merielle, Meriol, Meryl** et al.

MERIT Latin. "Deserved." **Meritt, Merrit, Merritt**

MERLE French. "Blackbird." **Merl, Merla, Merlina, Merline, Merola, Meryl, Murl, Myrleen, Myrlene, Myrline**

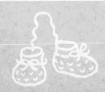

MERRILY Old English. "Joyously."

MERRY Old English. "Joyous." Also short form of **Meredith. Meri, Merie, Merree, Merri, Merrie, Merrita**

MERYL Variant of **Meriel. Meral, Merel, Merelle, Merrall, Merrell, Merril, Merrilee, Merrili, Merrill, Merryl, Meryle, Meryll**

MESSINA Latin. "Middle." Also a city in Sicily. **Messalina, Messitia, Messita**

META German variant of **Margaret.** Greek, "pearl." **Metta, Mette, Meyta**

METUKA Hebrew. "Sweet."

MIA Italian. "Mine."

MICHAELA Feminine form of **Michael.** Hebrew, "Who is like the Lord?" **Mica, Micaela, Michael, Michaelina, Michaeline, Michaila, Michal, Michalin, Micky** et al., **Miguela** et al., **Mikaela, Mikayla, Mikhaila, Mikhayla**

MICHELLE Feminine form of **Michael.** Hebrew, "Who is like the Lord?" **Machelle, Mechelle, Michele, Michelina, Micheline, Michell, Micky** et al., **Misha, Mishelle, Shelley** et al.

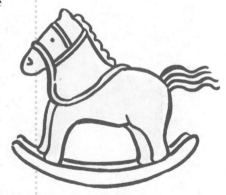

MICHIKO Japanese. "The virtuous path." **Michee, Michi**

MICKY Diminutive of **Michaela, Michelle. Mickee, Mickey, Micki, Mickie, Miki, Mikie, Miky**

MIDGE Short form of **Margaret.** Greek, "pearl."

MIETTE French. "Little sweet one." **Mietta**

MIGNON French. "Delicate." **Mignonette, Mignot, Minyonne, Minyonette**

MIGUELA Spanish feminine form of **Michael.** Hebrew, "Who is like the Lord?" **Miguelina, Miguelita, Miguella**

MILADA Czechoslovakian. "My love." **Lada**

MILAGROS Spanish. "Miracles." **Mila, Milagritos, Milagrosa, Milagrosita**

MILDRED Old English. "Strength." **Mil, Milda, Mildrid, Milly** et al.

MILENA Old German. "Mild." **Lena**

MILLICENT Old German. "High-born power." **Lissa, Mel, Meli, Melicent, Melisent, Melita, Mellecent, Melli, Mellicent, Mellie, Mellisent, Melly, Milicent, Milissent** et al., **Millisent, Millissent, Milly** et al., **Missy** et al.

MILLY Diminutive of **Amelia, Camille, Emily, Mildred, Millicent. Mille, Milli, Millie**

MIMI Diminutive of **Mary, Miriam, Wilhelmina.**

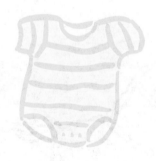

MINA Short form of **Adamina, Wilhelmina,** etc. **Min, Minna, Minetta, Minette, Minne, Minnie** et al.

MINDY Diminutive of **Melinda.** Latin, "honey." **Mindee, Mindi, Mindie**

MINERVA Latin. Roman goddess of wisdom. **Minnie** et al.

MINNIE Diminutive of **Mary, Minerva, Wilhelmina. Minee, Mini, Minni, Minny, Miny**

MINTA Short form of **Araminta.** English, "defender." **Mintha, Minty**

MIRA Short form of **Almera, Amira, Elmira, Mirabel, Miranda, Mirella. Mirah, Miri, Myra, Myrah, Myri**

MIRABEL Latin. "Admirable." **Mira, Mirabell, Mirabella, Mirabelle, Mirella**

MIRANDA Latin. "Amazed." **Marenda, Mira** et al., **Miran, Myranda, Randy** et al.

MIRELLA Hebrew. "God spoke." **Mira, Miranda, Mirela, Mireya, Mirielle, Mirilla, Myrella, Myrilla, Myrla**

MIRI Short form of **Miriam**, variant of **Mira. Myri**

MIRIAM Variant of **Mary.** Hebrew, "bitter." **Mariam, Maryam, Mimi, Mirham, Miri, Mirjam, Mirriam, Miryam, Mitzi** et al., **Myri**

MISSY Diminutive of **Melissa, Millicent. Misi, Misie, Missi, Missie, Misy**

MISTY Old English. "Of the mist." **Misti, Mistie**

MITZI English variant of **Miriam. Mitsee, Mitsey, Mitsi, Mitsie, Mitzie, Mitzy**

MIYUKI Japanese. "Tranquility."

MODESTY Latin. "Modesty." **Modesta, Modeste, Modestia, Modestina, Modestine**

MOINA Celtic. "Gentle." **Moyna**

MOIRA Celtic variant of **Mary. Maurya, Moyra, Myra**

MOLLY English variant of **Mary. Moll, Mollee, Molley, Molli, Mollie**

MOMI Hawaiian. "Pearl."

MONA Short form of **Ramona. Monah, Monna**

MONICA Disputed origin. St. Monica. **Mona, Monca, Mónica, Monicka, Monika, Monike, Monique, Monnica**

MONTANA Spanish. "Mountain." Also the forty-first U.S. state. **Montaña, Montanya**

MORASHA Hebrew. "Inheritance."

Accentuate the positive

Giving a person names whose initials spell out or usually stand for something odious—*SAP* or *SOB*, for instance—might do worse than make the person the butt of jokes for a lifetime. Two researchers at the University of San Diego examined some four million death certificates dating from 1969 through 1995. They came to the conclusion that men with embarrassing initials such as *BUM* or *UGH* died, on average, three years younger than men with innocuous initials. Even more amazing, men whose initials spelled out positive words such as *JOY* or *WOW* lived almost four-and-a-half years longer than average.

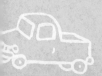

MORELA Polish. "Apricot."

MORGAN In legend, Morgan le Fay was the wicked fairy sister of King Arthur; she tried to have him murdered. **Morgana, Morgance, Morganella, Morganne, Morgen**

MORIAH Hebrew. "The Lord is my teacher." **Mariah, Moria**

MORIT Hebrew. "Teacher."

MORNA Irish. "Beloved." **Maurna, Mornah, Mourna, Myrna** et al.

MORRIGAN Irish. In myth, the goddess of battle.

MOSELLE Hebrew. Feminine form of **Moses.** Hebrew, possibly "savior." **Mozelle**

MOUNA Arabic. "Wish, desire." **Mounia, Muna**

MURIEL Irish. "Sea-bright." **Meriel** et al., **Miriel, Mirielle, Murial, Murielle**

MUSETTA Old French. "Thoughtful." **Musette**

MUSIDORA Greek. "Gift of the muses."

MYRA Feminine form of **Myron.** Greek, "fragrant oil." Also variant of **Moira.**

MYRNA Irish. "Beloved." **Merna, Mirna, Moina, Morna, Moyna, Muirna, Myrnna**

MYRTLE English. Any of numerous evergreen shrubs of the genus *Myrtle;* also periwinkle (*Vinca*). **Merta, Mertis, Mertle, Mirtle, Myrta, Myrtella, Myrtia, Myrtice, Myrtie, Myrtilla, Myrtis**

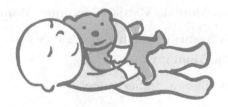

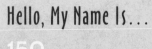

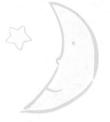

NAAVAH Hebrew. "Lovely." **Naama, Naamah, Naamana, Naava, Nama, Nava**

NABILA Arabic. "Noble." **Nabeela, Nabilah, Nabilla**

NADIA Slavic. "Hope." **Nada, Nadege, Nadezhda, Nadie, Nadiya, Nadja, Nadji, Nady, Nadya, Nadyenka, Nadzia, Nata, Natka**

NADINE French variant of **Nadia**. Slavic, "hope." **Nadeen, Nadena, Nadene, Nadenya, Nadina, Nadyna, Nadyne, Naydeen**

NAIDA Greek. "Water nymph." **Naia, Naiad, Naila, Nalya, Nayad, Nyad**

NAIRNE Scottish. "From the river."

NALANI Hawaiian. "Calm heavens."

NAN Variant of **Ann, Hannah, Fernandah**. **Nana, Nancy** et al., **Nanette** et al., **Nanine, Nann, Nanna, Nanne, Nanney, Nanni, Nannie, Nanny, Nanon**

NANCY Variant of **Ann**. Hebrew, "grace." **Nainsi, Nance, Nancee, Nanci, Nancie, Nancsi, Nanice, Nanncey, Nanncy, Nansee, Nansey, Nansi, Nansy**

NANETTE French variant of **Nan**. **Nanete, Nannette, Nettie, Netty**

NAOMI Hebrew. "Pleasant." **Naoma, Naomia, Naomie, Navit, Noami, Noemi, Noemie**

NAPEA Latin. "From the woods."

NARA Celtic. "Happy." **Narra**

NARCISSA Greek. "Daffodil." **Narcisa, Narcisse, Narcyssa, Narkissa, Narkita**

NARDA Latin. "Scented ointment."

NARIKO Japanese. "Gentle child."

NASIA Hebrew. "Miracle." **Nacia, Nasiya, Nasya**

NASTASIA Short form of **Anastasia.** Greek, "resurrection." **Nastacia, Nastassia, Nastassiya, Nastassja, Nastassya, Nastya, Nastyenka, Stacia, Stacy** et al.

NATALIE Latin. "Birth" or "birthday." **Nat, Nata, Natala, Natalee, Natalene, Natalia, Nataline, Natalja, Natalya, Natasha** et al., **Natelie, Nathalia, Nathalie, Natilie, Natividad, Nattilie, Nattie, Nettie**

NATANYA Feminine form of **Nathan.** Hebrew, "gift of God." **Natania, Nataniella, Natanielle, Nathana, Nathanella, Nathania, Nathaniella, Nathanyella, Netania, Netanya, Nethania, Nethanya**

NATASHA Russian variant of **Natalie.** Latin, "birth" or "birthday." **Nastaliya, Nastalya, Natacha, Natascha, Natashenka, Tasha, Tashua**

NATIVIDAD Spanish. "Birth," "Christmas."

NAYER Persian. "Sunshine."

NEALA Feminine form of **Neal.** Irish, "champion." **Neila, Neile, Neilla, Neille**

NEBULA Latin. "Smoke" or "darkness."

NEDA Feminine form of **Edward.** Old English, "wealthy defender." **Nedda, Neddie, Nedi**

NEGAR Persian. "Image."

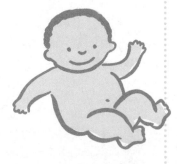

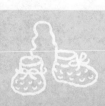

It's important for kids to stand out a little

Allison Glock is a magazine writer and author of a book about her grandmother, Beauty Before Comfort, *which contains the wonderful line, "Puberty hit my grandmother like a dropped piano." Allison lives in Knoxville, Tennessee.*

"We named our daughters *Dixie Jean* and *Matilda Mercy*. I liked the name *Dixie* from the time I was a little girl, and *Jean* is a family name. People's reactions to *Dixie* depend on where they are. I live in Tennessee, and people here think it is fine—they never say anything about it. My friends in New York, however, think it is very quirky.

"When I was pregnant the second time, I sent an email questionnaire to about twenty friends listing names and asking them to pick one. I told them that the winner could be present at the birth. We wound up not using any of those names, but it was fun to hear from friends.

"My husband is from Australia—you know, 'Waltzing Matilda' and all that. He chose that name. *Matilda* means 'warrior,' so I tempered that by adding *Mercy*.

"My mother didn't approve of these names, but I think kids need to stand out a little. These names let them do that. If we'd had a boy, his name would have been *Hieronymous,* which would have really given my mother something to fret about."

NEHEED Persian. Goddess of water.

NELIA Short form of **Cornelia.** Latin, "like a horn." **Neelia, Neelie, Neelya, Nela, Nila**

NELL Short form of **Eleanor, Cornelle, Danielle, Helen. Nel, Nella, Nelle, Nellette, Nelley, Nelli, Nellianna, Nellianne, Nellie, Nelly**

NEMA Hebrew. "Thread." **Nima**

NEOLA Greek. "Young."

NERINE Greek. "Sea nymph." **Nerice, Nerida, Nerina, Nerissa, Neryssa**

NESSIE Greek. "Lamb." Also diminutive of **Vanessa. Nesha, Nessa, Nesta, Neta, Netia**

NETTIE Diminutive of **Henrietta, Janet, Nanette. Net, Neti, Netta, Nette, Netti, Netty, Nety**

NEVADA Spanish. "Snowy." Also the thirty-sixth U.S. state. **Neva**

NIAMH Irish. In myth, a lover of the hero Cuchulain. Pronounced "nee-av."

NICOLE Feminine form of **Nicholas.** Greek, "victory of the people." **Colette** et al., **Cosetta, Cosette, Nicci, Nichelle, Nichola, Nichole, Nicholle, Nicia, Nickola, Nickole, Nicola, Nicolea, Nicoleen, Nicolene, Nicoleta, Nicoli, Nicolie, Nicolina, Nicoline, Nicolla, Nicolle, Nicolyne, Niki, Nikki** et al., **Nikola, Nikolia**

NIKE Greek. "Victory." Goddess of victory. **Nika**

NIKKI Diminutive of **Nicole. Nicki, Nickie, Nicky, Nikkey, Nikkie, Nikky**

NINA Spanish. "Girl." Also variant of **Annina, Gianina. Neena, Nena, Niña, Ninacska, Nineta, Ninete, Ninetta, Ninette, Ninnette, Ninon, Ninochka, Ninotchka**

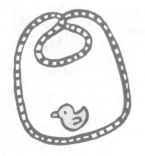

NIOBE Greek. "Fern."

NIRIT Hebrew. "Flower." **Nurit**

NITA Spanish. Short form of **Anita, Juanita,** etc.

NIXIE Old German. "Water sprite."

NOELANI Hawaiian. "Angel."

NOELLE French. "Christmas." **Noel, Noela, Noeleen, Noelene, Noelie, Noeline, Noella, Noelleen, Noelynn, Nowel, Noweleen, Nowell**

NOLA Short form of **Fionnula, Magnolia. Nolah, Nolla, Nollah**

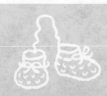

NOLETA Latin. "Unwilling." **Nolita**

NONA Latin. "Ninth." Also variant of **Ann, Helen. Nonah, Noni, Nonie, Nonna, Nonnah**

NORA Short form of **Eleanor, Honora, Leonora. Norah, Noreen** et al., **Norry**

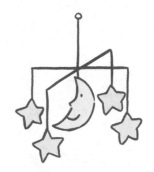

NORBERTA Feminine form of **Norbert.** Old German, "renowned northerner."

NOREEN Irish variant of **Nora**; short form of **Eleanor. Noirin, Norene, Norina, Norine, Noryne, Nureen**

NORMA Latin. "Pattern." **Norm, Normie**

NOVA Latin. "New."

NOVIA Spanish. "Girlfriend."

NOYA Hebrew. "Covered with jewels."

NUALA Short form of **Fionnula.** Irish, "white shoulder." **Nola, Nula**

NUNZIA Variant of **Annunciata.** Italian, "messenger." **Nunciata**

NUR Arabic. "Light." **Noor, Nurina**

NYDIA Latin. "Nest." **Neda, Nedda, Nidi, Nydya**

NYSA Latin. "Purpose." **Nissa, Nisse, Nyssa**

NYX Greek. "Night."

OBEDIENCE Latin. "Submission."

OBELIA Greek. "Indicator." **Obelya**

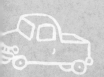

OCTAVIA Latin. "Eighth." **Octavie, Otavia, Ottavia, Tave, Tavi, Tavia, Tavie**

ODEDA Hebrew. "Courageous."

ODELIA Greek. "Song." **Oda, Odeelia, Odele, Odelet, Odelette, Odelinda, Odell, Odella, Odelle, Odilia, Othelia, Othilie**

ODESSA Greek. "Extended voyage." Also a city in the Ukraine.

ODETTE French, from German. "Wealthy." **Odetta** Odetta, an Alabama native trained as an opera singer, became a popular blues, folk, and gospel singer in the 1960s.

ODILE French, from German. "Wealthy." **Odila, Odilia**

OFIRA Hebrew. "Gold."

OFRA Old English. "Gift." **Ofrena, Ofrenya**

OFRAH West African. "Moon."

OLA Old Norse. "Protector." Also short form of **Olesia.**

OLEANDER Latin. A plant of the genus *Nerium,* especially the ornamental evergreen shrub *Nerium oleander.* **Oleandra, Oliana**

OLENA Russian variant of **Helen.** Greek, "light." **Alena, Lena, Lenya, Olenya**

OLESIA Greek. "Man's defender." **Ola, Olesa, Olessa**

OLETHEA Variant of **Alethea.** Greek, "truth." **Oleta, Olitia**

OLGA Russian. "Holy." **Elga, Helga, Ola, Olenka, Olia**

OLIANA Polynesian, from Latin. "Oleander."

OLINDA Latin. "Scented."

OLIVIA Latin. "Olive tree." **Liv, Liva, Livia, Livvie, Livvy, Livy, Oli, Olia, Oliva, Olive, Olivet, Olivette, Olivine, Ollie, Olly, Olva**

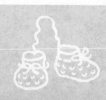

OLWEN Welsh. "White footprint." **Olwenn, Olwin, Olwyn**

OLYMPIA Greek. "Mount Olympus." In myth, the home of the gods. **Olimpe, Olimpia, Olympe, Olympie**

OMA Arabic. "Leader."

OMARA Feminine form of **Omar.** Arabic, "highest."

OMEGA Greek. "Final."

ONDINE Latin. "Little wave." **Ondina, Ondyne, Undine** et al.

ONDREA Slavic. "Strong," "courageous." Also a variant of **Andrea. Ohndrea, Ohndreea, Ohndria, Ondrea, Ondreea, Ondria, Onndrea, Onndreea, Onndria**

ONEIDA Native American. **Onida, Onyda**

ONELLA Greek. "Light." **Honella**

ONORA Variant of **Honora.** Latin, "honor." **Annora, Anora, Anorah, Onoria, Onorine, Ornora**

OONA Irish variant of **Una.** Latin, "one." **Oonagh**

OPAL Sanskrit. "Gem." **Opalina, Opaline**

OPHELIA Greek. "Aid." In Shakespeare's *Hamlet,* the daughter of Polonius. **Filia, Ofelia, Ofilia, Ophelie, Phelia**

OPHIRA Hebrew. "Gold." **Ofira**

OPRAH English variant of **Orpah.** Hebrew, "fawn." Oprah Winfrey, contemporary talk-show host. **Opra**

ORA Latin. "Prayer." Also short form of **Aurora. Orah, Orra**

ORABELLE Combination of **Ora** and **Belle. Orabel**

ORALEE Hebrew. "My light." **Orali, Oralit, Orlee, Orli, Orly**

ORALIE French variant of **Aurelia.** Latin, "gold." **Ora, Oralee, Orali, Oralia, Orel, Orelee, Oreli, Orlena**

Hapro just wouldn't sound as good

*O*rpah is one of the more obscure Biblical names. Born in the land of Moab and the sister-in-law of Ruth, Orpah is mentioned only twice in the Good Book. But when a female baby was born in rural Mississippi in 1954, the little girl's aunt chose the name *Orpah.* The name was difficult to pronounce, so family and friends began calling her *Oprah.* Now her name is *Oprah Winfrey,* and the name of the company that produces her television show is *Oprah* spelled backwards, or *Harpo.*

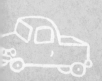

ORANE French feminine form of **Orion.** In Greek myth, a giant and mighty hunter who became, after his death, a constellation. **Orania**

ORELA Latin. "Announcement from the gods." **Orella, Orelya**

ORETA Variant of **Areta.** Greek, "woman of virtue." **Orete, Oretha, Oretta**

ORIANA Feminine form of **Orion.** Greek, "son of fire." **Oria, Oriande, Oriane, Orianna, Oriona**

ORINA Variant of **Irene.** Greek, "peace." **Oryna**

ORIOLE Latin. "Golden." Also a brightly colored bird. **Auriel** et al., **Oriel, Oriella, Orielle, Oriola**

ORIONA Feminine form of **Orion.** In Greek myth, a giant and mighty hunter who became, after his death, a constellation.

ORLA Celtic. "Light." **Aurla, Urla**

ORLANDA Feminine form of **Orlando,** Spanish variant of **Roland.** Old German, "famous land." **Orlande**

ORNA Latin. "To decorate." **Ornetta**

ORPAH Hebrew. "Fawn." **Oprah** et al.

ORQUIDEA Spanish. "Orchid." **Orquicia, Orquita**

ORSA Variant of **Ursula.** Latin, "bear." **Orsala, Orsaline, Orsela, Orselina, Orseline, Orsola, Orsolla**

ORSZEBET Hungarian variant of **Elizabeth.** Hebrew, "devoted to God."

ORTENSIA Italian variant of **Hortense.** Latin clan name.

OTTHILD Old German. "Prospers in battle." **Ottila, Ottilia, Ottilie, Ottiline, Ottoline**

OVA Latin. "Egg."

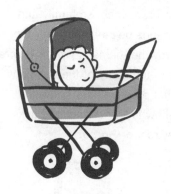

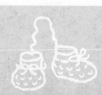

PADMA Hindi. "Lotus." **Padhma, Padmah**

PAGE French. "Young messenger." **Padget, Padgett, Paget, Pagett, Paige, Payge**

PALLAS Greek. "Goddess." Usually refers to **Athena**.

PALMA Latin. "Palm tree." **Pallma, Pallmirah, Pallmyra, Palmeda, Palmella, Palmera, Palmia, Palmira, Palmyra**

PALOMA Spanish. "Dove." **Palloma, Palometa, Palometta, Palomita, Peloma**

PAMELA Greek. "All-honey." **Pam, Pamala, Pamalla, Pamelia, Pamelina, Pamella, Pamilla, Pammela, Pammi, Pammie, Pammy**

PANDORA Greek. "Gift of all." In myth, Pandora opened the box that released all the world's evil, and with it hope. **Panndora, Pandorra**

PANPHILA Greek. "All-loving." **Panfila, Panfyla, Panphyla**

PANSY Middle French. "Thought." A large-blossomed hybrid violet. **Pansey, Pansi, Pansie**

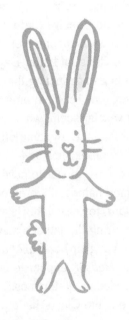

PANTHEA Greek. "All the gods." **Pantheia, Pantheya**

PAQUITA Nickname for **Francisca**. Spanish, from Latin, "from France."

PARI Persian. "Fairy."

PARISE French. "From Paris."

PARTHENIA Greek. "Virginal." **Partheenia, Parthenie, Parthinia, Pathina**

Must be something in all that Jell-O

Salt Lake City has long had the highest per-capita consumption of Jell-O in America, and, as it turns out, Utah has a goodly number of very unusual names. Cari Bilyeu Clark and her husband, Wesley, graduated from Brigham Young University in Utah. While living in the Beehive State, they noticed the unusual names among members of the Church of Jesus Christ of Latter-Day Saints. The Clarks began collecting these unusual names, and they now list them on a Web site, http://wesclark.com, where they write, "The quintessential Utah name often has a French-sounding prefix such as *Le-, La-, Ne-,* or *Va-.* Often names appear to have genesis in the combined names of the parents—*Veradeane* or *GlenDora,* for example. Related is the practice of feminizing the father's name—as in *Vonda* (dad is Vaughan) or *Danetta.* Others, such as *Snell* or *Houser,* appear to be surnames called into service as first names."

Here is the Clarks' list of extraordinary Utah names:

The new parents couldn't be happier: Gladell & Delightra (sisters), Luvit, Delecta, Delite, Joyette, Joi, Joyia, Joyellen, Joycell, Hallah Lujah, Bliss, Joyanne, Evol (*love* spelled backwards)

Cleanliness is next to godliness: Zestpoole, Sparkle

The choir director's daughters: Aria, Audia, Aurel, Choral, LaVoice, Tonilee, Capella, Chime, Rocksan Violin

Jewels every one: Amulet, Pearlette, Pearlene, Emerald, JewlyAnn, Ahmre Jade, Treasure Tonya, Turquoise Nova, Sequin, Amethist

Maybe they're in the Klingon Ward: Tchae, Xko, Corx, G'ni, Vvhs, Garn, Ka, Deauxti, Xymoya, Sha'Kira, Zy, Xela, Nivek, Zon'tl, Zagg, Xan, Judziah Datz (a female, named after a character in Star Trek), K'lar (ditto), Jarna Nazhalena, Chod, Xarek, Grik, Stod, T'Shara, Tral, Sherik, Curg

Astronomical: LeVoid, Sunan, Moonyene, Starlene, Sunelly, Luna, Lunia, Solinda, Sunirae, Staryl, Marandastarr, Aries, Starlyn, Cressent, Celestial Starr, Summerlyn, Astrolena

Parents were BYU math majors: Alpha Mae, Prime, Omega Lee, Jennyfivetina, Seven, Seavenly, Sevenly, Eighta, Ninea, Tenna, Elevena, Twenty, Datus

You can name a kid this, but you shouldn't ingest it: Cola, Vinyl, Orlon, Chlorine, Clorene, Florene, Florine, Lexann, Dow, Tide, Downy, Codiene, Daquari, DeCon, Starbuck, Crayon, Radon

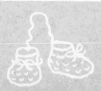

Names inspired by the family car: Audi, Fairlene, Celecta, Pontiac, Vonda, Vonza, Auto, Cherokee, Lexus, Porsche, Skylark, Truckston, Avis, Chevrollette, Chevonne, Caprice, Dodge

Wishful thinking: Darlin', Courage, Winsome, Justan Tru, Pictorianna, Paradise Sunrise, Angelic, Breed, Godlove, Myrth, LaVirgin, DeFonda Virtue, Chastice, Normalene, Lovie Angel, Precious Blessing, Heavenly Melanie, Glee, Mormon Beauty, Pledger, Jentill, Devota, Coy, Fondd, Bridella, Verna Noall, Vervine, Viva, Golden Noble, MarVel, MemRee, Brunette, Merrily, Merry Ann, Celestial, Cherrish, Kash, Cashelle, Teton, Forever, Luvit, Mystiq, Worthy, Truly, Speedy, Hereditary, Shrudilee, Halo, Gentry, Truthanne, Finita, Mavryck, Amen, Marvelous Man

Possible indications of birthplace: Arizonia, Floria, Montania, Utah, Utahna, Idahana, Idaho, Mauntana, Michigan, Nevadna, Okla, Vermont, Wyoming, Wyoma, Cache, Jordana, Payson, Vernal, Boise, Brookelynn, Lexington, Demoyn, Fredonia, Leremy, Platte, Salina, Seattle, Takoma, Tulsa, Tustin, Vail, Lundyn, Londyn, Irelynd, Irelan, Madrid, Manila, Cairo, Damascus, Tyre, Desert, Shahara, Trinidad, Houston, Cachelyn, D'Asia, Edon, Takoda, Orem, Shannon doah, Davenport Shore, Hollan

Possible indications of birthdates: Juneth, Junola, LaJune, Julyn, Halloween, Novella, Summerisa, Winnter, Christmas Holiday, Merrienoel, Kris Miss, Tuesdee, Aprella

I hope the computer will accept apostrophes in the name fields: D'Ann, D'Aun, D'Bora, D'Dee, D'Elise, D'Loaf, D'Shara, E'all, L'Deane, L'orL, Ja'mon, J'Costa, J'dean, J'Leen, J'net, J'Shara, J'Vonna, La'Donis, Me'shell, M'Jean, M'Kaaylie, M'Kenna, Mi'Lara, M'Lisa, M'Liss, M'Lu, M'Recia, O'lea, R'dell, R'lene, Shan'l, Young'n, B'andra, De'lys, D'Dree, J'l

Future names of prescription drugs: Lyravin, Monalaine, Nyleen, Merlaine, Monease, Naquel, Ronalene, Nylan, Rolayne, Tyron, Lexine, Lyrin, Mikatin, Artax, Xtrin, Tylene, Qedrin, Tamrin, Denilyn, Kevrin, Nicolin, Xylan, Tolex, Zylan, Daycal, Falycid, Zerin, Davon, Sydal, Dynevore

Commemorating something or another: Welcome Exile, Confederate American, Southern Justice, Diksi, Liberty Lulu, Young Elizabeth, Genesis, MistiNoele, Imagine, Thankful Flood, Friends Forsaken, Joyous Noel, Tennyson, Knight Train, Miracles Precious One, Sunday's Hoseana, Disney, Blessing Ream, Stormy Shepherd, Denim Levi, Vernal Independence, Sincere Devotion, Elvoid, Noah-Lot, Mormon Miracles, MyLae, Nightrain Lane, Zion Anakin, Jeopardee, Statehood, Timberland Miner, Lucky Blue

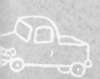

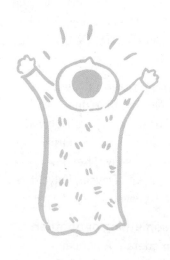

PARVANEH Persian. "Butterfly."

PASCALE French. "Of Easter." **Pascalette, Pascaline, Pascalle, Pascha, Paschal, Paschale, Pashel**

PATIENCE English. "Patience." **Paciencia, Patia**

PATRICIA Feminine form of **Patrick.** Latin, "upper class." **Pat, Patia, Patreece, Patrica, Patrice, Patricka, Patriece, Patrisia, Patrizia, Patsy, Patty** et al., **Tricia** et al.

PATRONELA Romanian. "Rock."

PATSY Diminutive of **Patricia,** feminine form of **Patrick.** Latin, "upper class."

PATTY Diminutive of **Patricia,** feminine form of **Patrick.** Latin, "upper class." **Patte, Pattee, Pattey, Patti, Pattie**

PAULA Feminine form of **Paul.** Latin, "small." **Paola, Paolina, Paule, Pauletta, Paulette, Paulie, Paulina, Pauline, Paulita, Paulla, Paullette, Paully, Pauly, Pavia**

PAULINE French feminine form of **Paul.** Latin, "small." **Pauleen, Paulene, Paulyne, Polline**

PAZ Spanish. "Peace." **Pas**

PAZIA Hebrew. "Golden." **Paza, Pazice, Pazit**

PEACE Middle English. "Peace."

PEARL English, from Latin. "Pearl." Pearl Buck, twentieth-century American novelist. Pearl Bailey. **Pearla, Pearle, Pearleen, Pearlette, Pearlie, Pearline, Perl, Perla, Perle, Perlette, Perley, Perline, Perlline**

PEGEEN Irish nickname for **Margaret.** Greek, "pearl."

PEGGY Nickname for **Margaret.** Greek, "pearl." **Peg, Pegeen, Peggie**

PEKE Old German. "Lustrious."

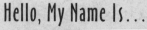

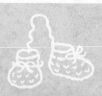

PELAGIA Greek. "Sea." **Pelage, Pelageia, Pelagie, Pelajya, Pellagia**

PEMA Tibetan. "Lotus."

PENELOPE Greek. "Weaver." In the *Odyssey*, Odysseus's faithful wife. **Pen, Peneli, Penelopa, Penina, Penna, Pennelope, Penny** et al.

PENINAH Hebrew. "Pearl." **Penina, Peninit**

PENNY Diminutive of **Penelope. Penney, Penni, Pennie**

PENTHEA Greek. "Fiftieth."

PEONY Greek. "Peony," a flowering perennial plant of the genus *Paeonia.* **Peoni**

PEPITA Spanish diminutive of **Josefa,** feminine form of **Joseph.** Hebrew, "the Lord provides." **Pepa, Pepi, Peta**

PERDITA Latin. "Lost."

PERFECTA Spanish. "Flawless."

PERNELLA French feminine form of **Peter.** Greek, "rock." **Parnella, Pernelia, Pernelle, Pernelya**

PERPETUA Latin. "Everlasting." St. Perpetua.

PERRY French. "Pear tree." **Perrey, Perri, Perrie**

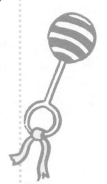

PERSEPHONE Greek. "Dazzling." In myth, Persephone's return from the underworld causes spring and the cycle of the seasons. **Persephoneia, Persephonie**

PERSIS Latin. "From Persia." **Perssis**

PETRA Feminine form of **Peter.** Greek, "rock." **Pat, Patra, Perrin, Perrine, Perry, Pet, Peta, Peterina, Petrina, Petronel, Petronela, Petronella, Petronelle, Petronia, Petronija, Petronilia, Petronilla, Petronille, Petrova, Petrovna, Pietra, Pitri, Pitry**

PETULA Latin. "Bold speaker." **Petulah, Petulla, Petullah**

PETUNIA New Latin. "Petunia." **Petunya**

PHEDRA Greek. "Bright." In myth, Phedra killed herself for unrequited love of her stepson. **Faydra, Phaedra, Phaedre, Phaidra, Phedre**

PHEMIA Greek. "Speech." **Femia, Phemie, Phemya**

PHEODORA Russian feminine form of **Theodore**. Greek, "gift of God." **Fedora, Feodora, Fyodora, Pheodorna**

PHILA Greek. "Love."

PHILANA Greek. "Loving humanity." **Filania, Filanna, Filanya, Phila, Philene, Philina, Philine, Phillana, Phillane**

PHILANTHA Greek. "Lover of flowers." **Philanthe**

PHILBERTA Middle English. "Bright loving." **Filberta, Filiberta, Philiberta**

PHILIPPA Feminine form of **Philip**. Greek, "lover of horses." **Felipa, Filipa, Filippa, Pelipa, Phil, Philipa, Philippe, Philippine, Philli, Phillie, Phillipa, Phillipina, Philly, Pip, Pippa, Pippy**

PHILOMELA Greek. "Lover of song." In myth, her brother-in-law cut out her tongue, but she told the story wordlessly through a weaving. The gods saved her from murder by turning her into a swallow. **Filomela, Philomelania**

PHILOMENA Greek. "Beloved." **Filimena, Filomena, Philomène, Philomina,**

PHOEBE Greek. "Shining, brilliant." **Fibi, Fibie, Pheabe, Phebe, Pheby, Phoebey**

PHOENIX Greek. In myth, a bird that rose from burning ashes.

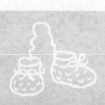

PHYLLIDA Variant of **Phyllis.** Greek, "leafy bough." **Fillida, Phillida, Phillyda**

PHYLLIS Greek. "Leafy bough." **Fillys, Fyllis, Philis, Phillida, Phillis, Philys, Phyl, Phylis, Phyliss, Phyllida, Phylliss, Phyllys, Phylys**

PIA Latin. "Pious."

PIEDAD Spanish. "Piety." **Piedadina**

PIER Feminine form of **Pierre.** French, from Greek, "rock." **Pierella, Pierena, Pieretta, Pierette, Pierina**

PILAR Spanish. "Pillar." From the Virgin of the Pillar, the patron saint of Spain.

PING Chinese. "Duckweed."

PIPER Old English. "Pipe player." **Phifer**

PLACIDIA Latin. "Serene." **Placida, Plasida**

PLEASANT Old French. "Pleasing." **Pleasance, Pleasante, Pleasence**

POLLY Old English variant of **Mary.** Hebrew, "bitter." **Poll, Polli, Pollie**

POLLYANNA Combination of **Polly** and **Anna.**

POMONA Latin. "Fruit." Roman goddess of orchards.

POPPY Latin. "Poppy." **Poppi, Poppie**

PORA Hebrew. "Fruitful."

PORSCHE German variant of **Portia.** Also the name of a luxury car.

PORSHA Contemporary American variant of **Porsche, Portia. Porshe**

PORTIA Latin. Clan name. Wife of Julius Caesar. Heroine of *Merchant of Venice.* **Porsha, Porsche, Porshe**

PRIMA Latin. "First." **Primalia, Primetta, Primi, Primina, Priminia**

PRIMAVERA Italian, Spanish. "Spring." **Vera**

PRIMROSE Middle English. "First rose," perennial plant of the genus *Primula.*

PRISCILLA Latin. "Ancient." **Cilla, Pris, Prisca, Priscella, Prisilla, Prissie, Prissy**

PROSPERA Latin. "Prosperous." **Prosperia**

PRUDENCE Latin. "Sound judgment." **Pru, Pruda, Prudencia, Prudentia, Prudie, Prudy, Prue**

PRUNELLA Latin. "Small plum."

PSYCHE Greek. "Breath" or "spirit." In myth, the beloved wife of Cupid.

PULCHERIA Latin. "Beauty." **Pulcherya**

PURITY Middle English. "Purity." **Pura, Pureza**

PYRALIS Greek. "Fire." **Pyra, Pyrena**

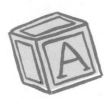

QUALIA Contemporary English. "A mental experience." **Quale**

QUEENIE Old English. "Queen." **Queena, Queenya, Quyen**

QUELLA Old English. "Killer." **Quellia**

QUERIDA Spanish, from Latin. "Dear one." **Quericia**

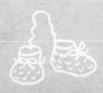

QUIANA Contemporary American. **Kiana, Quianna**

QUINANNA Contemporary American. **Quinanne**

QUINN Irish. "Wise leader." **Quina, Quinna, Quinne**

QUINTA Latin. "Fifth." **Quintella, Quintilia, Quintilla, Quintina**

QUITA Contemporary American, short form of **Poquita.** Spanish, "very little." **Laquita, La Quita**

RABAB Arabic. "Pleasant wind." **Rabia, Rabiah**

RACHEL Hebrew. "Ewe." **Rachael, Racheal, Rachele, Racheli, Rachelle** et al., **Rachie, Rachil, Rae** et al., **Rahel, Rahil, Rakel, Raquel** et al., **Raychel, Raychelle, Shelley** et al.

RACHELLE French variant of **Rachel.** Hebrew, "ewe." **Rachele, Rashell, Rashelle**

RADMILLA Slavic. "Industrious for the people." **Radmella, Radmila**

RAE Short form of **Rachel.** Hebrew, "ewe." **Ray, Raye**

RAEANN Combination of **Rae** and **Ann. Raeanne, Rayann, Rayanne**

RAFA Arabic. "Prosperity." **Rafah, Rafalya**

RAGNILD Teutonic. "All-knowing power." **Ragnhild, Ragnhilda, Ragnhilde, Ragnilda, Ragnilde, Ranild, Ranilde, Ranillda, Reinheld, Renilda, Renilde**

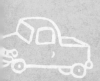

CHINESE NAMES

In recent years, thousands of American families have adopted baby girls from China. Many of these adoptive parents want their daughters to have some connection to their homeland's heritage, so they give the child at least one Chinese name.

Americans delight in naming children creatively and spelling names in any way that strikes our fancy. Although fine in the land of Aronns and Britannees, these practices will not fly in China or among Chinese people. Chinese naming is very complicated. For example, Chinese individuals often receive three names—one, a "milk name," upon birth, another upon entering school, and another when taking a job.

Making up a name that sounds Chinese to American ears or paying little attention to the juxtaposition of Chinese names can result in a child's bearing a moniker that, while sounding fine to Americans, may make Chinese people laugh out loud. For this reason, non-Chinese parents planning to give a child a Chinese name should first check the name with a helpful Chinese person. Often adoption-agency personnel can assist in the naming process.

Chinese babies usually come with names they have received in their orphanages, and these names are a good place to begin. Many adoptive parents give their child an American first name and a Chinese middle name. Children want to fit in with others, and having a more conventional first name will allow the child to do so. Perhaps your child may choose to go by the Chinese name later in life.

Another consideration is how the name sounds. If the child will grow up in this country, the Chinese name should be something that Americans can pronounce. Having a name that is hard to say is a burden for any child—in any language. The lists below contain names that Americans can readily say.

These are some Chinese boys' names:

An	"peace"
Chang	"prosperity"
Chen	"great" or "fast"
Ho	"good"
Jin	"gold"
Kong	"glorious"
Kun	"mountain range"
Lei	"thunder"
Lin	"forest"
Lok	"happy"
Long	"dragon"
Ming	"shining" or "clear"

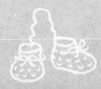

San	"three" or "third child"	Li	"beautiful"
Shaiming	"sunshine"	Li Wei	"beautiful rose"
Tai	"very big"	Lin ("leen")	"beautiful jade"
		Ling	"tinkling jade"

And here are some Chinese girls' names:

		Mei	"plum"
Fen ("fun")	"fragrant"	Ping	"duckweed"
Jia Li	"good, beautiful"	Shan	"coral"
Jing	"sparkling"	Wan	"gentle, gracious"
Jiao (rhymes with *meow*)	"beautiful"	Wei	"rose"
Lei	"flower bud"	Xia ("see-ah")	"glow of sunrise"

RAIN English, from French or Spanish. "Queen." **Raenah, Raene, Rainah, Raine, Rane, Raya, Rayna, Rayne**

RAISA Yiddish. "Rose." **Raissa, Raiza**

RAJA Arabic. "Hope."

RAMONA Spanish feminine form of **Raymond.** Old German, "guardian." **Monna, Mona, Ramonda, Ramonde, Ramonna, Raymonda, Romona, Romonda, Romonde**

RANA Latin. "Frog." Also variant of **Rani,** short form of **Veronica.**

RANDA Feminine form of **Randall.** Old German, "wolf." **Ronda**

RANDY Diminutive of **Miranda.** Latin, "amazed." **Randa, Rande, Randee, Randene, Randi, Randie**

RANI Sanskrit. "Queen." **Rana, Ranee, Rania, Ranya**

RANITA Hebrew. "Song." **Ranit, Ranite, Ranith, Ranitta**

RAPA Hawaiian. "Moonbeam."

RAPHAELA Feminine form of **Raphael.** Hebrew, "God heals." **Rafa, Rafaela, Rafaele, Rafaelia, Rafaella, Rafella, Rafelle,**

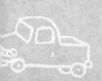

Raffaela, Raffaele, Raphaelle, Raphela, Raphelia, Raphelya

RAQUEL Spanish variant of **Rachel.** Hebrew, "ewe." **Raquela, Raquella, Raquelle**

RASHIDA Feminine form of **Rashid.** Turkish, "rightly guided." **Rasheda, Rasheeda, Rasheida, Rashidah**

RASOHERINA Madagascarian. A queen.

RAVEN English. "Raven." **Ravenne**

RAVENNA Italian. A city in Italy, on the Adriatic Sea.

RAWNIE English Gypsy. "Lady." **Rawnee, Rawny, Roni, Ronie, Ronni, Ronnie**

RAYA Hebrew. "Friend." **Reya**

RAYETTE Contemporary American.

RAYLEEN Contemporary American. **Raeleen, Raelene, Rayleen, Rayleine, Rayline**

RAYNELLE Contemporary American.

RAZ Hebrew. "Secret."

READE Old English. "To advise." **Read**

REBA Short form of **Rebecca.** Hebrew, "joined." **Rebe, Reeba, Reyba, Rheba**

REBECCA Hebrew. "Joined." **Becca, Becka, Beckie, Becky, Bekka, Bekki, Reba** et al., **Rebeca, Rebecka, Rebeka, Rebekah, Rebekkah, Rheba, Riva, Rivah, Rivi, Rivka, Rivkah, Rivy**

REESE Welsh. "Enthusiasm." **Reece**

REGAN Irish. "Little king." **Raigan, Raigen, Raygan, Rayggen, Reagan, Regen**

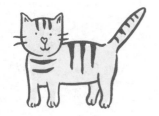

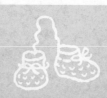

REGINA Latin. "Queen." **Gina, Reggi, Reggie, Reggy, Regine, Rina**

REIKO Japanese. "Gratitude."

REINA Spanish. "Queen." **Reyna**

REINE French. "Queen."

REMEDIOS Spanish. "Help." **Remedia, Remedina, Remi**

REMY French. "From Rheims." **Remi, Remie**

RENA Hebrew. "Melody." Also variant of **Irene**; short form of **Serena, Sirena. Reena**

RENATA Latin. "Reborn." **Renae, Renate, Renée** et al., **Renette, Renie, Renita, Rennie**

RENE Short form of **Irene.** Greek, "peace." **Renie, Rennie, Renny**

RENÉE French. "Reborn." **Renae, Renay, René, Renie, Rennie, Renny**

RENELLE Contemporary American. **Renel, Renele, Renell**

RENITA Disputed origin. **Reneeta, Renicia**

RESEDA New Latin. "Magnonette." *Reseda odorata,* a sprawling annual plant with a strong fragrance.

RETA Variant of **Rita.** Greek, "pearl." **Reeta, Rheta, Rhetta**

RETHA Short form of **Aretha.** Greek, "woman of virtue."

REUBENA Feminine form of **Reuben.** Hebrew, "behold, a child." **Reubenya**

REXANA Latin, "Regally graceful." **Rex, Rexanna, Rexanne**

RHEA Greek. "Earth mother." **Rea, Rhia, Ria**

RHETA Greek. "Eloquent."

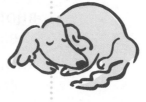

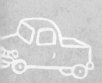

RHIANNON Welsh. "Witch" or "goddess." **Rhianna, Rhianon, Rianon, Riannon, Rignon**

RHODA Greek. "Rose." **Rhode, Rhodea, Rhodeia, Rhodia, Rhodie, Rhody, Roda, Rodi, Rodie, Rodina**

RHODANTHE Greek. "Rose blossom." **Rhodante, Rhodanthia, Rhodanthya**

RHONA Old Norse. "Rough island." **Rhona, Roana, Rona**

RHONDA Irish. "Strong river." **Rhonnda, Rhonnie, Ronda**

RIA Latin, "victor." Spanish, "fjord." **Rea**

RIANE Feminine form of **Ryan.** Irish, disputed meaning. **Rhiane, Rhianna, Riana, Rianna, Rianne, Ryann, Ryanne**

RICA Short form of **Erica, Ricarda, Roderica, Ulrica. Ricca, Rieca, Riecka, Rieka, Rika, Riqua, Rycca**

RICARDA Feminine form of **Richard.** Old German, "great ruler." **Rica, Richanda, Richarda, Richel, Richela, Richele, Richella, Richelle, Richenda, Richenza, Richia, Richilene, Richmal, Richmalle, Ricka**

RICKIE Diminutive of **Erica, Frederica. Ricci, Riccie, Rickey, Ricki, Ricky, Ricquie, Riki, Rikki, Rikkie, Rikky, Ryckie**

RICKMA Hebrew. "Woven." **Rikma**

RIKU Japanese. "Land."

RILLA Middle German. "Small brook." **Rilletta, Rillette**

RIMA Arabic. "Antelope."

RINA Variant of **Irene, Regina. Reena, Rena**

RISA Latin. "Laughter." **Riesa, Rise, Rysa**

RISHONA Hebrew. "First." **Rishana, Rishanah, Rishonah**

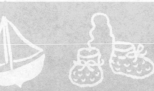

RITA Short form of **Marguerita**. Greek, "pearl." **Reatha, Reeta, Reita, Reta, Rheeta, Riet, Rieta, Ritha, Ritta**

RITIKA Sanskrit. "On the move."

RITSA Short form of **Alexandra**, feminine form of **Alexander**. Greek, "man's defender."

RIVA Latin. "Riverbank." Also a variant of **Rebecca. Ree, Reeva, Rivalee, Rivi, Rivka, Rivkah, Rivy**

RIVABELLE Latin. "Beautiful riverbank." **Rivabel, Reevabel**

RIVER English. "River." **Rivana, Rivanya, Rivera, Riverine**

ROANNA Variant of **Rosanne. Ranna, Roana, Roani, Roanne, Ronni, Ronnie, Ronny**

ROBBIE Diminutive of **Roberta, Robin. Robbee, Robbey, Robbi, Robby**

ROBERTA Feminine form of **Robert**. Old English, "bright fame." **Berta, Bertie, Berty, Bobbette, Bobbie** et al., **Bobette, Bobi, Bobina, Bobine, Bobinette, Robbie** et al., **Robertena, Robertene, Robertina, Robi** et al., **Robin**

ROBIN Variant of **Roberta**, feminine form of **Robert**. Old English, "bright fame." **Robbie** et al., **Robbin, Robbyn, Robeena, Robena, Robene, Robenia, Robi, Robina, Robine, Robinet, Robinett, Robinette, Robinia, Robyn, Robyna, Robynna, Robynette**

ROCHELLE Old French place name. "Little rock." **Roch, Rochel, Rochelia, Rochell, Rochella, Rochelle, Roshelle, Shelley** et al.

RODERICA Feminine form of **Roderick**. Old German, "renowned ruler." **Rica, Roddie, Roderiqua, Roderique, Rodica, Rodika, Rory** et al.

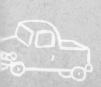

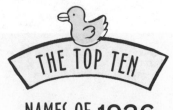

THE TOP TEN

NAMES OF 1936

The Year Jesse Owens Won Four Gold Medals at the Summer Olympics

BOYS

Robert
James
John
William
Donald
Richard
Charles
Ronald
George
Joseph

GIRLS

Mary
Shirley
Barbara
Betty
Patricia
Maria
Dorothy, Nancy (tie)
Joan
Margaret

ROHANA Sanskrit. "Sandalwood." **Rohanna**

ROISIN Celtic. "Rose." **Roisa, Rosheen, Roshine**

ROLANDA Feminine form of **Roland.** Old German, "famous land." **Orlanda, Orlande, Rolande, Rollanda, Rollande**

ROLINE Short form of **Caroline,** feminine form of **Carl, Charles.** Old German, "man." **Roelene, Rolaine, Roleen, Rolene, Rolina**

ROMA Latin. "Rome." Also a variant of **Romia. Romina, Romma**

ROMAINE French. "Roman." **Romayne, Romeine, Romene**

ROMANA Spanish. "Roman."

ROMELDA German. "Roman warrior." **Romhilda, Romhilde, Romilda, Romilde**

ROMIA Hebrew. "Glorious." **Roma**

ROMOLA Latin. "Woman of Rome." **Romella, Romelle, Rommola, Romolla, Romula, Romy**

RONA Old Norse. "Rough island." **Rhona, Ronella, Ronelle, Ronna**

RONNI Feminine form of **Ronald,** diminutive of **Veronica.** Old English, "powerful ruler." **Ronee, Ronette, Roni, Ronie, Ronna, Ronnee, Ronney, Ronnie, Ronny**

RORY Short form of **Aurora, Roderica. Rori, Rorie**

ROSA Latin. "Rose." **Arrosa, Rosina, Rosita**

ROSABEL Latin. "Beautiful rose." **Rosabella, Rosabelle**

ROSALBA Latin. "White rose."

ROSALIA Italian. "Rose garden." **Rosalina, Roselia, Rozalia, Rozellia**

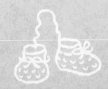

ROSALIE French variant of **Rosalia.** Italian, "rose garden." **Rosalee, Rosaleen, Rosaley, Rosaline, Rosalyne, Rosel, Rosella, Roselle, Rozali, Rozalie, Rozele, Rozelie, Rozella, Rozelle, Rozely**

ROSALIND English variant of **Rosalinda.** Spanish, "pretty rose." Daughter of the banished duke in Shakespeare's *As You Like It.* **Ros, Rosalen, Rosalin, Rosalinde, Rosaline, Rosalinn, Rosalyn, Rosalynd, Rosalynda, Rosalynn, Rosalynne, Roseleen, Roselin, Roselina, Roselind, Roselinda, Roselinde, Roseline, Roselinn, Roselyn, Roselynda, Roselynde, Roselynn, Roselynne, Rosina, Rosinda, Roslyn, Roslynn, Roslynne, Roz, Rozalin, Rozalind, Rozalinda, Rozaline, Rozalyne, Rozalynn, Rozalynne, Rozelin, Rozelind, Rozelinda, Rozelyn, Rozelynd**

ROSALINDA Spanish. "Pretty rose."

ROSAMOND Old German. "Mounted protector." **Ros, Rosamonde, Rosamund, Rosamunda, Rosamunde, Rosemond, Rosemonda, Rosmund, Rosmunda, Rosomund, Roz, Rozamond**

ROSARIO Spanish. "Rosary."

ROSE English, from French. "Rose." **Rasia, Rasine, Rasja, Rasya, Roesa, Roese, Roesia, Rosa** et al., **Roselia, Roselina, Roseline, Rosella, Roselle, Rosena, Rosenah, Rosene, Rosenja, Rosenya, Rosetta, Rosette, Rosie, Rosy, Roza, Roze, Rozele, Rozella, Rozina, Rozsi, Rozsika, Rusena, Rusenja, Rusenya, Ruzena**

ROSEANNE Combination of **Rose** and **Anne. Ranna, Roanna** et al., **Rosan, Rosanna, Rosannah, Rosanne, Roseann, Roseanna, Rozanna, Rozanne, Rozeanna**

ROSEBUD English. "Rosebud."

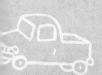

ROSEMARY English. "Rosemary," a perennial herb used in cooking. From Latin, "dew of the sea." **Rosemaree, Rosemarey, Rosemaria, Rosemarie, Rosmarie, Rozmary**

ROWENA Irish. "Slender and fair." **Roweena, Roweina, Rowenya, Rowina**

ROXANNE Persian. "Dawn." **Roksanne, Roxana, Roxane, Roxann, Roxanna, Roxene, Roxey, Roxie, Roxine, Roxy**

ROYALE Old French. "Royal." **Royal, Royalene, Royall, Royalle, Royalyn**

RUBY Latin. "Red." **Rubee, Rubet, Rubetta, Rubette, Rubey, Rubi, Rubia, Rubie, Rubina, Rubinia, Rubyna**

RUDELLE Old German. "Renowned." **Rudelia, Rudella, Rudellya**

RUFINA Latin. "Red-haired." **Rufeena, Rufine, Ruphina, Ruphyna**

RUMER Romany. "Gypsy."

RUNA Old Norse. "Flowing." **Runja, Runya**

RUTH Hebrew. "Friend," "companion." **Ruthe, Ruthelle, Ruthetta, Ruthi, Ruthie, Ruthina, Ruthine**

RUTHANN Combination of **Ruth** and **Ann**. **Ruthanna, Ruthanne**

SAADA Hebrew. "Support." **Saadah**

SABA Greek, "from Sheba," an ancient country in southern Arabia. Arabic, "morning." **Sabah, Sheba** et al.

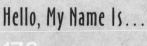

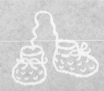

SABINA Latin. "Sabine," of an ancient tribe of central Italy, conquered by the Romans. **Bina, Sabine, Sabinna, Sabinya, Sabyna, Savina, Savine, Sebina, Sebinah**

SABRA Unknown origin. **Sabrah, Zabra**

SABRINA A mythical princess of ancient Britain. Also Arabic, "white rose." **Brina, Sabreena, Sabrinah, Sabrinna, Sabryna, Zabrina, Zabrinah**

SACAGAWEA Shoshone. Disputed meaning; "boat pusher" or "bird woman." Guide and interpreter for the Lewis and Clark expedition. **Sacagaweah, Sacajawea, Sacajaweah**

SACHI Japanese. "Child of joy." **Sachiko**

SADELLE Variant of **Sarah.** Hebrew, "princess." **Sadella, Sadellia, Saydell, Sydelle** et al.

SADIE Variant of **Sarah.** Hebrew, "princess." **Sada, Sadah, Saidee, Saydi, Saydie, Sadelle** et al., **Sydelle** et al.

SADIRA Persian. "Lotus tree."

SAFFRON Arabic. "Saffron," a crocus prized for its stigma, used as a flavoring and dye. **Saffren, Saffronia, Saphron**

SAGE Latin. "Wise." Also an herb once associated with wisdom. **Saige, Sayge**

SAHAR Hebrew. "Moon."

SAHARA Arabic. The world's largest desert.

SAKURA Japanese. "Cherry blossom."

SALENA Variant of **Selina.** Greek goddess of the moon.

SALIMAH Arabic. "Healthy." **Salima**

SALLY Variant of **Sarah.** Hebrew, "princess." **Sal, Saletta, Sallee, Salletta, Sallette, Salley, Salli, Sallie**

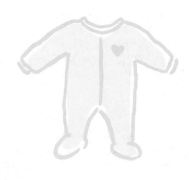

SALOME Hebrew. "Peace." **Saloma, Salomey, Salomi, Shalom**

SALVADORA Spanish. "Savior." **Salvadorna**

SALVIA Latin. "Whole," "well," "safe." Also the botanical name for sage. **Sallvia, Salvina**

SAMALA Hebrew. "Requested of God." **Samale, Sammala**

SAMANTHA Aramaic. "Listener." **Sam, Samentha, Sammantha, Sammee, Sammey, Sammie, Sammy, Semantha, Semanntha, Simantha, Symantha**

SAMARA Hebrew. "Under God's rule." **Samaria, Sammara**

SAMIRA Feminine form of **Samir.** Arabic, "entertainer." **Sameerah, Samirah**

SAMUELA Feminine form of **Samuel.** Hebrew, "told by God." **Samella, Samelle, Samuelia, Samuella, Samuelle, Samuelya**

SANCTA Latin. "Sacred." **Sancha, Sanchia, Santa** et al., **Santsha, Santshia, Santsia, Sanzia**

SANDRA Short form of **Alexandra, Cassandra. Sahndra, Sandera, Sandrah, Sandreea, Sandria, Sandrina, Sandrine, Sandy** et al., **Sanndra, Sanndria, Saundra, Sondra** et al., **Zandra** et al.

SANDY Diminutive of **Alexandra, Cassandra, Sandra. Sandee, Sandi, Sandie**

SANTA Spanish, Italian variant of **Sancta.** Latin, "sacred." **Santalina, Santaline, Santha, Santina**

SAPPHIRE Hebrew. "Sapphire." **Safira, Saphira, Sapir, Sapira, Sapphira, Sephira**

SARAH Hebrew. "Princess." **Sada, Sadelle** et al., **Sadie** et al., **Sally** et al., **Sara, Sarette, Sari, Sarice, Sarika, Sarita, Sarra,**

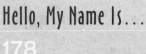

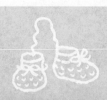

Sarrah, Sasa, Serita, Shara, Sherry et al., **Socha, Sorali, Soralie, Sydelle** et al., **Zara** et al.

SARALEE Combination of **Sarah** and **Lee. Sarahlee, SarahLee, Sarah Lee, SaraLee, Sara Lee**

SASHA Russian variant of **Alexandra,** feminine form of **Alexander.** Greek, "man's defender." **Sacia, Sacha, Sascha, Saschenka, Sashah, Sashenka**

SATURNIA Latin. "Of Saturn" or Cronus, the ruler of all the gods until he was dethroned by Zeus; also the sixth planet from the sun. Saturn was associated with the sowing of seeds. **Saturna, Saturnina, Saturnya**

SAVANNAH Spanish, from Taino. "Grassy plain with few trees." Also a city in Georgia. **Savana, Savanna**

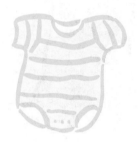

SAYO Japanese. "Born in the night."

SCARLETT Middle English. "Deep red." **Scarlet, Scarlette**

SEASON Contemporary American. "Season."

SEBASTIANE Feminine form of **Sebastian.** Latin, "revered." **Sebastiana, Sebastienne**

SECUNDA Latin. "Second." **Segunda**

SEEMA Greek. "Symbol." **Cima, Cyma, Seemah, Sema, Semah, Sima, Simah, Sina**

SELDA Old English. "Rare." Also short form of **Griselda. Zelda**

SELENA Greek goddess of the moon. Selena Quintanilla Perez, popular Tejana musician murdered in 1995. **Celena** et al., **Saleena, Salena, Salina, Saline, Sela, Selene, Selia, Selie, Selina, Selinda, Seline, Sena, Silena, Silina, Zena**

SELIMA Hebrew. "Tranquil." **Selimah**

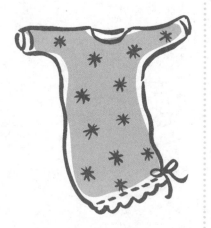

SELMA Short form of **Anselma.** Old German, "godly helmet." **Sellma, Selmah, Zelma**

SEMELE Greek. "Beautiful mortal." In myth, the mother of Dionysus. **Semel, Semell, Semelle**

SEMIRAMIS Hebrew. "Highest heaven." **Semira, Semiramida, Semiramide**

SENALDA Spanish. "Sign."

SENGA Variant of **Agnes.** Greek, "pure" or "virginal." **Sengassa**

SEPTEMBER Middle English, from Latin. The ninth month of the year (the seventh month of the Roman year).

SEPTIMA Latin. "Seventh."

SERAPHINA Hebrew. "Ardent." In the Bible, the Seraphim were fiery six-winged angels who guarded God's throne. **Sarafima, Sarafina, Serafima, Serafina, Serafine, Seraphe, Seraphine**

SERENA Latin. "Serene." Serena Williams, professional tennis player. **Reena, Rena, Sareen, Sarene, Sarina, Sarine, Saryna, Serene, Serenia, Serenity, Serenya, Serina, Seryna**

SERENITY English, from Latin. "Serenity."

SERILDA Old German. "Armed fighting woman." **Sarilda, Serhilda, Serhilde, Serrilda**

SETAREH Persian. "Star."

SHAINA Hebrew. "Beautiful." **Shaine, Shana, Shaney, Shani, Shanie, Shayna, Shaynah, Shayne**

SHAKA Zulu. "Great king." A nineteenth-century Zulu king who led wars against neighboring tribes. **Chaka, Chakira, Shakaina, Shakeela, Shakeera, Shakeita, Shakette, Shakila, Shakina, Shakira, Shakitra, Shaqua, Shaque, Shaquina, Shaquita**

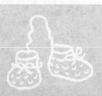

SHAN Chinese. "Coral."

SHANA Short form of **Shannon, Shoshana;** variant of **Shaina, Shawn. Shanah, Shanna**

SHANDEY Contemporary American. **Shandee, Shandeigh**

SHANEIKA Contemporary American. **Shanecka, Shaneikah, Shanequa, Shaneyka, Shanika, Shanique, Sheniqua, Shonyce**

SHANELLE Contemporary American, from French. Possibly inspired by the Parisian fashion designer Gabrielle (Coco) Chanel and, especially, by perfume sold under the Chanel label. **Chanel, Chanelle, Channel, Channelle, Chenel, Chenelle, Chennel, Chennelle, Shanel, Shanella, Shannel, Shanita, Shenelle, Shonelle**

SHANICE Contemporary American. **Shaneese, Shaniece, Shanisse, Shanniece, Shannise, Sheneese, Shenice, Sheniece, Shenisse, Shoneese, Shonice, Shoniece, Shonisse, Shonyce**

SHANINGO Algonquin. "Beautiful one."

SHANNON Irish. "Ancient." Also a river in Ireland. **Channa, Chanon, Shana** et al., **Shanen, Shanin, Shannen, Shanon, Sinann, Sionnan**

SHANTAL American variant of **Chantal,** feminine form of **Chanticleer.** Middle English, from Old French, "to sing clearly." **Shanta, Shantalle, Shantay, Shante, Shantee, Shantel, Shantella, Shantelle, Shanti, Shantial, Shantialle, Shantie, Shontal, Shontalle, Shontelle**

SHARLA Variant of **Sharlene,** feminine form of **Charles.** Old German, "man." **Charla**

When Hennessy met Shalimar

An increasing number of parents are giving babies brand names. *Tiffany* and *Mercedes* have been girls' names for so long that people who hear them don't automatically think of the famous products, but what about *Lexus, Armani,* and *Chanel?* Or the boys' names *Timberland, Guinness,* and *Corvette?*

The owners of these trade names don't seem to mind parents piggybacking on the trademark. So far, no companies have forced parents to put ™ beside a child's name.

When parents pick commercial names, it seems they consistently go upscale. There may be kids named *Wal-Mart, Hyundai,* and *Schlitz* out there, but you're far more likely to run into *Infiniti, Gucci,* and *Courvoisier.*

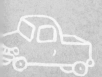

NAMES FOR GIRLS

181

SHARLENE Feminine form of **Charles.** Old German, "man." **Cherline, Cherleen, Sharla, Sharleen, Sharleyne, Sharlina, Sharline, Sharlyne, Sherleen, Sherlene, Sherline, Sherlyne, Shurleen, Shurlene, Shurline, Shurlyne**

SHARMAN Old English. "Just distributor." **Sharmen, Sharmon**

SHAROLYNN Combination of **Sharon** and **Lynn. Sharolynne**

SHARON Hebrew place name. "A plain." **Charin, Cheron, Shaaron, Shara, Sharan, Shareen, Sharen, Shari, Sharie, Sharin, Sharona, Sharonda, Sharren, Sharrin, Sharronne, Sharyn, Sheran, Sherina, Sherry** et al.

SHAVONNE American variant of **Siobhan,** Irish variant of **Joan.** Hebrew, "the Lord is gracious." **Shavan, Shavanne, Shavaun, Shavaune, Shavaunne, Shavon, Shevan, Shevanne, Shevonne, Shivaun, Shivaunne, Shivonne, Shovonne, Shyvon, Shyvonne**

SHAWN Feminine form of **Sean,** Irish variant of **John.** Hebrew, "the Lord is gracious." **Seana, Shana, Shanna, Shaun, Shauna, Shauni, Shaunie, Shauny, Shawna, Shawnee, Shawneen, Shawnette, Shawny, Shona** et al., **Sianna**

SHEA Irish. "Fairy mound." **Shae, Shai, Shay, Shayla, Shaylyn, Shy, Sid**

SHEBA An ancient country in southern Arabia. Also short for **Bathsheba. Saba, Sabah, Sebah, Shebah**

SHEENA Irish feminine variant of **Jane,** feminine variant of **John.** Hebrew, "the Lord is gracious." **Sheenagh, Sheenah, Sheina, Shena, Shene, Shiona, Sine, Sinead**

SHEILA Irish variant of **Cecilia.** Latin, "blind." **Seila, Selia, Selya, Shelia, Shayla, Shaylah, Sheela, Sheelagh, Sheelah, Sheilagh, Sheilah, Shela, Shelagh, Shelia, Shelly, Shiela, Shielah**

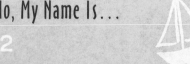

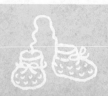

SHELBY Old English. "Estate on the ledge." **Shelbee, Shelbey, Shelbi, Shelbie, Shellbi, Shellbie, Shellby**

SHELLEY Old English. "Meadow's edge." Also diminutive of **Michelle, Rachelle, Rochelle. Shelle, Shellee, Shellie, Shelly**

SHERILYN Combination of **Sheryl**, or **Sharon**, and **Lynn. Cherilyn** et al., **Sharalin, Sharalyn, Sharalynn, Sharalynne, Sharelyn, Sharelynn, Sharelynne, Sheralin, Sheralyn, Sheralyne, Shereline, Sherileen, Sherilynn, Sherilynne, Sherylin, Sheryline, Sherylyn, Sherylynne**

SHERRY Variant of **Chère**; diminutive of **Sarah, Sharon, Sheryl. Cheree, Cheri, Cherrie, Cherry, Sharee, Shari, Sharie, Sheree, Sherey, Sheri, Sherice, Shericia, Sherie, Sherina, Sherita, Sherree, Sherrey, Sherri, Sherrie, Sherye**

SHERYL Variant of **Cheryl**, feminine form of **Charles**. Old German, "man." **Sharel, Sharell, Sharil, Sherill, Sherryl, Sheryll**

SHIFRA Hebrew. "Beautiful." **Schifra, Shifrah**

SHIMRA Hebrew. "To protect." **Shimria, Shirmrah, Shirmya**

SHINAKO Japanese. "Faithful child."

SHIR Hebrew. "Song." **Shira, Shirah, Shiri, Shirit**

SHIRLENE Combination of **Shirley** and **Charlene. Sherleen, Sherlene, Sherline, Shirleen, Shirline, Shurleen, Shurlene, Shurline**

SHIRLEY Old English. "Shire's meadow." **Sher, Sheree, Sheri, Sherlee, Sherlie, Shirl, Shirlee, Shirlley, Shirly, Shurlee, Shurley, Shurlie, Shurly**

SHIZU Japanese. "Quiet." **Shizue, Shizuka, Shizuki, Shizuko**

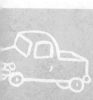

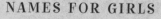

SHONA Feminine form of **Sean**, Irish variant of **John**. Hebrew, "the Lord is gracious." **Shawn** et al., **Shonee, Shoni, Shonie, Shonna, Shonny, Shony**

SHONALEE Combination of **Shona** and **Lee**. **Shonnalee**

SHOSHANA Hebrew. "Lily." **Oshana, Shana, Shosha, Shoshan, Shoshanah, Shoshannah, Shushana, Susan** et al.

SHULAMITH Hebrew. "Peacefulness." **Shelomith, Shula, Shulamit, Sula, Sulamit, Sulamith**

SIBLEY Middle English. "Sibling." **Siblina, Sibline**

SIBYL Greek. "Seer." **Sabilla, Sabylla, Sib, Sibbell, Sibel, Sibell, Sibella, Sibelle, Sibette, Sibil, Sibill, Sibilla, Sibille, Sibyll, Sibylla, Sybel, Sybella, Sybelle, Sybil, Sybill, Sybilla, Sybille, Sybyl**

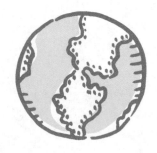

SIDONIE Latin. "Sacred shroud." **Sidaine, Sidonia, Sidony, Sidonya, Sydonia, Syndonia, Syndie**

SIDRA Latin. "Of the stars."

SIERRA Spanish. "Steep mountain range." **Sierrah**

SIGFREDA Old German. "Victory peace." **Freda, Frida, Fridha, Sigfreida, Sigfrid, Sigfrida, Sigfrieda**

SIGISMONDA Italian, from Old German. "Victorious protector." **Sigismunda, Sigmonda, Sigmunda**

SIGNA Latin. "Signal." **Signe, Signild, Signilda, Signilde, Signy**

SILVER Old English. "Silver." **Sylver**

SILVIE Variant of **Sylvia**. Latin, "from the woods." **Silvee, Silvi, Sylvee, Sylvi, Sylvie, Sylvy**

SIMA Aramaic. "Treasure." **Simi**

SIMCHA Hebrew. "Joy."

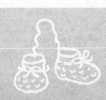

SIMONE Feminine form of **Simon.** Hebrew, "one who listened." Simone de Beauvoir, twentieth-century French writer and existentialist. **Simeona, Simona, Simonetta, Simonette, Simonia, Simonina, Simonne, Symona, Symone**

SINANN Irish. The river Shannon. Pronounced "SHIN-on."

SINEAD Irish variant of **Jane,** feminine form of **John.** Hebrew, "the Lord is gracious." Pronounced "shi-NADE." **Seonaid, Sheena** et al.

SIOBHAN Irish variant of **Joan,** feminine form of **John.** Hebrew, "the Lord is gracious." Pronounced "zhuh-VON." **Chavonne** et al., **Shavonne** et al., **Siobahn**

SIRENA Greek. "Siren." In myth, the singing of sirens lured sailors to their deaths. **Reena, Rena, Sireena, Sirena, Sirenia, Siryna, Syrena**

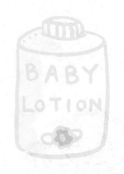

SIRIUS Greek. "Burning brightly." The Dog Star, the brightest in the sky. **Sirios**

SISSY Diminutive of **Cecilia.** Latin, "blind." **Cissey, Cissi, Cissie, Cissy, Sissee, Sissey, Sissi, Sissie**

SKYE Scottish. An island in northwest Scotland. **Skai, Sky**

SKYLER Dutch. "Giving shelter." **Schuylar, Schuyler, Schyler, Skyla, Skylar, Skyllar**

SOCORRA Spanish. "Aid."

SOLACE Latin. "Comfort." **Solasse, Solice, Solicia**

SOLANGE French. "Without equal." **Souline, Zeline**

SOLEDAD Spanish. "Solitude."

SOLVEIG Scandinavian. "Woman of the house." **Solvag**

SOMA Greek. "Body." Also a drug in Aldous Huxley's *Brave New World.*

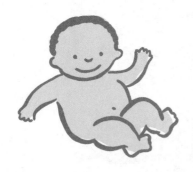

SONA Latin. "To make a sound." **Sonara, Sonarra**

SONDRA Short form of **Alexandra**. Greek, "man's defender." **Saundra, Sohndra, Sondre, Sonndra, Zohndra, Zondra**

SONIA Variant of **Sophia**. Greek, "wisdom." **Sonja, Sonnja, Sonny** et al., **Sonya, Zonia, Zonya**

SONNY Diminutive of **Sonia, Sophia. Sonni, Sonnie**

SOPHIA Greek. "Wisdom." **Saffi, Sofi, Sofia, Sófia, Sofie, Sofy, Sonia** et al., **Sonny** et al., **Sophey, Sophie, Sophy, Zofia** et al., **Zsofia**

SOPHRONIA Greek. "Sensible, prudent." **Sofronia, Sofronya, Sophronya, Zofronia, Zophronia**

SORCHA Irish. "Bright, shining." **Sorca**

SORREL English. "Chestnut-colored." **Sorrell, Sorrelle**

SOUSAN Persian. "Flower."

SPERANZA Italian. "Hope." **Esperanza** et al., **Sperancia, Speransa**

SPRING Old English. "Springtime."

STACY Irish variant of **Anastasia**; short form of **Eustacia. Stace, Stacee, Stacey, Staci, Stacie, Stasey, Stasi, Stasie, Stasy**

STAR Old English. "Star." **Staria, Starla, Starlene, Starr, Starry**

STELLA Latin. "Star." **Estella, Estelle, Estrella, Stelle**

STEPHANIE Feminine form of **Stephen**. Greek, "crowned." **Stefa, Stefania, Stefanida, Stefanie, Stefenie, Stefenney, Steffaney, Steffanie, Steffie, Steffy, Stefinney, Stepfanie, Stepha, Stephana, Stephania, Stephanine, Stephannie, Stepheny, Stephine, Stevana, Stevena, Stevey, Stevie**

STINA Short form of **Christina**. Greek, "Christian." **Stine, Tina** et al.

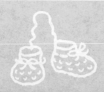

STORM Old English. "Storm." **Stormie, Stormy**

SUKEY Diminutive of **Susan**. Hebrew, "lily." **Sukee, Suki, Sukie, Suky**

SULA Short form of **Ursula, Shulamith. Seula**

SUMMER Old English. "Summer."

SUNNY English. "Sunny." Also diminutive of **Sunshine. Sunni, Sunnie**

SUNSHINE English. "Sunshine." **Sunny** et al.

SUSAN Hebrew. "Lily." **Shoshana** et al., **Soosan, Soosen, Su, Sue, Suesann, Suezanne, Sukey** et al., **Susanetta, Susanette, Susann, Susanne, Susette, Susi, Susie, Susy, Suzan, Suzane, Suzannah** et al., **Suzanne, Suze, Suzee, Suzette, Suzie, Suzy, Suzzanne, Zsa Zsa**

SUSANNA Hebrew. "Lily." **Soosanna, Sosanna, Suesanna, Susana, Susannagh, Susannah, Suzanna, Suzannah, Zana, Zanna, Zsusanna**

SWAN Old English. "Swan." **Swana, Swann, Swanne**

SYBIL Variant of **Sibyl**. Greek, "seer."

SYDELLE Variant of **Sarah**. Hebrew, "princess." **Sadelle** et al., **Sydel, Sydell, Sydella**

SYDNEY Old French. "St. Denis." **Sid, Sidne, Sidney, Sydne, Sydni, Sydnie**

SYLVIA Latin. "From the forest." **Silva, Silvaine, Silvana, Silvanna, Silvannah, Silvia, Silviana, Silvianne, Silvie** et al., **Sylva, Sylvana, Sylvanna, Sylvette, Sylviana, Sylvianne, Sylvine, Sylwia, Zilve, Zilvia, Zylvia**

SYRILLA Variant of **Cyrilla**, feminine for **Cyril**. Latin, "lordly." **Siri, Sirilla**

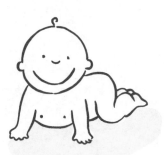

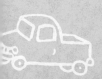

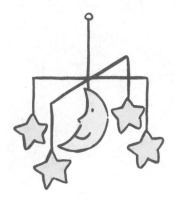

TABINA Arabic. "Muhammad's follower." **Tabeena**

TABITHA Aramaic. "Gazelle." **Tabatha, Tabbee, Tabbey, Tabbi, Tabbie, Tabbitha, Tabby, Tabetha, Tabethe, Tabithe, Tabytha**

TACITA Latin. "Silent." **Tace, Tacey, Tacye**

TAFFY Welsh. "Loved one." **Taafe, Tavi, Tevi**

TAHIRA Arabic. "Pure."

TAJA Arabic. "Crown." **Taj**

TAKARA Japanese. "Treasured object."

TALIA Hebrew. "Heaven's dew." Also variant of **Thalia. Tal, Tali, Talley, Talli, Tallia, Tallie, Tally, Tallya, Talya**

TALITHA Aramaic. "Young girl." **Taleetha, Taletha, Talita**

TALLULAH Choctaw. "Leaping water." Pronounced "ta-LOO-lah." **Talley, Tallie, Tallou, Tallula, Tallullah, Tally**

TALMA Hebrew. "Hill." **Talmit, Talmita**

TALOR Hebrew. "Morning dew." **Talora**

TAMARA Arabic, Hebrew. "Palm tree." **Tama, Tamah, Tamar, Tamarah, Tamarra, Tamary, Tamera, Tamma, Tammara, Tammy** et al., **Temira, Thamar, Thamara, Thamarra**

TAMARIND Arabic. "Tamarind," a leguminous tropical tree with tart-fleshed seed pods.

Hello, My Name Is...

188

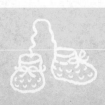

TAMIKA Contemporary American. **Tameeka, Tamicka, Tamickah, Tamiecka, Tamieka, Tamike, Tamiqua, Tamiquah, Tammy** et al., **Timeeka, Timika, Timikah, Tomeeka, Tomika, Tomikah**

TAMIKO Japanese. "People child."

TAMMARIE Combination of **Tamara,** or **Tammy,** and **Marie.**

TAMMY Short form of **Tamara, Tamika, Thomasina. Tami, Tammee, Tammey, Tammi, Tammie**

TAMSIN Cornish. "Free person." **Tamzen, Tamzin**

TANIA Short form of **Letania, Tatiana, Titania. Tanya** et al.

TANISHA Contemporary American. **Taneesha, Tanicia, Taniesha, Tanishah, Tanitia, Tannicia, Tanniece, Tannisha, Tannishah, Teneesha, Tinecia, Tiniesha, Tynisha**

TANITH Irish. "Estate." **Tanitha, Tanithe**

TANSY Greek. "Everlasting life." Also a diminutive of **Anastasia,** and a yellow-flowered perennial plant. **Tandie, Tansee, Tansey, Tansi, Tansie, Tanzey**

TANYA Short form of **Letania, Tatiana, Titania. Tana, Tahnee, Tahnya, Taneea, Tania, Tanita, Tanja, Tawnya, Tonya, Tonyah**

TAO Chinese. "Peach."

TARA Irish. "Rocky hill." Tara Meath was the seat of the ancient High Kings of Ireland; Tara was also the plantation home of Scarlett O'Hara in Margaret Mitchell's *Gone with the Wind.* **Tarah, Tarra, Tarrah, Taryn, Temair**

TARYN Variant of **Tara.** Irish, "rocky hill." **Taran, Tarin, Tarina, Tarren, Tarrin, Tarryn, Teryn**

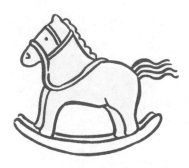

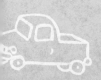

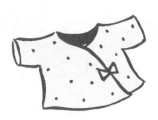

TASHA Short form of **Anastasia, Natasha. Tahsha, Tasia, Tasla, Tasya**

TATIANA Feminine form of **Tatius**, a Roman clan name. **Tania, Tanya** et al., **Tatenya, Tati, Tatie, Tatyana, Tatyanna**

TAUBA Old German. "Dove." **Taubena, Taubi, Taubina, Tobie, Toby**

TAYLOR Middle English. "Tailor." **Tailor, Taillor, Tayler**

TECIA Greek. "Immortal fame." **Tesha, Thecia, Thekla** et al.

TEGAN Celtic. "Doe." **Taigan, Taigen, Tayggen, Teggan**

TEMIRA Hebrew. "Tall." **Temora, Timora**

TEMPERANCE Latin. "Moderation."

TEMPEST Old French. "Storm."

TEOFILA Romanian. "Divinely loved."

TERENA Latin. Feminine form of **Terence**, a Roman clan name. **Tereena, Terina, Terrena, Teryna**

TERI Short form of **Theresa**. Greek, "harvest." **Tere, Teree, Terella, Teri, Terie, Terrey, Terri, Terrie, Terry, Terrye**

TERRANDA Latin. "Land." **Terra**

TERTIA Latin. "Third." **Tertiara**

TESSA Short form of **Theresa**. Greek, "harvest." **Tess, Tesse, Tessey, Tessi, Tessie, Tessy**

TET Nickname for **Elizabeth**. Hebrew, "pledged to God." **Tetty**

THADDEA Feminine form of **Thaddeus**. Greek, "gift of God." **Thada, Thadah, Thadda, Thaddeah**

THALASSA Greek. "Sea."

THALIA Greek. "Blooming." In myth, the Grace of good cheer and the Muse of comedy. **Talia, Talie, Talley, Tally, Thala, Thalie, Thalya**

THANA Arabic. "Thanksgiving."

THEA Greek. "Goddess." Also short form of **Dorothea.**

THEKLA Greek. "Immortal fame." **Tecia** et al., **Tecla, Tecle, Tekli, Telca, Telka, Thekle**

THELMA Greek. "Will." **Telma, Thelme**

THEODORA Feminine form of **Theodore.** Greek, "gift of God." **Dora, Fedora** et al., **Ted, Tedda, Teddey, Teddie, Teddy, Tedra, Teodora, Teodory, Theadora, Theda, Theo**

THEODOSIA Greek. "Gift of God." **Feodosia, Theda, Teodosia**

THEOLA Greek. "Divine." **Theolia, Tiola**

THEONE Greek. "Name of God." **Theoni, Theonie**

THEOPHANIA Greek. "God's appearance." **Theophanie**

THEOPHILA Greek. "God-loving." **Theofila**

THERESA Greek. "Harvest." **Taresa, Tera, Terasa, Teresa, Terese, Teresia, Teresina, Teresita, Teressa, Tereza, Terezinha, Terezsa, Terrasa, Terresa, Terresia, Terrosina, Terry** et al., **Terrya, Terza, Tessa** et al., **Thérèse, Theresina, Theresita, Tiersa, Tierza, Tracy** et al., **Treesa, Tresa, Tressa, Tressella, Trescha, Treza, Zita**

THOMASINA Feminine form of **Thomas.** Greek, "twin." **Tamasin, Tamasina, Tamasine, Tammy** et al., **Tamzina, Thomasa, Thomasin, Thomasine, Thomazine, Toma, Tomasina, Tomasine, Tommi, Tommie, Tommy**

THORA Old Norse. "Thunder." **Thodia, Thordia, Thordis, Thyra, Tyra**

Keeping the name but switching the gender

The parents of Thora Birch, an actress, were sure they would have a son, whom they planned to name *Thor,* after the Norse god. When their baby turned out to be a girl, they simply feminized *Thor* by adding an *a* at the end.

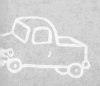

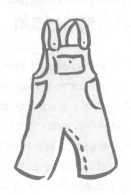

THRINE Greek. "Pure." **Thrina**

THURAYYA Arabic. "Star." **Thuraia, Thuraya, Thurayah**

TIA Spanish. "Aunt." **Tiana**

TIARA Latin. "Tiara," an ornamented headdress.

TIBERIA Latin. "Of the Tiber River." **Tibbie, Tibby, Tiberya**

TIFFANY Greek. "God's appearance." **Teffan, Teffany, Thefania, Theophanie, Thifania, Thiffanie, Tifennie, Tiffaney, Tiffani, Tiffanie, Tiffenie, Tiffie, Tiffiny, Tiffney, Tiphanie, Tyffany**

TILDA Short form of **Matilda**. Old German, "battle-mighty." **Thilda, Thilde, Tilde, Tildie, Tildy, Tilley, Tillie, Tilly**

TIMOTHEA Feminine form of **Timothy**. Greek, "reverent." **Thea, Timmie**

TINA Short form of **Augustina, Celestina, Christina, Clementina, Constantina, Martina, Valentina. Teena, Teenie, Teina, Tena, Teyna, Tinah, Tine, Tiny**

TIRA Hebrew. "Safe camp."

TIRZA Hebrew. "Desirable woman." **Thersa, Thirsa, Thirza, Thirzah, Thursa, Thurza, Tierza, Tirzah, Tyrzah**

TITA Spanish. Short form of **Margarita**, etc.

TITANIA Greek. "Giant." **Tania, Tita, Titanya, Titiana, Tityana, Tiziana**

TOBY Hebrew. "God is good." Also a variant of **Tauba. Toba, Tobe, Tobee, Tobelle, Tobey, Tobi, Tobia, Tobye, Tova, Tovah, Tove**

TOMAKO Japanese. "Jewel child." Pronounced "to-mah-ko."

TONI Short form of **Antoinette**. Latin, "beyond price." **Tonee, Toney, Tonie, Tony**

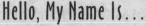
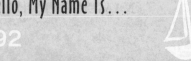
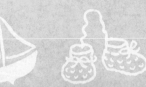

The baby of ten thousand dreams

In the past decade, Americans have adopted some 22,000 abandoned Chinese baby girls. Peggy Livingston first laid eyes on her Chinese daughter in June of 2002.

"I named my daughter *Lisa.* I wanted something that goes well with my last name. *Livingston* has three syllables, and I thought a three-syllable first name would make quite a mouthful. I also wanted a name that is not too common for someone of her age.

"For Lisa's middle name, I wanted something to reflect her Chinese heritage. Since most of the Chinese babies who are adopted were originally abandoned, we do not know what names their birth parents gave them—if they gave them a name at all. For this reason, the caregivers in the orphanages name them. As a surname, they may have the name of the orphanage, the name of the town, or even the name of the official who heads the orphanage. In China, the surname comes first.

"For her middle name, I used her two Chinese names. She came to me as *Wan Meng*—the latter pronounced 'mung'—a name that means 'ten thousand dreams.' Several children in her orphanage had the surname *Wan.* There was *Wan Feng,* meaning 'ten thousand virtues,' and *Wan Ting,* meaning 'ten thousand graces.'

"So her name is *Lisa Wan Meng Livingston.* I call her *Lisa,* and I love her very much."

TONIA Short form of **Antoinette, Antonia.** Also variant of **Tanya. Tonya, Tonyah**

TOPAZ Latin. "Topaz." **Topaza**

TORI Japanese. "Bird." Also short form of **Victoria.**

TORY Short form of **Victoria.** Latin, "victory." **Torey, Tori, Toria, Torie, Torrey, Torri, Torrie, Torry, Torrye**

TOYA Contemporary American. **Toia, Toyah, Latoya** et al.

TRACY Short form of **Theresa. Tracee, Tracey, Traci, Tracie, Trasey**

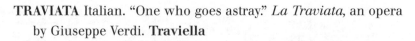

TRAVIATA Italian. "One who goes astray." *La Traviata*, an opera by Giuseppe Verdi. **Traviella**

TRICIA Short form of **Patricia**, feminine form of **Patrick**. Latin, "upper class." **Treasha, Trichia, Trish, Trisha**

TRILBY The heroine of an eponymous novel by Daphne DuMaurier. **Trilbi, Trilbie, Trillby**

TRINA Short form of **Katrina**. Greek, "pure." **Treena, Treina, Trine, Trinetta**

TRINIDAD Spanish. "(Holy) trinity." **Trinity, Trini, Trinidade**

TRINITY English, from Latin. "Triad." **Trini**

TRISTA Latin. "Sad." **Tristella**

TRISTAN Celtic. In legend, a knight of King Arthur's court and lover of Isolde. **Tristam, Tristen, Tristin, Tristine, Tristram, Trystan, Trystin**

TRIXIE Diminutive of **Beatrice**. Latin, "bringer of gladness." **Trix, Trixi, Trixy**

TRUDY Short form of **Gertrude**. Old German, "spear wielder." **Truda, Trude, Trudey, Trudi, Trudie**

TRYPHENIA Greek. "Delicate." **Tryphella, Tryphena**

TSIFIRA Hebrew. "Crown."

TUESDAY Old English. "Tiw's day," the day of the week named for the ancient Germanic god of war.

TWYLA Middle English. "Weave." Twyla Tharp, ballet dancer and choreographer. **Twila**

TYBAL Old English. "Holy place." **Tybalia, Tyballa**

TZIGANE Hungarian. "Gypsy." **Tsigana, Tsigane**

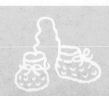

UALANI Hawaiian. "Heavenly rain."

UDELE Old German. "Wealthy." **Uda, Udella, Udelle, Yudella, Yudelle**

ULA Celtic. "Gem of the sea." **Eula, Ulla, Yulla**

ULANI Hawaiian. "Cheerful."

ULIMA Arabic. "Astute." **Ulema, Ulima, Ullima**

ULLA Old French. "The proper amount." Also variant of **Ula.**

ULRICA Feminine form of **Ulric.** Old German, "power of the wolf." **Rieka, Rica, Ricka, Ulka, Ullrica, Ullricka, Ulricha, Ulrika, Ulrike**

ULTIMA Latin. "Final."

ULVA Old German. "Wolf." **Ulfa**

UMA Sanskrit. "Flax."

UMBERTA Italian. "Famous warrior."

UNA Latin. "One." **Oona, Oonagh**

UNDINE Latin. "Little wave." **Ondine** et al., **Undeen, Undene, Undina, Undyne**

UNICE Variant of **Eunice.** Greek, "victorious." **Uniss**

UNITY Middle English. "Oneness." **Unita**

UPALA Sanskrit. "Sandy coast."

URAEUS Greek, from Egyptian. "Cobra."

URANIA Feminine form of **Uranus.** Greek, "heavenly." **Urainia, Uraniya, Uranya**

URBANA Latin. "Of the city." **Urbanna**

URIT Hebrew. "Brightness." **Urith, Urithe**

URLA Variant of **Earla,** feminine form of **Earl.** Old English, "nobleman."

URSULA Latin. "Female bear." St. Ursula. **Orsa, Seula, Sula, Ulla, Ursa, Ursala, Ursel, Ursella, Ursie, Ursina, Ursola, Ursule, Ursulina, Ursuline, Ursy, Urszuli**

UTA Unknown derivation. **Yuta**

UTENDE Kiswahili. "Witchcraft."

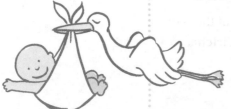

VAL Short form of **Valentina, Valerie.**

VALA Old German. "Singled out." **Valla**

VALDA Feminine form of **Waldemar.** Old German, "renowned ruler." **Vallda, Velda**

VALENTINA Feminine form of **Valentine.** Latin, "strong." **Tina** et al., **Val, Vale, Valeda, Valena, Valencia, Valentia, Valentijn, Valentine, Valenzia, Valera, Valida, Valina, Vallera, Valli, Vallie, Vally, Valora, Velora**

VALERIE Latin. "Strong." **Val, Valaree, Valarey, Valari, Valaria, Valarie, Valeree, Valeria, Valery, Valerye, Valie, Vallarie, Vallee, Valleree, Vallerie, Vallery, Vallie, Valry**

VALESKA Feminine form of **Vladislav.** Russian, "splendid ruler."

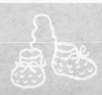

VALHALLA Variant of **Wahalla.** Scandinavian, "hall of immortal warriors."

VALONIA Latin, from Greek. A species of oak or its dried acorn cups, which are used in tanning. **Vallonia**

VALORA Latin. "Courageous." **Valori, Valoria, Valorie, Valory, Valorya**

VANDA Variant of **Wanda.** Old Norse, "slender rod." **Vannda**

VANESSA Invented by Jonathan Swift in his poem "Cadenus and Vanessa." Vanessa Redgrave, contemporary actress. **Nessa, Nessi, Nessie, Nessy, Van, Vanesa, Vanesse, Vanetta, Vanna, Vannessa, Vannie, Venesa, Venessa**

VANETTA Contemporary American. **Van, Vanna, Vannetta, Vannie, Venetta**

VANIA Russian. "God's gift." **Vanija, Vanya**

VANNA Khmer. "Golden." Also short form of **Vanessa, Vanetta. Vannah**

VANORA Celtic. "White wave." **Vannora**

VARDA Arabic. "Rose." **Vardia, Vardina, Vardis, Vardit**

VARVARA Variant of **Barbara.** Greek, "stranger." **Varenka, Verina, Varinka, Varya**

VASHTI Persian. "Lovely." **Vashtee**

VEDA Sanskrit. "Knowledge, wisdom." **Vedis, Veeda, Veida, Vida**

VEDETTE Italian. "Sentry" or "scout." **Vedetta**

VEDIS Singhalese. "Hunter."

VEGA Arabic. "Falling."

VELA Latin. "To sail." **Vella**

VELDA Old German. "Open field." **Velde**

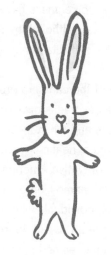

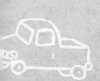

NATIVE AMERICAN NAMES

Despite having treated our aboriginal population so badly, Americans have a continuing fascination with Native American lore and names. A staple summer-camp activity for generations of children was receiving an "Indian" name, usually some mishmash of syllables supposed to inspire the happy camper to follow the way of the noble savage. The winds of political correctness have all but blown this practice away, although many of the camps themselves still retain multisyllabic "Indian" names.

Some of the campers grew up to become New Age devotees, lovers of crystals and aromatherapy, and when these people discovered sweat lodges, healing ceremonies, and other elements of Native American culture and religion, Indian name kleptomania began anew. This time, individuals who had no Indian ancestors at all began adopting real Native American names and passing themselves off as healers and shamans.

Among true Native Americans, as among other ethnic groups, contemporary parents are much more likely than their forebears to choose ethnic names for their children. A look at the Web site of just one tribe, the Navajo Nation, gives evidence of this trend. None of the Nation's executive officers listed on the site have Navajo names—at least not ones they choose to list. In a recent Navajo high-school track meet, however, running alongside Melissa, Amber, and Brianna were Shi-Tawana, Nishoni, Latasha, and Calah.

Many Native American names have numerous syllables—*Atakullakulla,* for instance, the name of an eighteenth-century Cherokee leader, and the famous *Sacajawea.* As distinguished as these names are, they would be difficult for any child carry into an American classroom. The choices listed below have positive meanings and fewer syllables, and sound pleasing to the ear besides.

These are Native American names for boys:

Annawan	an Algonquin chief	Algonquin
Hosa	"young crow"	Arapaho
Kohana	"swift"	Sioux
Mankato ("man-kay-to")	"blue earth"	Sioux
Mato	"bear"	Mandan
Nashoba	"wolf"	Chocktaw
Niwot ("NIGH-watt")	"left hand"	Arapaho

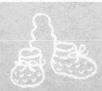

Onacona	white owl	Cherokee	**Hialeah** ("HI-ah-lee-ah")	"pretty prairie"	Creek
Ouray ("you-ray")	"arrow"	Ute	**Hiawassee**	"meadow"	Cherokee
Samoset	"traveler"	Algonquin	**Kaya**	"older sister"	Hopi
Sequoyah	"sparrow"	Cherokee	**Kimi**	"secret"	Algonquin
Tanase, Tanasi ("tah-NAH-see")	river in Tennessee	Cherokee	**Kiminela** ("kih-mee-neh-la")	"butterfly"	Sioux
Tadoka	variant of *Dakota,* "friend"	Sioux	**Mansi**	"plucked flower"	Hopi
Tecumseh	"panther passing across"	Shawnee	**Shaningo**	"beautiful one"	Algonquin
			Tallullah ("ta-LOO-lah")	"leaping water"	Chocktaw

And here are some Native American names for girls:

			Weeko	"pretty"	Sioux
Ama	"water"	Cherokee	**Winona**	"firstborn daughter"	Sioux
Anamosa	"white fawn"	Sauk	**Wyome** ("wy-o-mee")	"large plain"	Algonquin
Cheyenne	"people of different speech"	Sioux			
Eyota ("EE-yo-tah")	"greatest"	Sioux			

VELIKA Slavic. "Great, wondrous."

VELMA Short form of **Wilhelmina,** feminine form of **Wilhelm.** Old German, "will-helmet." **Valma, Vellma**

VELVET Middle English. "Velvet."

VENEZIA Italian. "Venice." **Venda, Venecia, Veneta, Venetia, Venice, Venise, Venita, Venitia, Venize, Vinetia, Vinita, Vonitia, Vonizia**

VENTURA Feminine form of **Venturo.** Spanish, "luck."

VENUS Latin. "True." In myth, goddess of love and beauty. **Venusa, Venusina**

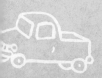

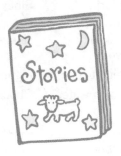

VERA Slavic. "Faith." Also short form of **Veronica. Veera, Veira, Verah, Vere, Verena** et al., **Verla, Verochka, Veroshka, Veruka, Verushka**

VERBENA Latin. "Holy branch." **Verbeena, Verbina, Verbyna**

VERDAD Spanish. "Truth."

VERDI Latin. "Green, vibrant." **Verda**

VERENA Latin. "Truthful." **Vereena, Verene, Verina, Verinka, Veruchka, Veruschka, Veryna**

VERITY English, from Latin. "Truth." **Verita, Veritee, Veriti, Veritie**

VERNA Latin. "Springtime." **Verne, Vernee, Vernelle, Verneta, Vernetta, Vernette, Verni, Vernice, Vernie, Vernis, Vernise, Vernisse, Vernita, Virna**

VERONA A city in northern Italy. **Veron, Verone**

VERONICA Latin. "True image." **Rana, Ranna, Ronica, Ronni** et al., **Ronnica, Vera** et al., **Veranica, Veranique, Verohnica, Verohnicca, Veronice, Veronicka, Veronika, Veronike, Veroniqua, Veronique, Vonnie, Vonny**

VESPERA Latin. "Evening star." **Hesper** et al.

VESTA Latin. In myth, goddess of the hearth. **Vesti**

VICTORIA Feminine form of **Victor.** Latin, "victory." **Vic, Vicci, Vici, Vickee, Vickey, Vicki, Vickie, Vicky, Victorie, Victorina, Victorine, Vika, Viki, Vikie, Vikkey, Vikki, Vikkie, Vikky, Viktoria, Viktorija, Viktorina, Viktorine, Vita, Vitoria, Vittoria**

VIDA Spanish. "Life." Also short form of **Davida,** variant of **Veda. Veeda, Vidette, Vieda, Vita** et al.

VIDONIA Portuguese. "Branch of a vine." **Veedonia, Vidonya**

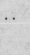

VIGDIS Old Norse. Goddess of war. **Vigdess**

VIGILIA Latin. "Wakefulness." **Vigila, Vigilla**

VILHELMINA Variant of **Wilhelmina**. **Vilhelmine, Villhelmina**

VILLETTE French. "Small town." **Villa**

VILMA Russian feminine form of **Wilhelm**. Old German, "will-helmet." **Wilma** et al.

VINA Short form of **Alvina, Davina, Elvina**. **Veena, Vena, Vinetta, Vinette, Vinita, Vinni, Vinnie, Vinny, Vyna, Vynetta, Vynette**

VINCENTIA Feminine form of **Vincent**. Latin, "conquering." **Vicencia, Vincenta, Vincentena, Vincentina, Vincentine**

VINIA Latin. "Grapevines."

VIOLA Latin. "Violet color," "violet flower."

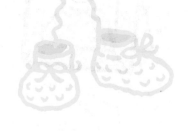

VIOLET English, from Latin. "Violet color," "violet flower." **Vi, Viola, Violaine, Violanta, Violante, Violanthe, Viole, Violeine, Violeta, Violetta, Violette, Voletta, Vyolet, Vyoletta, Vyolette**

VIORELA Romanian. Unknown meaning.

VIRGINIA Latin. "Virgin." **Gene** et al., **Gina** et al., **Ginella, Ginelle, Ginger** et al., **Gingia, Ginia, Ginny** et al., **Ginya, Jinia, Verginia, Virginie, Verginya, Virge, Virgenya, Virgie, Virgine, Virginie, Virginnia**

VIRIDIS Latin. "Green." **Veradis, Veredissa, Virdis, Viridia, Viridian**

VITA Latin. "Life." Also short form of **Davida, Victoria**. **Veeta, Vitel, Vitella, Vitia, Vitka, Vitta**

VIVA Latin. "Alive." Also short form of **Aviva**. **Veeva, Viveca, Vivva**

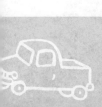

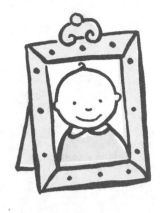

VIVECA Scandinavian. "Alive." **Vivecka, Viveka**

VIVIAN Latin. "Full of life." **Bibiana** et al., **Vevay, Vi, Vibiana, Viv, Vivee, Vivi, Vivia, Viviana, Viviane, Vivianna, Vivianne, Vivie, Vivien, Vivienne, Vivyan, Vivyana, Vivyanne, Vivyen, Vivyenne, Vyvyan, Vyvyana, Vyvyanne**

VONDA Variant of **Wanda.** Old Norse, "slender rod." **Vondi, Vondie**

WAHALLA Old Norse. "Hall of immortal warriors." **Valhalla, Walhalla**

WAKENDA Old Norse. "To rise."

WALBURGA Old German. "Strong protection." St. Walburga, whose feast is on May Day. **Walberga, Waliburga, Walpurgis**

WALDA Feminine form of **Waldo.** Old German, "ruler." **Wallda, Welda, Wellda**

WALIDA Arabic. "Newborn child."

WALKER Old English. "One who thickens cloth." **Wallker**

WALLIS Variant of **Wallace.** Old English, "from Wales." **Wallie, Walliss, Wallissa, Wallisse, Wally, Wallys**

WAN Chinese. "Gentle, gracious."

WANDA Old Norse. "Slender rod." **Vanda, Vandis, Vonda** et al., **Wahnda, Wandah, Wandie, Wandis, Wandy, Wannda, Wonda, Wonnda**

WANETTA Old English. "Pale-skinned." **Wanette**

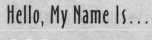

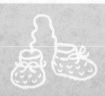

WARDA Feminine form of **Ward.** Old German, "guardian." **Wardia, Wardine**

WARRENE Feminine form of **Warren.** Old French, "stockyard." **Warrine, Warryne**

WASILA Middle English. "Be healthy." A toast, festive drink, or revelry. **Wasilla**

WEI Chinese. "Rose."

WENDY English. Diminutive of **Guinevere, Gwendolyn.** **Wenda, Wendaline, Wendall, Wendee, Wendeline, Wendey, Wendi, Wendie, Wendye, Windy**

WESLEY Old English. "Western meadow." **Weslee, Wesli, Weslie, Wesly, Westley**

WHITNEY Old English. "White island." **Whit, Whitnee, Whitnie, Whitny**

WHOOPI Contemporary American. "Gleeful shout." Whoopi Goldberg, contemporary American actress. **Whoopie, Whoopy**

WILDA Old English, Old German. "Wild." **Willda, Wylda**

WILFREDA Feminine form of **Wilfred.** Old English, "determined protector." **Freda**

WILHELMINA Feminine form of **Wilhelm.** Old German, "will-helmet." **Billa, Billie** et al., **Ellma, Elma, Guglielma, Guillelmina, Guillelmine, Guillema, Guillemette, Guillemine, Guillerma, Helma** et al., **Mimi, Mina** et al., **Velma** et al., **Vilhelmina** et al., **Vilma, Wileen, Wilene, Wilhelmine, Willa, Willamina, Willamine, Willeen, Willemina, Willene, Willetta, Willette, Willi, Williamina, Willie, Willit, Willmina, Willmine, Willy, Wilma** et al., **Wilmina, Wilna**

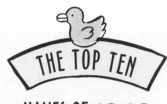
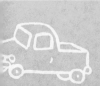

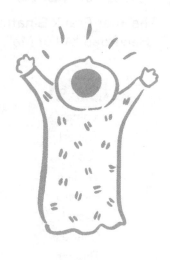

WILLA Feminine form of **William.** English, from Old German, "will-helmet."

WILLOW English. "Willow."

WILMA Feminine form of **William.** English, from Old German, "will-helmet." **Willma, Wilmette, Wylma**

WILONA Old English. "Desired."

WINIFRED Welsh. "Good friend." **Freda** et al., **Wina, Winafred, Winefred, Winefride, Winefried, Winfreda, Winfrieda, Winiferd, Winiford, Winifryd, Winnie** et al., **Winniferd, Winniford, Winnifred, Wynafred, Wynifred, Wynn, Wynnifred**

WINNIE Diminutive of **Guinevere, Gwendolyn, Winifred, Winona. Win, Winona, Winnie, Winny, Wynne** et al.

WINOLA Old German. "Charming friend."

WINONA Sioux. "First-born daughter." **Wenona, Wenonah, Winnie, Winonah, Wynnona, Wynona, Wyomia**

WINTER Old English. "Winter."

WREN Old English. "Wren."

WYNNE Welsh. "Fair, pure." **Gwynn** et al., **Wyn, Wynn, Wynnie**

WYOME Algonquin. "Large plain." Pronounced "wy-o-mee."

XAMIRA Farsi. "Diamond."

XANDRA Dutch variant of **Alexandra.** Greek, "man's defender."

XANTHE Greek. "Yellow." **Xantha, Xanthia, Zanthe**

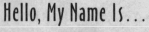
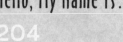

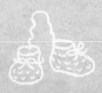

XAVIERA Feminine form of **Xavier**. Basque, "new house."
Javiera, Xavera, Xavyera, Zaviera

XENIA Greek. "Hospitable host." **Cena, Xeenia, Xena, Xene, Zena** et al.

XIA Chinese. "Glow of sunrise."

XIAO Chinese. "Heaven."

XIMENIA Feminine form of **Ximenes**, Spanish variant of
Simon. Hebrew, "one who listened." **Jimena** et al., **Ximena,
Ximenya**

XINA Short form of **Christina**. **Xena**

XYLIA Greek. "Forest dweller." **Xylina, Xylona**

YAFFA Hebrew. "Beautiful." **Jafit** et al., **Yaffah, Yafit, Yafite**

YAKIRA Hebrew. "Precious."

YAMINAH Arabic. "Suitable, proper." **Yamina**

YARA Australian Aboriginal. "Seagull."

YARINA Variant of **Irene**. Greek, "peace."

YARROW English. A biennial plant with umbelliferous flowers.

YASMIN Arabic. "Jasmine." **Jasmine** et al., **Yasmeen,
Yasmeena, Yasmena, Yasmene, Yasmina, Yasmine**

YASU Japanese. "Peaceful."

YEHUDIT Hebrew. "Praised." Also a variant of **Judith**. **Jehudit,
Jehudith, Yudith** et al.

Mayflower monikers

The Puritans, those wonderful folks who roasted turkeys and burned witches, loved to bestow on their children names that suggested favorable moral qualities. In his *God's Secretaries,* Adam Nicholson gives examples of names for little Puritans: *Eschew-evil, Lament, Sorry-for-sin, Learn-wisdom, Faint-not,* and the very popular *Sin-deny.*

When the Mayflower famously ferried Puritans from England to America in 1620, some of the younger passengers reflected this fad. Four children of William Brewster were named *Fear, Love, Patience,* and *Wrestling.* Isaac and Mary Allerton had a daughter named *Remember.* William and Susana White had sons named *Peregrine* and *Resolved.* Others on board included Humility Cooper, Desire Minter, and Degory Priest. The prize for best name on the Mayflower, however, has to go to a baby who was born while the ship was at sea. Stephen and Elizabeth Hopkins named their son *Oceanis.*

YEIRA Hebrew. "Light."

YEMINA Arabic. "Dove." **Yemimah, Yenina, Yonina**

YENTE Yiddish variant of **Henriette**. Old German, "estate ruler." Also a general Yiddish term for a gossip. **Yenta**

YESHISHA Hebrew. "Old."

YETTA Short form of **Harriet, Henrietta**. Old German, "estate ruler." **Yette**

YLESHA Variant of **Aisha**. Arabic, "woman." **Yleshah**

YNEZ Spanish variant of **Agnes**. Greek, "pure" or "virginal." **Inez** et al., **Ynes, Ynesa, Ynesita, Ynessa**

YOKO Japanese. "Good, positive." Yoko Ono, contemporary visual artist and musician, and widow of John Lennon.

YOLANDA Greek. "Violet flower." **Eolande, Eolantha, Iolanthe** et al., **Jolan** et al., **Yalonda, Yola, Yoland, Yolande, Yolantha, Yolanthe, Yollande, Yulanda**

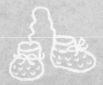

YONINA Hebrew. "Dove." **Jona** et al., **Yona, Yonah, Yoninah, Yonit, Yonita**

YOSEPHA Feminine form of **Joseph.** Hebrew, "the Lord provides." **Josephine** et al., **Yosefa, Yosifa, Yuseffa**

YOVELA Hebrew. "Ram's horn."

YSABEL Variant of **Isabel,** Spanish variant of **Elizabeth.** Hebrew, "pledged to God." **Ysabella, Ysobel, Yzabelle**

YSANNE Contemporary American. **Ysande, Ysanna**

YUKIKO Japanese. "Snow child."

YULIYA Russian variant of **Julia,** feminine form of **Julius.** Latin, "youthful." **Yulenka**

YULLIS Old Norse. Mid-winter festival. **Yule, Yulis**

YVETTE French. "Little archer." **Evette, Ivette, Yevette, Yvetta**

YVONNE Old German. "Yew wood." **Evonne** et al., **Ivonne**

ZABRA Variant of **Sabra.** Unknown origin.

ZADA Syrian. "Fortunate, prosperous." **Zaida, Zayda, Zayeeda**

ZAHARA Swahili. "Flower."

ZAHAVAH Hebrew. "Gilded." **Zachava, Zachavah, Zahava, Zechava, Zehavah, Zehavit**

ZAHIRA Arabic. "Brilliant, shining." **Zaheera, Zahirah**

ZAHRA Arabic. "Flower." **Zahrah**

ZAIDA Arabic. "Good fortune."

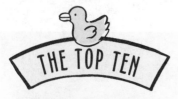

BOYS

Michael
Robert
David
James
John
William
Richard
Mark
Thomas
Steven

GIRLS

Mary
Susan
Debra
Linda
Deborah
Patricia
Karen
Maria
Barbara
Donna

ZALLEH Persian. "Dew."

ZANDRA Short form of **Alexandra.** Greek, "man's defender." **Zahndra, Zanndra, Zohndra, Zondra**

ZANNA Short form of **Susanna.** Hebrew, "lily." **Zana**

ZARA Hebrew. "Dawn." Also a variant of **Sarah. Zahra, Zaira, Zarah, Zaria, Zarita, Zariza, Zayeera**

ZAZA Hebrew. "Movement."

ZEHIRA Hebrew. "Safe."

ZELDA Short form of **Griselda.** Old German, "gray fighting maid." **Selda, Zelde, Zellda**

ZELIA Old French. Disputed meaning. **Zele, Zelie, Zelle**

ZELMA Variant of **Anselma,** feminine form of **Anselm.** Old German, "godly helmet." **Sellma, Selmah**

ZENA Variant of **Xenia, Zenobia. Zeena, Zeenia, Zeenya, Zenia, Zenya, Zina**

ZENDA Persian. "Sacred."

ZENOBIA Greek. "Power of Zeus." **Cenobia, Cenobie, Zeba, Zeena, Zena, Zenaida, Zenaïde, Zenayda, Zenina, Zenna, Zenobie**

ZEPHYR Greek. "West wind." **Zefeera, Zefir, Zefira, Zefiryn, Zephira, Zephyra**

ZERLINDA Hebrew/Spanish. "Beautiful dawn." **Zerlina**

ZETTA Hebrew. "Olive." **Zeta, Zetana**

ZEVIDA Hebrew. "Gift."

ZIA Latin. "Grain." **Zea**

ZIGANA Hungarian. "Gypsy." **Tsigana, Tsigane, Tzigana, Tzigane**

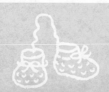

ZILLA Hebrew. "Shade." **Zillah, Zylla**

ZILPHA Hebrew. Unknown meaning. **Zilpah, Zillpha, Zylpha**

ZINNIA New Latin. "Zinnia," a showy flowering plant of the genus *Zinnia*, named for the German physician and botanist Johan G. Zinn. **Zinia, Zinnya, Zinya**

ZIPPORA Hebrew. "Bird." **Zipora, Ziporah, Zipporah**

ZITA Greek. "Seeker." Also short form of **Teresita. Zeeta, Zyta**

ZIVA Hebrew. "Brilliance, brightness." **Zeeva, Ziv, Zivit**

ZOE Greek. "Life." **Zoë, Zoee, Zoelie, Zoeline, Zoelle, Zoey, Zoie, Zoya** et al.

ZOFIA Variant of **Sophia.** Greek, "wisdom." **Zofi, Zophia, Zsofia**

ZOLA Italian. "Lump of earth." **Zoela**

ZONA Latin. "Belt." **Zonia, Zonya**

ZORA Slavic. "Dawn's light." Also a variant of **Aurora. Zarya, Zohra, Zorah, Zorana, Zorina, Zorine, Zorra, Zorrah, Zorya**

ZOYA Russian variant of **Zoe. Zoia, Zoyenka, Zoyya**

ZSA ZSA Slavic variant of **Susan.** Hebrew, "lily."

ZSOFIA Hungarian variant of **Sofia.** Greek, "wisdom."

ZSUSANNA Slavic variant of **Susanna.** Hebrew, "lily."

ZULEIKA Arabic. "Lovely girl."

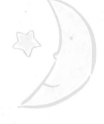

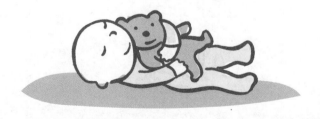

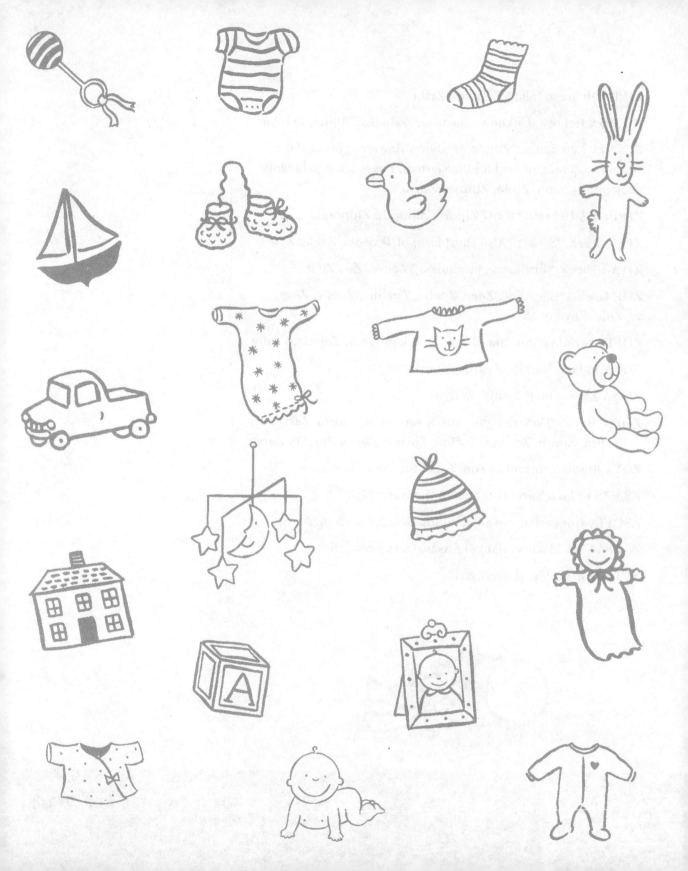

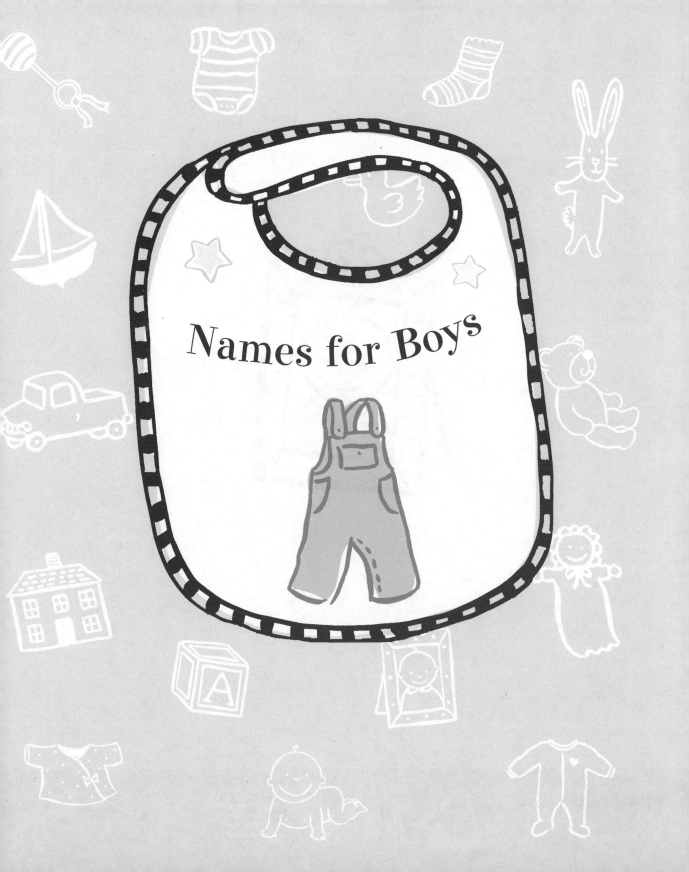

Names for Boys

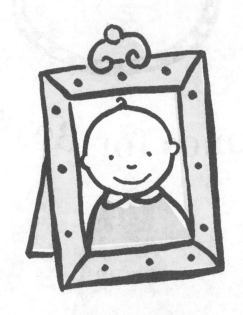

AADIL Arabic. "Just, upright."

AAHIL Arabic. "Prince."

AARIZ Arabic. "Respectable man."

AARON Hebrew. "Exalted." **Aaran, Aaren, Aarron, Aeron, Aharon, Ari, Arin, Arnie, Arny, Aron, Arran, Arron, Erin, Ron, Ronnie, Ronny**

ABBA Aramaic. "Father." **Aba, Abad, Abbas, Abbe, Abboid**

ABBEY Diminutive of **Abbot, Abelard, Abner. Abbie, Abby**

ABBOTT Hebrew. "Father." **Ab, Abad, Abba, Abbe, Abe, Abbey, Abbie, Abbot, Abby, Abot, Abott**

ABDA Arabic. "Servant."

ABDIAS Arabic variant of **Obadiah.** Hebrew, "servant of God."

ABDUL Arabic. "Servant of." **Ab, Abdal, Abdel, Abdiel, Abdullah, Del**

ABE Short form of **Abel, Abelard, Abraham, Abram. Abey, Abie**

ABEL Hebrew. "Breath." Also short form of **Abelard. Abe** et al., **Able**

ABELARD Middle English. "Guard of the abbey." **Ab, Abbey, Abby, Abe** et al., **Abel**

ABIAH Hebrew. "My father is the Lord." **Abia, Abija, Abijah**

ABIDA Hebrew. "God knows."

ABIEL Hebrew. "My father is God."

ABIMELECH Hebrew. "My father is king."

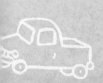

ABIR Hebrew. "Strong."

ABISHA Hebrew. "Gift of God." **Abishai**

ABNER Hebrew. "My father is light." **Ab, Abna, Abnar, Abnor, Avner, Eb, Ebbie, Ebby**

ABRAHAM Hebrew. "Father of many." **Abarran, Abe** et al., **Abrahamo, Abrahan, Bram, Ibrahim**

ABRAM Hebrew. "He who is high is father." **Abe** et al., **Abrami, Abramo, Avram, Avrom, Bram**

ABSALOM Hebrew. "Father is peace." **Absolom**

ACAYIB Turkish. "Peculiar."

ACE English. "Expert." **Acelet, Acelin, Acer, Acey, Acie**

ACHILLES Greek. In the *Iliad*, the chief Greek hero in the siege of Troy. **Achill, Achille, Achillea, Akil, Akilles**

ACHIM Hebrew. "God will judge." **Acim**

ACKERLEY Middle English. "Oak meadow." **Accerly, Ackerlea, Ackerleigh, Ackerly, Acklea, Ackleigh, Ackley, Acklie**

ACTON Old English. "Oak tree town."

ADAIR Scottish. "Oak tree crossing." **Adaire, Adare**

ADALFIERI Italian. "Noble oath."

ADALRIC Old German. "Highborn ruler." **Adelric**

ADAM Hebrew. "Son of the red earth." **Ad, Adamo, Adams, Adan, Adao, Addam, Addams, Addie, Addis, Addy, Ade, Adhamh, Adnet, Adnot**

ADAMSON Old English. "Son of Adam." **Adamsson, Addamson**

ADAR Hebrew. "Noble." **Addar, Addi, Addie, Adin, Adino, Adir**

ADDISON Old English. "Son of Adam." **Ad, Addie, Addy, Adison, Adisson**

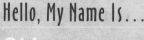

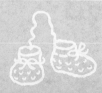

ADDY Teutonic. "Awe-inspiring." Also short form of **Adair, Addison. Addie, Ade, Ado**

ADEL Old German. "Noble." Also short form of **Adelard. Adal, Adelino**

ADELARD Old German. "Noble eagle." **Ad, Adal, Adalar, Adalard, Addler, Adelar, Adler, Adlar**

ADELINO Portuguese and Spanish variant of **Adel.**

ADELPHE French, from Greek. "Brother." **Adelphus**

ADEN Variant of **Aidan, Alden.**

ADER Hebrew. "Flock."

ADHAM Arabic. "Black."

ADLAI Hebrew. "My ornament." Adlai Ewing Stevenson, U.S. vice president, 1893–1997. His grandson of the same name, presidential nominee, 1952. **Ad, Addie, Addy, Adley**

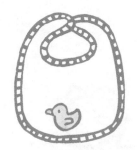

ADLER Variant of **Adelard.** Old German, "noble eagle." **Addler, Adlar**

ADNAH Hebrew. "Ornamented."

ADNEY Old English. "The noble's island."

ADOLPH Old German. "Noble wolf." **Ad, Adolf, Adolfo, Adolfus, Adolphe, Adolpho, Adolphus, Dolf, Dolph, Dolphus**

ADON Phoenician. "Lord."

ADONIS Greek. In myth, the handsome lover of Venus.

ADRIAN Latin. "From Adria," a city in northern Italy. **Ade, Adiran, Adriano, Adrien, Adryan, Hadrian, Hadrien**

AEGIR Old Norse. God of the sea.

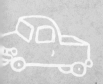

AENEAS Greek. "He who is praised." In the *Aeneid*, a Trojan warrior who went to Italy after the fall of Troy. **Eneas, Enné**

AFIF Arabic. "Chaste."

AFTON Old English. "Behind." A place name. **Affton**

AGNOLO Italian. "Angel."

AHAB Hebrew. "Father's brother." In Melville's *Moby Dick*, the captain who pursued the whale.

AHEARN Irish. "Horse lord." **Ahearne, Aherin, Ahern, Aherne, Hearn, Hearne, Herin, Hern**

AHMED Arabic. "Greatly praised." **Achmad, Achmed, Ahmad**

AHSAN Arabic. "Compassion." **Ehsan, Ihsan**

AIDAN Irish. "Fiery one." **Aiden, Edan, Eden**

AIKEN Old English. "Made of oak." **Aicken, Aikin, Ayken, Aykin**

AIMÉ French. "Much loved."

AIMERY Teutonic. "Hardworking ruler." **Aimerey, Aimeric, Amerey, Aymeric, Aymery**

AINSLEY Scottish. "His meadow." **Ainsley, Ainsleigh, Ainslie, Ansley, Aynslee, Aynsley, Aynslie**

AJANI Nigerian. "Victorious."

AKBAR Arabic. "Great."

AKELO Ugandan. "Bring forth."

AKIHIKO Japanese. "Bright."

AKIM Russian variant of **Joachim**. Hebrew, "God will judge."

AKIRA Japanese. "Smart."

AKMAL Arabic. "Perfect."

 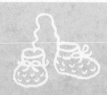

ALAIRE French variant of **Hilary**. Latin, "joyful." **Alair, Hilary, Larie, Lary**

ALAN Irish. "Rock." **Ailean, Ailin, Al, Alain, Aland, Alann, Alano, Alen, Alin, Allan, Allayne, Allen, Alley, Alleyn, Alleyne, Allie, Allin, Allon, Allyn, Alon, Alun**

ALARD Old German. "Noble and steadfast." **Al, Allard**

ALARIC Old German. "Ruler of all." **Al, Alarick, Alarico, Aleric, Alerick, Allaric, Allarick, Alleric, Allerick, Alric, Alrick**

ALASTAIR Scottish variant of **Alexander**. Greek, "man's defender." **Al, Alaisdair, Alaistair, Alaister, Alasdair, Alasteir, Alaster, Alastor, Aleister, Alester, Alistair, Alistar, Alister, Allaistair, Allaistar, Allaster, Allastir, Allistair, Allister, Allistir, Allysdair, Allysdare, Allystair, Allystar, Alysdair, Alysdare, Alystair, Alyster, Lester, Lister, Lyster**

ALBAN Latin. "From Alba," a city in northwest Italy. **Al, Albain, Alban, Albany, Albie, Albin, Albinet, Alby, Alvan, Alvy, Auban, Auben**

ALBERIC Middle German. "Clever ruler." **Aelric, Aiberik, Alberi, Alberich, Alberick, Auberi**

ALBERN Old German. "Noble courage."

ALBERT Old English. "Brilliant." **Adalbert, Adalbrecht, Adelbert, Adelbrecht, Ailbert, Al, Alberto, Albie, Albrecht, Albrekt, Aubert, Bert, Bertie, Berty, Elbert, Ulbricht**

ALBERTO Spanish variant of **Albert**. Old English, "brilliant."

ALBIN Latin. "Pale-skinned." **Al, Aubin**

ALBION Latin. "From Gaul" or "white."

ALCANDER Greek. "Strong." **Alcinder**

ALCOTT Old English. "Old cottage." **Alcot, Alkott, Allcot, Allcott**

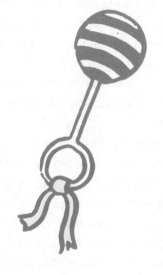

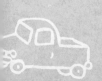

NAMES FROM AFRICA

Many are the stories of immigrants to America whose names—first as well as last—got changed by low-echelon clerks at Ellis Island and other entry points. Of all the people who came to this country, however, those who arrived in slave ships and their descendants received the worst treatment, in naming and in other matters. Stripped of their African names, they were given the last names of their owners. At one time in the American South, it was fashionable to give slaves the first names of Romans, those classical slave owners.

With the 1960s rise of Black Muslims, Black Power, and the civil rights movement, African-Americans gained a heightened appreciation of their ancestral homeland. Some began rejecting their "slave names" and adopting names from Africa or Arabic-speaking countries. In the most famous of these name changes, the boxer Cassius Clay became Muhammad Ali.

In turning to Africa, seekers of new names tapped into the most linguistically rich continent in the world, a place with more than eight hundred languages, from Ashanti to Zulu. Individuals fortunate enough to know from which area their ancestors came could narrow their choice of names, but many felt free to choose from the entire continent or even to invent names that sound African. In these ways, African names have immeasurably enriched the pool of American names.

Here are some African names for boys, with their meanings and sources:

Akelo	"bring forth	Uganda
Amir	"prince"	Arabic
Chaka, Shaka	"great king"	South Africa
Dakar	capital of Senegal	Senegal
Jamal	"beautiful"	Arabic
Kamali	"spirit"	Zimbabwe
Lumumba	"gifted"	Congo
Mandela	from Nelson Mandela	South Africa
Nasir	"helper" or "friend"	Arabic
Radama	a king of Madagascar	Madagascar
Samori	a Mandinka king	Mali
Selassie	"trinity"	Ethiopia
Tem	unknown	Togo
Tessema	"he has been heard"	Ethiopia
Zuri	"good"	South Africa

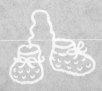

Following are some African names for girls:

			Imani	"faith"	Tanzania and Kenya
Aaliyah	"high, exalted"	Arabic	**Jada**	"goodness"	Arabic
Asante, Ashanti	"thank you"	Ghana and Ivory Coast	**Malkia**	"queen"	South Africa
			Nabila	"noble"	Arabic
Bria	a city	Central African Republic	**Ofrah**	"moon"	West Africa
			Rasoherina	a queen	Madagascar
Didessa	a river	Ethiopia	**Tanisha**	"born on Monday"	West Africa
Ebiere	unknown	Nigeria			
Falashina	a language	Ethiopia	**Zahra**	"flower"	Arabic

ALDEN Old English. "Old friend." **Al, Aldin, Aldon, Aldwin** et al., **Elden** et al., **Eldwin** et al.

ALDO Italian variant of **Aldous**. "Old."

ALDOUS Old German. "Old." Aldous Huxley, 1894–1963, British writer, author of *Brave New World.* **Al, Aldis, Aldivin, Aldo, Aldon, Aldus, Eldin, Eldis, Eldon, Eldous**

ALDRED Old English. "Old counsel." **Alldred, Eldred, Elldred**

ALDRICH Old English. "Old leader." **Al, Aldric, Aldridge, Aldrige, Aldritch, Alldrich, Alldridge, Allric, Alrick, Audric, Eldrich, Eldridge** et al., **Rich** et al.

ALDWIN Old English. "Old friend." **Alden** et al., **Aldwyn, Aldwynn, Elden** et al., **Eldwin** et al.

ALEM Arabic. "Wise man." **Alerio**

ALERON Latin. "On the flank."

ALEX Short form of **Alexander**. Greek, "man's defender." **Alix**

ALEXANDER Greek. "Man's defender." **Al, Alastair** et al., **Alec, Aleck, Alejandro, Alejo, Alek, Aleksander, Aleksandr, Alessandre, Alessandri, Alessandro, Alex, Alexandre,**

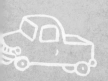

Alexandro, Alexandros, Alic, Alick, Alik, Alisander, Alissander, Alissandre, Alix, Alsandair, Alsandare, Iskander, Lex, Sacha et al., **Sander** et al., **Sandy** et al., **Sikander, Xan, Zindel, Zindil**

ALEXIS Greek. "Helper." **Alejo, Alexei, Alexey, Alexi, Alexio, Alexy**

ALFORD Old English. "Old river-ford." **Aldford**

ALFRED Old English. "Counsel from the elves." **Ailfrid, Ailfryd, Al, Alf, Alfeo, Alfie, Alfredo, Alfy, Alured, Fred, Freddie, Freddy, Fredo**

ALGER Old English. "Noble spear." **Al, Algar, Allgar, Allger, Elgar, Elger, Ellgar, Ellger**

ALGERNON Old French. "Wearing a mustache." **Al, Alger, Algey, Algie, Algy**

ALGIS Old German. "Spear."

ALI Arabic. "Elevated" or "noble." **Aalee, Aly**

ALIM Arabic. "Wise." **Alem**

ALISON Old English. "Son of the highborn." **Allison, Allisoun, Allson, Allyson**

ALLARD Old English. "Courageous." **Allerd**

ALON Hebrew. "Oak tree." **Allon**

ALONZO Variant of **Alphonse.** Old German, "ready for battle." **Alonso, Lon, Lonas, Lonnie, Lonny, Lonzo**

ALOYSIUS Old German. "Renowned warrior." **Alois, Aloisio, Aloisius, Aloys, Lewis** et al., **Louis** et al., **Lucho, Ludovicus** et al., **Ludwig** et al., **Luigi**

ALPHEUS Hebrew. "He who follows after." **Alpheaus, Alpheius, Alphoeus**

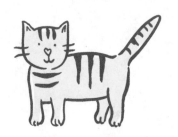

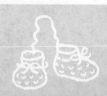

ALPHONSE Old German. "Ready for battle." **Afonso, Aphonso, Al, Alfie, Alfo, Alfons, Alfonso, Alfonsus, Alfonzo, Alfonzus, Alfy, Alonzo** et al, **Alphie, Alphonso, Alphonsus, Alphonzo, Alphonzus, Alphy, Fons, Fonsie, Fonz, Fonzie**

ALPIN Latin. "Tall mountains." **Alpine**

ALROY Irish. "Redheaded."

ALSTON Old English. "Town of nobles." **Allston**

ALTMAN Old German. "Old man." **Altmann**

ALTON Old English. "Old town." **Allton, Alten, Elton, Ellton**

ALUPH Hebrew. "Leader."

ALURED Variant of **Alfred.** Old English, "counsel from the elves."

ALVA Hebrew. "Brilliance." **Alba, Alvah, Alvan**

ALVAR Old English. "Army of elves."

ALVIN Old English. "Of the elves." **Ailwyn, Al, Aloin, Aluin, Aluino, Alva, Alvan, Alven, Alvie, Alvy, Alvyn, Elvin** et al.

ALVIS Old Norse. "Wise." **Alvys, Elvis, Elvys**

ALWIN Old English. "Handsome." **Alwin, Alwyn, Alwynn, Aylwin, Elwin, Elwyn, Elwynn**

AMADEO Spanish. "Loved by God." **Amadée, Amadei, Amadeus, Amadi, Amadieu, Amadis**

AMADO Spanish, Portuguese. "Beloved."

AMADOUR French. "Lover." **Amadis, Amado, Amadore**

AMANDO Spanish. "Loving."

AMASA Hebrew. "Bearing a burden."

AMBROSE Greek. "Ever-living." Ambrose Bierce, satiric American writer, 1842–c. 1914. **Ambie, Ambrogio, Ambroise, Ambros, Ambrosi, Ambrosio, Ambrosius, Amby, Brose**

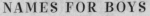

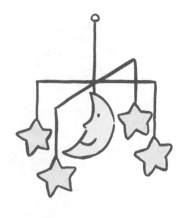

AMERIGO Italian variant of **Amory, Emery.** Old German, "home ruler." Amerigo Vespucci, Italian navigator for whom America is named.

AMI Hebrew. "My people." **Amiel**

AMIEL Hebrew. "God of my people."

AMIN Arabic. "Affirmation." **Amen, Ammon, Amnon, Amon**

AMIR Arabic, "prince." Hebrew, "strong." **Aamir, Emir**

AMORY Old German. "Home ruler." **Aimory, Amerigo, Amery, Amorey, Emery** et al.

AMOS Hebrew. "Carried." St. Amos. **Amós**

AMRIT Sanskrit. "Immortal one."

AMYAS Latin. "Loved by God." **Amias**

AN Chinese. "Peace."

ANAN Hebrew. "Cloud."

ANASTASIUS Greek. "Resurrection." **Anastas, Anastase, Anastasio, Anastatius, Anastice, Anastius, Anasto, Anstas, Anstice, Stasio, Stasius**

ANATOLE Greek. "From the east." **Anatol, Anatolio, Anatoly, Antal**

ANCEL Old German. "Godlike." **Ancelin, Ancelot, Ansela, Ansell, Ansellus, Ansila**

ANCHER Greek. "Anchor."

ANDER Variant of **Andrew, Leander.**

ANDERS Scandinavian variant of **Andrew.** Greek, "manly."

ANDERSON Scandinavian. "Son of Anders." **Andersen, Andersson**

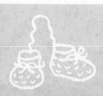

ANDRÉ French variant of **Andrew**. Greek, "manly." **Andras, Andres, Andris**

ANDREW Greek. "Manly." **Aindrea, Aindreas, Ander, Anders, Andie, Andonis, André, Andrea, Andreas, Andrej, Andres, Andresj, Andrey, Andrezj, Andriy, Andro, Andy, Drew, Dru, Drod, Drugi**

ANEURIN Welsh. "Honor." **Aneirin**

ANGEL Greek. "Messenger." **Ange, Angell, Angelo, Angelus, Angie, Angy**

ANGUS Irish, Scottish. "Sole choice." In Irish myth, a chief of the Tuatha De Danann, an ancient people or fairy folk. **Aonghus, Ennis, Gus** et al., **Oenghus, Oengus**

ANNAN Scottish. "From the brook."

ANNAWAN Algonquin. An Algonquin chief.

ANNIBAL Variant of **Hannibal**. Carthaginian general.

ANOOSH Persian. "Joyful."

ANSCOM Old English. "Valley of the noble one." **Anscomb, Anscombe**

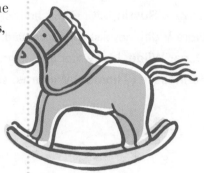

ANSEL Old French. "Follows nobility." Ansel Adams, twentieth-century photographer of landscapes in the American West. **Ancell, Ansell**

ANSELM Old German. "God-helmet." St. Anselm **Anse, Ansel, Anselme, Anselmi, Anselmo, Anshelm, Elmo**

ANSLEY Old English. "Nobleman's meadow." **Anslea, Ansleigh, Anslie, Ansly**

ANSON English. "Son of Andrew." **Annson, Ansson**

ANTHONY Latin. "Beyond price." **Anntoin, Antin, Antione, Antjuan, Antoine, Anton, Antone, Antonello, Antoney,**

Gay guys with great names

Sergei Diaghileff, Russian Ballet impresario

Elton John, rocker, balladeer, and royal musical eulogist

W. Somerset Maugham, British novelist

Harvey Milk, San Francisco politician and martyr

Vaslav Nijinsky, the Russian ballet dancer

Rudolf Nureyev, the Mick Jagger of ballet

Cole Porter, delightful, delicious American composer

Bayard Rustin, Civil Rights activist

Gore Vidal, novelist who once said, "A narcissist is someone better looking than you are"

Oscar Wilde, Irish writer and epigrammatist

Tennessee (Thomas) Williams, some say the best American playwright

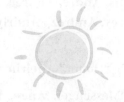

Antoni, Antonin, Antonino, Antonio, Antonius, Antons, Antony, Antuan, Antuwain, Antuwaine, Antuwayne, Antuwon, Antwahn, Antwain, Antwaine, Antwan, Antwaun, Antwohn, Antwoin, Antwoine, Antwon, Antwone, Toney, Toni, Tony

ANTOINE French variant of **Anthony.**

ANWAR Arabic. "Light." Anwar al-Sadat, president of Egypt 1970–1981, winner of the Nobel Peace Prize.

ANWELL Welsh. "Loved one." **Anwel, Anwil, Anwill, Anwyl, Anwyll**

APOLLO Greek. "Manly." **Apollinaire, Apollinaris, Apollon, Apollonian, Apollos**

AQUILA Latin. "Eagle." **Acquila, Acquilla, Aquilla**

ARAM Assyrian "High place."

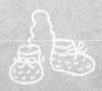

ARCHARD Old English "Holy." **Archerd**

ARCHELAUS Greek. "Ruler of the people."

ARCHER Old French. "Bowman."

ARCHIBALD Old German. "Valorous." **Arch, Archaimbaud, Archambault, Archibaldo, Archibold, Archie, Archimbald, Archy**

ARDEN Latin. "Burning." **Ard, Arda, Ardie, Ardin, Ardy**

ARDLEY Old English. "Home-lover's meadow." **Ardly, Ardsley, Ardsly**

ARDMORE Latin. "Zealous."

ARDON Hebrew. "Bronze."

ARES Greek. In myth, the god of war, and the despised son of Zeus and Hera.

ARGUS Greek. "Vigilant guardian." In myth, a monster with many eyes. **Argos**

ARGYLE Scottish. Place name. **Argyll**

ARIC Old German. "Ruler." **Arick, Arric, Arrick, Eric** et al.

ARIEL Hebrew. "Lion of God." Ariel Sharon, current prime minister of Israel. **Aeriell, Airel, Airyel, Airyell, Arel, Arie, Ariell, Aryel, Aryell**

ARIES Latin. "Ram." The first sign of the zodiac. **Arese, Ariese**

ARISOPHANES Greek. Writer of comedy, fifth to fourth century B.C.

ARISTO Greek. "The best." **Ari**

ARISTOTLE Greek. "Superior." **Ari, Arie, Arri, Ary**

ARLEDGE Old English. "Lake with the hares." **Arlidge, Arlledge**

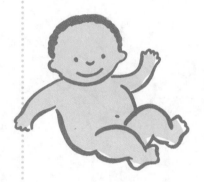

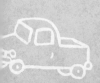

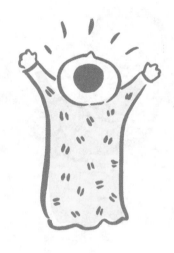

ARLEN Hebrew. "Oath." **Arlan, Arles, Arlin, Arlyn, Arllen, Arrlen**

ARLES French. A city in Provence.

ARLEY Old English. "Meadow of hares." **Arlea, Arleigh, Arlie, Arly**

ARLO Spanish. "Barberry." Arlo Guthrie, contemporary American musician and storyteller.

ARMAN Persian. "Ideal."

ARMAND French variation of **Herman.** Old German, "soldier." Armand Hammer, 1898–1990, American industrialist and art collector. According to his biographer, he was named by his father, the founder of the American Communist Party, for the arm-and-hammer symbol of the Socialist Labor Party. **Arman, Armande, Armando, Armin, Armon, Armond, Armonde, Armondo, Orman, Ormand, Ormond, Ormonde, Ormondo**

ARMSTRONG Old English. "Strong arm."

ARNE Old German. "Eagle." **Arney, Arni, Arnie**

ARNETT Old French diminutive of **Arne.** Old German, "little eagle." **Arnat, Arnet, Arnot, Arnott**

ARNO Old German. "Eagle-wolf." **Arnoe, Arnou, Arnoux**

ARNOLD Old German. "Strength of an eagle." **Arnaldo, Arnaud, Arnault, Arney, Arni, Arnie, Arnoldo, Arny**

ARRAN Scottish. An island in Scotland. **Arren, Arrin, Arron**

ARRIGO Variant of **Henry.** Old German, "estate ruler."

ARSEN Greek. "Strong."

ARTEMUS Greek. Masculine variant of **Artemis,** goddess of the moon. **Art, Artemas, Artemis, Artey, Artie, Artimas, Artimis, Artimus, Arty**

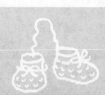

ARTHUR Scottish. "Rock." **Art, Artair, Arte, Artey, Arthor, Arthuro, Artie, Artor, Artur, Arturo, Artus, Arty**

ARUNDEL Old English. "Eagle valley."

ARVA Latin. "Countryside." **Arv, Arvada, Arval, Arwa**

ARVAD Hebrew. "Voyager." **Arpad, Arv, Arvid, Arvie, Arvy, Arvyd**

ARVIN Old German. "People's friend." **Arv, Arve, Arvie, Arvy, Arwin, Arwyn**

ASA Hebrew. "Doctor." **Ase**

ASAN Variant of **Hassan.** Arabic, "handsome." **Assan**

ASAPH Hebrew. "Gathering." **Asaf, Asaff, Asoph**

ASCOT Old English. "Eastern cottage." **Ascott**

ASHBROOK English. "Ash-tree brook."

ASHBURN Old English. "Ash-tree brook."

ASHBY Old English. "Ash-tree farm." **Ash, Ashbey, Ashbie, Ashburn**

ASHER Hebrew. "Felicitous." **Ash**

ASHFORD Old English. "Ford near ash trees." **Ash, Ashenford**

ASHLEY Old English. "Ash-tree meadow." **Ash, Ashely, Asheley, Ashelie, Ashlan, Ashleigh, Ashlen, Ashlie, Ashlin, Ashling, Ashlinn, Ashly, Ashlyn, Ashlynn**

ASHTON Old English. "Ash-tree settlement."

ASHUR Assyrian. In myth, the ruler of the gods. **Ashir, Ashshur, Asshur, Assur, Asur**

ASTON Old English. "Eastern town."

ASWIN Old English. "Spear-friend." **Aswinn, Aswyn, Aswynn**

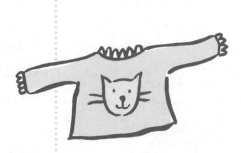

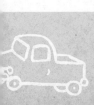

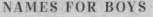

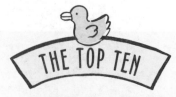

THE TOP TEN

NAMES OF 1963

The Year the Beatles Released "I Want to Hold Your Hand"

BOYS

David
John, Michael (tie)
James
Robert
Mark
Richard, William (tie)
Thomas
Kevin

GIRLS

Lisa
Mary
Maria
Susan
Karen
Patricia
Linda
Donna
Sandra
Deborah

ATHELSTAN Old English. "Rock of the highborn."

ATHENE Masculine variant of **Athena**. Greek goddess of wisdom. **Athens, Athien, Attene, Attien**

ATHERTON Old English. "Town by the spring."

ATHOL Scottish. A district in Scotland. **Athole, Atholl**

ATLAS Greek. In myth, Atlas is the Titan forced to carry the world on his shoulders. **Etlas**

ATLEY Old English. "From the meadow." **Atlea, Atlee, Atleigh, Attlee, Attleigh, Attley**

ATTILA King of the Huns, a Mongolian tribe. **Atili, Atli, Atoy, Attilio**

ATWATER Old English. "At the river."

ATWELL Old English. "At the well."

ATWOOD Old English. "At the wood."

ATWORTH Old English. "At the farmstead."

AUBERON Old German "Bear-like." **Auberron, Oberon, Oberron, Oeberon**

AUBREY Old French. "Elf ruler." **Aube, Aubry, Avery** et al.

AUDLEY Old English. Place name.

AUDRIC Old German. "Noble ruler."

AUGUSTUS Latin. "Worthy of respect." **Agostino, Agosto, Aguistin, Agustin, Agustino, Augie, August, Auguste, Augustin, Augusto, Augy, Austin** et al., **Gus** et al., **Gustus**

AURELIUS Latin. "Golden." Roman clan name. **Aurea, Aurel, Aurelio, Aurelo, Aury**

AUSTIN English variant of **Augustus**. Latin, "worthy of respect." **Austen, Austyn**

 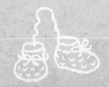

AVENALL Old French. "Oat pasture." **Aveneil, Aveneill, Avenel, Avenell, Avenil, Avenill**

AVERILL Old English. "Boar-fighter." **Ave, Averel, Averell, Averil, Averyl, Averyll, Avrel, Avrell, Avrill, Avryll**

AVERITT Variant of **Everett**. Old English, "boar hardness."

AVERY Old English. "Elf-ruler." **Aubrey** et al., **Averey, Averie**

AVI Hebrew. "Father." **Abi, Av, Avodal**

AXEL Old German. "Father of peace." **Aksel, Ax, Axe, Axell, Axil, Axill**

AYAAN Arabic. "God's gift."

AYLMER Old English. "Highborn and renowned." **Ailemar, Aillmer, Ailmer, Allmer, Ayllmer, Aylmar, Aymer, Elmer** et al.

AYLWARD Old English. "Great guardian."

AZURIAH Hebrew. "Helper." **Azaria, Azariah, Azriel, Azul, Azur, Azuria, Ezra** et al.

BADGER English. "Badger."

BAILEY Middle English. "Bailiff." **Bail, Bailie, Baillie, Baily, Bayley, Bayly**

BAINBRIDGE Irish. "Pale bridge." **Bain, Baynbridge, Bayne, Baynebridge**

BAIRD Scottish, Irish. "Bard." **Bar, Bard, Barde, Barr, Bayerd, Bayrd**

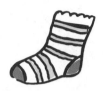

BAKER Old English. "Baker."

BALBO Latin. "Babbler." **Bailby, Balbi, Ballbo**

BALDEMAR Variant of **Valdemar**. Old German, "renowned leader." **Baumar, Baumer**

BALDER Old Norse. In myth, the most beloved of the gods. **Baldur, Baldwin, Ball, Baudier, Baudoin**

BALDRIC Old German. "Brave ruler." **Baldri, Baldrick, Baudrey, Baudri, Baudric**

BALDWIN Old German. "Brave friend." **Bald, Baldewin, Baldovino, Balduin, Baldwinn, Baldwyn, Baldwynn, Ball, Balldwin, Baudoin**

BALFOUR Scottish. "Grazing land." **Balfor, Balfore**

BALINT Hungarian. "Strong." **Balin, Baline**

BALLARD Old German. "Brave and strong."

BALTHASAR Greek. "God save the king." In Christian folklore, one of the Magi. **Baldassare, Baltasar, Baltazar, Balthasaar, Balthazar, Belshazzar**

BAMDAD Persian. "Morning."

BANCROFT Old English. "Bean field." **Ban, Bancrofft, Bank, Binky**

BANFIELD English. "Bean field."

BANNING Irish. "Fair one."

BAPTIST Greek. "Dip." **Baptista, Baptiste, Bautista**

BARAK Hebrew. "Light." **Barac, Barack**

BARBER Latin. "Beard." **Barbour**

BARCLAY Old English. "Meadow where birches grow." **Bar, Barcley, Barklay, Barkley, Barklie, Barrclay, Berkeley** et al.

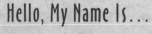

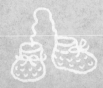

BARDEN Middle English. "Valley of barley." **Bardon, Borden, Bordon**

BARDOLF Old English. "Axe-wolf." **Bardolph, Bardou, Bardoul, Bardulf, Bardulph**

BARDRICK Teutonic. "Axe-ruler." **Bardric**

BARKER Old English. "Birch." **Birc, Birk, Birke, Burc, Burcke, Burk, Burke**

BARKSDALE English. "Valley of birches."

BARLOW Old English. "Bare hillside." **Barlowe, Barrlow**

BARNABAS Hebrew. "Son of comfort." In the Bible, Barnabas sold his land and gave the money to Christ's apostles. **Barna, Barnaba, Barnabé, Barnabee, Barnabey, Barnabie, Barnabus, Barnaby, Barnebas, Barnebus, Barney** et al.

BARNES Old English. "Barns." **Bairnes**

BARNETT Old English. "Blackened land." **Barnet, Barney** et al., **Baronet, Baronett, Barry** et al.

BARNEY Diminutive of **Barnabas, Barnett, Barnum, Bernard. Barnie, Barny**

BARNUM Old English. "Baron's home." **Barnham, Barney** et al.

BARON Old English. Title of nobility. **Barron, Barry** et al.

BARRA Irish. "Fair-headed."

BARRET Old German. "Bear-strength." **Baret, Barrat, Barratt, Barrett, Barry** et al.

BARRINGTON English. "Spear town." Place name.

BARRY Irish. "Sharp." Also diminutive of **Barret** and **Barnett. Bari, Barrie, Baris**

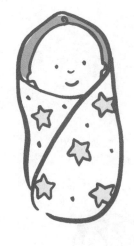

BARTHOLOMEW Hebrew. "Farmer's son." **Bart, Bartel, Barth, Barthelemy, Bartho, Bartholomaus, Bartholome, Bartholomeo, Bartholomeus, Bartlet, Bartlett, Bartolome, Bartolomeo, Bartolommeo, Bartome, Bartt, Bat, Meo, Mewes, Tholy, Tolly, Tolomey, Tolomieu**

BARTON Old English. "Barley settlement." **Bart, Barrton**

BARTRAM Old English. "Bright raven." **Barthram**

BARUCH Hebrew. "Blessed." **Barush**

BASIL Greek. "Royal." **Basile, Basilio, Basilius, Bazil, Bazyli**

BASSETT Old English. "Little person." **Basset**

BAVOL Romany. "Wind." **Beval, Bevol**

BAXTER Old English. "Baker." **Bax**

BAYARD Old English. "Russet-haired." **Baiardo, Bay, Baye**

BEACHER Old English. "Near the beech trees." **Beach, Beachy, Beech, Beecher, Beechy**

BEAGAN Irish. "Small one." **Beagin**

BEAL Old French. "Handsome." **Beale, Beall, Beals**

BEAMAN Old English. "Beekeeper." **Beamann, Beamen, Beeman, Beemen**

BEAMER Old English. "Trumpet player."

BEATTIE Irish masculine form of **Beatrice**. Latin, "bringer of gladness." **Beatie, Beatty, Beaty**

BEAU French. "Handsome." **Bo**

BEAUFORT Old French. "Beautiful fort."

BEAUMONT Old French. "Beautiful mountain."

BEAUREGARD French. "Handsome." **Beau, Bo**

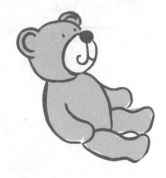

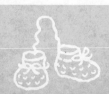

BEAUVAIS French. A city in France.

BECK Old English. "Small stream."

BEDE Old English. "Prayer." **Bedivere**

BEDIR Turkish. "Full moon."

BELDEN Middle English. "Pretty valley." **Beldon, Bellden, Belldon**

BELL Latin. "Handsome." **Bel, Bellini**

BELLAMY Latin. "Handsome friend." **Belamy, Bellaimy, Bellamey, Bellamie**

BELTON Latin. "Beautiful town." **Bellton**

BELVEDER Italian. "Handsome." **Belvedere, Belvidere**

BEN Hebrew. "Son." Also short form of **Benjamin, Benedict. Benn, Bennie, Benny, Benroy**

BENEDICT Latin. "Blessed." Benedict Arnold, fighter both for and against the fledgling United States in the 1770s. St. Benedict, early Christian monk and founder of the Benedictine order. **Ben, Bendick, Bendict, Benedetto, Benedick, Benedicto, Benedictus, Benedikt, Bengt, Benigno, Benito, Bennet, Bennett, Bennie, Bennt, Benoit, Bent**

BENJAMIN Hebrew. "Son of the right hand." **Ben, Benejamen, Beniamino, Benja, Benjaman, Benjamen, Benjamino, Benjamon, Benji, Benjie, Benjiman, Benjimen, Benjy, Bennie, Benyamin, Benyamino**

BENOIT French variant of **Benedict.** Latin, "blessed."

BENONI Hebrew. "Son of my sorrow."

BENSON "Son of Ben." **Bensen, Benssen, Bensson**

BENTLEY Old English. "Meadow with coarse grass." **Ben, Bentlea, Bentlee, Bentley, Bentlie, Bently, Lee**

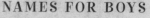

One name says it all

You know you have arrived in pop culture when you need only one name, like *Elvis, Bono, Cher, Prince, Sting, Roseanne, Houdini, Madonna, Sting, Liberace, Tarzan,* and *Eminem*. Others with more lasting fame have come down through history with one name: *Ramses, Moses, Aristotle, Homer, Jesus, Hannibal, Cleopatra, Buddha, Nostradamus, Charlemagne, Montezuma, Pocahontas,* and *Sacagawea*.

BENTON Old English. "Ben's town."

BEOWULF Old English. Hero of an Anglo-Saxon epic, a slayer of monsters and a dragon. **Beowolf**

BER Old Norse. "To live."

BERESFORD Old English. "Ford where barley grows."

BERG Old Norse, German. "Mountain." **Bergh, Bergin, Borg, Borje, Burg, Burgh**

BERGEN Scandinavian. "Hills." **Beagin, Birgin**

BERGER French. "Shepherd."

BERKELEY Old English. "Where birches grow." **Barclay** et al., **Berk, Berkie, Berkley, Berky**

BERLIN Teutonic. "Lime tree settlement." Capital of Germany. **Berlyn**

BERN Old German. "Bear." Also a city in Switzerland and short form of **Bernard. Berne, Bernie, Berny**

BERNAL Old German. "Strength of a bear." **Bernald, Bernhald, Bernhold, Bernold**

BERNARD Old German. "Courageous." **Barnard, Barnardo, Barney** et al., **Barnhard, Barnhardo, Barhardt, Bear, Bearnard, Bern, Bernardo, Bernarr, Bernhard, Bernhardo, Bernhardt, Bernie, Burnard**

BERRY English. "Berry."

BERSH Romany. "One year." **Besh**

BERT Old English. "Bright." Also short for **Dalbert, Delbert, Albert,** etc. **Bertie, Berty, Burt, Burtie, Burty**

BERTHOLD Old German. "Bright strength." **Bert, Berthoud, Bertold, Bertolde**

BERTON Old English. "Bright settlement." **Bert, Burt, Burton**

BERTRAM Old German. "Bright raven." **Bart, Bartram, Beltran, Beltrano**

BERTRAND Old German. "Bright shield." **Bertrando, Bertranno**

BERWYN Old English. Disputed meaning; "bear friend" or "bright friend." **Berwin, Berwynn, Berwynne**

BEVAN Welsh. "Son of Evan." **Beavan, Beaven, Bev, Beven, Bevin, Bevon**

BEVERLY Old English. "Beaver stream." **Beverlea, Beverleigh, Beverley, Beverlie**

BEVIS English variant of **Beauvais. Beafus, Beavis, Bevan, Bevin, Bivian, Bix.** *Beavis and Butthead,* animated television comedy, 1993–1997.

BIAGIO Italian variant of **Blaise.** Latin, "one who stutters." **Biaggio**

BIANCO Italian. "White."

BICKFORD Old English. "Axe-man's ford."

BING Chinese, "tea leaves." Old Norse, "heap" or "bin." Also short form of **Bingham.** Bing Crosby, twentieth-century popular American singer.

BINGHAM Old English. Disputed meaning. **Bin, Bing, Binnie**

BIRCH Old English. "Birch." **Birk, Burch**

BIRKETT Middle English. "Birch coastland." **Birket, Birkit, Birkitt, Burket, Burkett, Burkitt**

BIRKEY Middle English. "Island of birch trees." **Birkee, Birkie, Birky**

BIRLEY Old English. "Meadow with the cow byre." **Birlie, Birly**

But is just one name a good idea for you?

At this writing, Boulder County, Colorado, has eighteen people who had changed their names to one word. They are *Allessandra, Annatta, Candy, Chrystalynn, Florence, Holandia, ky, Lakey, Nyssa, Orfeo, Pax, Pua, Raven, Sandalphon, Shatar, Su-Mo-Ki, Truthsayer,* and *You.*

According to the *Daily Camera,* the local newspaper, people with one name have more than one headache. Annatta, for instance, has gotten credit cards bearing the name *Annatta Annatta.* The man known as ky took to writing *NLN*—for "no last name"—on forms, and now he has to endure hearing medical-office receptionists trying to pronounce *NLN* as if it were his name.

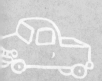

BIRNEY Old English. "Island in a stream." **Birnie, Birny, Burney, Burnie**

BIRTLE Old English. "Hill of birds."

BISHOP Old English. "Bishop."

BJORN Scandinavian. "Bear." **Bjarne, Bjornstjerne**

BLACK Old English. "Black."

BLACKBURN Old English. "Black brook."

BLAGDEN Old English. "Dark valley."

BLAINE Irish. "Slender." **Blane, Blayne**

BLAIR Scottish. "Plain." **Blaire, Blayr, Blayre**

BLAISE Latin. "One who stutters." **Biaggio, Biagio, Blás, Blase, Blasius, Blaze** et al., **Braz, Vlass.** St. Blás.

BLAKE Old Norse. "Bright, white."

BLAKELY Old English. "Light meadow." **Blakelee, Blakeleigh, Blakeley, Blakelie**

BLAKESLEY Old English. "Blake's meadow." **Blakeslee, Blakesly**

BLANCHARD Old French. "Whitish."

BLANCO Spanish. "White."

BLANFORD Old English. "Gray man's ford." **Blandford**

BLAZE English variant of **Blaise.** Latin, "one who stutters." **Blaize, Blase, Blayse, Blayze**

BLISS Old English. "Happiness."

BLYTHE Old English. "Happy." **Bligh, Blithe**

BO Old Norse, "householder." Chinese, "precious." Also variant of **Beau.**

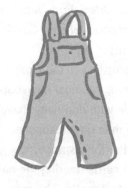

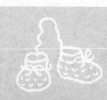

BOAZ Hebrew. "Swiftness." **Boas, Boase**

BOB Diminutive of **Robert.** Old English, "bright fame." **Bobbie, Bobby**

BODEN Old French. "One who brings news." **Bodin, Bowden, Bowdoin**

BOGART Old French. "Bow strength." **Bo, Bogey, Bogie, Bogy**

BOGDAN Slavic. "Gift of God." **Bodgan, Bohday, Bojan**

BOGUSLAW Slavic. "Glory of God." **Bohuslav**

BOND Old Norse. "Together." **Bondie, Bondon, Bondy**

BONIFACE Latin. "Do-gooder." St. Boniface. **Boneface, Boni, Bonifacio, Bonifacius, Bonyface, Facio, Fazio**

BOOKER Old English. "Writer" or "bookkeeper." Booker T. Washington, 1856–1915, African-American educator, founder of the Tuskegee Institute.

BOONE Old French. "Good." **Bon, Bone, Boon, Boonie, Boony**

BOOTH Old German. "Dwelling place." **Boot, Boote, Boothe, Boothy**

BORDEN Old English. "Valley of the boar."

BORIS Slavic. "Warrior." **Boriss, Borris, Borys**

BOTAN Japanese. "Peony."

BOTOLF Old English. "Messenger wolf." **Botolph, Botulf**

BOURNE Old English. "Brook." **Beirne, Bourn, Burne** et al.

BOWEN Welsh. "Son of the young one." **Bow**

BOWIE Scottish. Unknown meaning; possibly "bowl." **Bow**

BOYCE Old French. "Woods." **Boice, Boise**

BOYD Scottish. "Blond." **Boid**

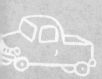

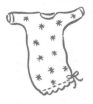

BOYNE Irish. "White cow."

BRAD Old English. "Broad." Also short form of **Bradley, Bradburn, Braden, Bradford, Bradshaw.**

BRADBURN Old English. "Wide stream." **Bradbourn, Bradbourne, Bradburne**

BRADEN Old English. "Wide valley." **Bradan, Bradin**

BRADFORD Old English. "Wide river-crossing." **Braddford, Bradfurd**

BRADLEY Old English. "Wide meadow." **Brad, Bradlea, Bradleigh, Bradlie, Bradly, Bradney, Lee, Leigh**

BRADSHAW Old English. "Broad forest."

BRADY Old English. "Wide island."

BRAGE Old Norse. In myth, the god of poetry and eloquence. **Braggo, Bragi**

BRAINARD Old English. "Courageous raven." **Brainerd**

BRAM Irish. "Raven." Also short form of **Abraham, Abram. Bramm, Bran, Brann**

BRAMWELL Old English. "Spring by the broom." **Brammell, Bramwel, Bramwyll**

BRAND Old English. "Torch." **Brander, Brandie, Brandt, Brant, Brantley, Brantlie**

BRANDON Old English. "Broom-covered hill." **Brand, Branden, Brandin, Brandyn, Brannon**

BRANT Old English. "Proud." **Brannt**

BRAXTON Old English. "Brock's town."

BRAWLEY Old English. "Field at base of a hill."

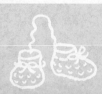

Notable botanists with nifty names

Botanists name the plants they discover, and some of them have names worthy of note themselves.

Liberty Hyde Bailey, founder of Cornell's College of Agriculture and Life Sciences

Gaspard Bauhin, originator of a binomial system of classification

Sir Jagadis Chandra Bose, Indian plant physiologist and physicist

Nathaniel Lord Britton, founder of the New York Botanical Garden

Luther Burbank, father of modern plant breeding

Ferdinand Cohn, one of the founders of bacteriology

Heinrich Anton De Bary, a founder of modern mycology and plant pathology

Augustin Pyrame De Candolle, originator of a structural criteria for determining natural relations among plants

Hugo De Vries, first to hypothesize the existence of genes

Asa Gray, author of the first *Manual of the Botany of the Northern United States*

Carolus Linnaeus, originator of the modern system of classification of plants and animals

André Michaux, eighteenth-century Frenchman who studied the plants of North America

Matthias Jakob Schleiden, co-founder of cell theory

Christian Konrad Sprengel, German whose studies of sex in plants led him to a general theory of fertilization

BRENDAN Irish. "Burning." **Brandon, Brennan, Brennen, Brennon**

BRENT Old English. "Steep."

BRENTON Old English. "Steep town." **Brentan, Brenten, Brentin, Brentyn**

BRETT Irish. "Briton." **Bret, Brette, Bretton, Brit, Britt, Britton**

BREWSTER Old English. "Brewer." **Brewer**

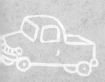

BREVARD Middle English. "Brief."

BRIAN Irish. "Strong one." **Briano, Briant, Brien, Brion, Bryan, Bryant, Bryen, Bryent, Bryon**

BRIDGELY Old English. "Meadow by the bridge." **Bridgeley**

BRIDGER Old English. "Lives near the bridge." **Bridge**

BRIGHAM Old English. "Little village near the bridge." **Brigg, Briggs, Brigman**

BRINLEY Old English. "Burnt meadow." **Brindley, Brindly, Brinlee, Brinleigh, Brinly, Brynly**

BROCK Old English. "Horse."

BROCKLEY Old English. "Meadow of the badger."

BRODERICK Old Norse. "Brother." **Brod, Broddy, Broderic, Brodric, Brodrick, Ric, Rick, Rickee, Rickey, Ricky**

BRODY Irish. "Ditch." **Brodee, Brodey, Brodie, Broedy**

BROMLEY Old English. "Broom meadow." **Brom**

BROMWELL Old English. "Broom well." **Brom**

BRONSON Old English. "Brown one's son." **Bron, Bronnson, Bronsen, Bronsin, Bronsonn, Bronsson**

BROOK Old English. "Stream." **Brooke, Brookes, Brookie, Brooks**

BROUGHTON Old English. "Settlement near the fortress."

BROWN Middle English. "Brown-skinned." **Brownie**

BRUCE Old French. "Brushwood thicket." **Brucey, Brucie, Bruis**

BRUIN Dutch. "Brown." The name of the bear in the old German animal epic *Reynard the Fox*. Often applied to brown bears in general.

BRUN French. "Brown."

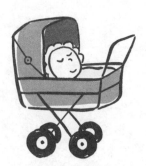

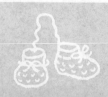

BRUNO Italian. "Brown."

BRUTUS Latin. "Brutish, stupid." In legend, the first king of Britain. **Brut**

BRYCE Variant of **Price.** Welsh, "prize." **Brice**

BUBBA Variant of **Bub.** Old English, "pal." The name **Bub** dates at least to the mid-nineteenth century.

BUCK Old English. "Stag." **Buckey, Buckie, Buckner, Bucky**

BUCKLEY Old English. "Meadow of the deer."

BUD English. Short form of **Buddy. Budd**

BUDDY English. "Friend." **Bud, Budd, Buddie, Buddy**

BUELL Middle English. "Bull." Many parents have been inspired to name their boys *Buell* after Don Carlos Buell, a Union general in the U.S. Civil War. **Buel**

BURCHARD Old English. "Fortification." **Burchardt, Burckhard, Burckhardt, Burgard, Burgaud, Burkhard, Burkhardt, Burkhart**

BURFORD Old English. "Crossing near the castle." **Burkeford, Burkford**

BURGESS Old English. "Citizen." **Burges, Burgiss, Burr**

BURKE Old French. "Castle." **Berk, Berke, Birk, Bourke, Burk**

BURLEIGH Old English. "Meadow with knotty-trunk trees." **Bierly, Burley, Burlie, Byrleigh, Byrley, Lee, Leigh**

BURNABY Old Norse. "Warrior's lands."

BURNE Variant of **Bourne.** Old English, "brook." **Bourne** et al., **Burn, Byrn, Byrne, Byrnes**

BURNELL Old French. "Small brown one." **Burnel**

BURNET Old English. "Brown." **Burnett**

Was Redneck Redneck Redneck already taken?

In 2003, a man living in Springfield, Illinois, had his named legally changed to *Bubba Bubba Bubba.* The 39-year-old formerly known as Raymond Allen Gray, Jr., worked at the time in the Illinois Secretary of State office. And what did Raymond Allen Gray, Sr., think of this? He and his wife, mercifully, were already deceased.

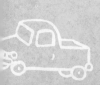

BURNEY Old English. "Island in a stream." **Birney** et al.

BURTON Old English. "Fortified enclosure." **Bert, Burt, Burtt, Burty**

BUSBY Norse. "Village in the thicket."

BUSTER English. "Lively, strong person" or "fellow." Usually a nickname. Buster Keaton, silent film actor and director.

BUTCH English. A nickname for tough boys.

BUTCHER Old English. "Butcher."

BYFORD Old English. "By the crossing."

BYRD Old English. "Birdlike." **Bird, Byrdie**

BYRON Old English. "Barn for cows." **Beyren, Beyron, Biren, Biron, Buiron, Byram, Byran, Byren, Byrom**

CADBY Old English. "Warrior's town."

CADDARIC English. "Battle leader." **Cad**

CADDOCK Welsh. "Eager for battle."

CADELL Welsh. "Battle." **Caddell, Cadel**

CADMAN Anglo-Saxon. "Warrior."

CADMUS Greek. "From the east." In myth, a Phoenician prince who slew a dragon, founded Thebes, and introduced the alphabet into Greece.

CADWALLER Welsh. "Battle commander." **Cadwaladar, Cadwalader, Cadwalladr, Cadwell**

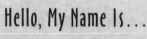 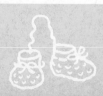

CAESAR Latin. "Long-haired." After Julius Caesar, the title of Roman emperors. **Caezar, Casar, César, Cesare, Cesaro, Cez, Seasar, Sezar**

CAHIL Turkish. "Inexperienced." **Kahil**

CAIN Hebrew. "Spear." In the Bible, Cain slew his brother Abel.

CAIUS Latin. "Rejoice." **Cai, Caio**

CAL Short form of **Calder, Caldwell, Caleb, Calvert, Calvin.**

CALDER Old English. "Stream." **Cal**

CALDWELL Old English. "Cold well." **Cal**

CALEB Hebrew. "Courageous." **Cal, Cale, Kal, Kale, Kaleb**

CALEY Irish. "Lean."

CALHOUN Irish. "Narrow woods." **Colhoun, Colquhoun**

CALVERT Old English. "Calf herder." **Cal, Calbert**

CALVIN Latin. "Hairless." **Caiv, Cal, Calvino, Kalvin, Vin, Vinnie, Vinny**

CAMDEN Scottish. "Winding valley." **Cam**

CAMERON Scottish. "Crooked nose." **Cam, Camron**

CAMILLUS Latin. Masculine form of **Camilla,** the fleet-footed queen of the Volscians in the *Aeneid*. **Camilio, Camillo, Camilo**

CAMILO Spanish, Portuguese variant of **Camillus.** Latin. Masculine form of **Camilla,** the fleet-footed queen of the Volscians in the *Aeneid*.

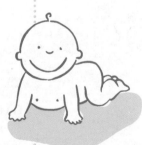

CAMLO Romany. "Beautiful."

CAMPBELL Irish, Scottish. "Curved mouth." **Cam, Camp, Campie, Campy**

Computers, security, and the bureaucratic mind versus middle names

C. Larkin Hosmer lives in Boulder, Colorado.

"My family has a tradition of going by our middle names. My father was Chester Craig Hosmer, and he always went by *Craig Hosmer*. For a formal signature, he would write *C. Craig Hosmer*. My name is *Craig Larkin Hosmer*, and I go by *Larkin*. I have two sons, and their names are *David Craig Hosmer* and *Larkin Wyatt Hosmer*. Everyone knows them as *Craig* and *Wyatt*.

"This sounds simple enough, but not when bureaucracies are involved. Over the years my wife and I have had several battles with schools. The teachers in the classrooms usually call our sons the names they prefer, but any thing coming from a computer—attendance lists, sports rosters, et cetera—shows only the first name and last name. Many computer programs have a 'Preferred Name' field, but most schools—unless they are asking alumni for money—don't seem to think this is important.

"It *is* important. Children in elementary schools may be teased when adults call them by names unfamiliar to the class, and when kids get older things can get more complicated. With all the security surrounding travel these days, you have to make sure that the name on the ticket matches the name on a driver's license or school I.D. card. I've known parents who have seriously thought about going to court to reverse their children's first and second names to avoid all these problems. They shouldn't have to do that—this issue isn't that complicated."

CANNING French. "Official of the church." **Cannan, Cannon, Canon**

CANUTE Scandinavian. "Knot." **Cnut, Knute** et al.

CARADOC Welsh. "Good-natured." **Caractacus, Caradawg, Caradog, Caratacos, Carthac, Carthage, Craddock**

CAREY Welsh. "Near the castle." **Cary**

CARL Old German. "Man." **Karl** et al.

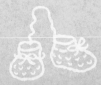

CARLETON Old English. "Freeman's town." Charlton Heston, popular Hollywood actor in the 1950s and 1960s, and later president of the National Rifle Association. **Carl, Carlton, Charleton, Charlton**

CARLIN Irish. "Little champion." **Carling, Carly**

CARLISLE Old English. "Fortified tower." **Carley, Carly, Carlyle**

CARLOS Spanish variant of **Charles.** Old German, "man." **Carlo**

CARLSON English. "Carl's son." **Karlsen**

CARLUS Irish variant of **Charles.** Old German, "man."

CARMEL Hebrew. "Vineyard." **Carmeli, Carmelo, Carmen, Carmi, Carmiel, Karmel** et al.

CARMICHAEL Scottish. "Follower of Michael."

CARMINE Latin. "Song." **Carman, Carmen**

CARNEY Irish. "Winner." **Carny, Kearney** et al.

CAROLLAN Irish. "Little champion." **Carlin** et al., **Carolan**

CARR Scandinavian. "Marsh." **Karr, Kerr**

CARROLL Variant of **Charles.** Old German, "man." **Carel, Carol, Carolus, Carrol, Caryl, Karel, Karol, Karoly**

CARSON Old English. "Son of the marsh-dwellers."

CARSTEN Variant of **Christian.** Greek, "Christian."

CARSWELL Old English. "Well where the watercress grows." **Cresswell**

CARTER Old English. "One who drives carts."

CARTHAGE English variant of **Caradoc.** Welsh, "good natured." Also an ancient city in North Africa.

CARVELL Old French. "Swampy dwelling." **Carvel**

Name it like Beckham

One variation on the name-the-child-after-a-place scheme is to choose the baby's name based on where the little tyke was conceived. David Beckham, a soccer superstar, and his wife, Victoria, a.k.a. Posh Spice, named their son *Brooklyn* for the place where his first cell came together.

In a *Vanity Fair* article, Ron Howard, the movie director, said that his twin daughters both have the middle name *Carlyle* because they were conceived in the Carlyle Hotel in New York City. Howard's son was named after Reed Cross, a street in London. Does this mean the director and his wife actually happened to "do it in the road"? The answer is no. "Volvo," according to Howard, "isn't a very good middle name."

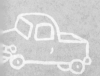

CARVER Old English. "One who carves wood."

CARY Old English. "Pretty stream." **Carey**

CASE English variant of **Casimir**. Slavic, "bringing peace." Also short form of **Cassius**.

CASEY Irish. "Vigilant." Also short form of **Casimir, Cassius**. **Cacey, Cayce, Caycey, Kasey**

CASH Short form of **Cassius**. Latin. "Vain."

CASIMIR Slavic. "Bringing peace." **Case, Casey, Casimire, Cass, Cassie, Cassy, Kazimierz** et al.

CASPER Persian. "Guard." **Caspar, Cass, Cassie, Cassy, Gaspar** et al., **Jaspar, Jasper, Josper, Kaspar**

CASSIDY Irish. "Clever." **Cass, Cassady, Cassie, Cassy**

CASSIUS Latin. "Vain." American boxer Cassius Clay, as he was known until he converted to Islam in the 1960s and changed his name to *Muhammad Ali*. **Case, Casey, Cash, Casius, Caskey, Cass, Cassie, Cassio, Cassy, Cazzie, Cazzy**

CASTOR Greek. "Beaver." **Caster**

CATALIN Hungarian masculine form of **Catherine**. Greek, "pure."

CATHBAD Irish. In myth, the chief druid of Ulster. Pronounced "cah-vah."

CATO Latin. "All-knowing." Cato the Elder, Roman statesman, 234–149 B.C. Cato the Younger, his grandson and a Roman Stoic philosopher and patriot, 95–46 B.C.

CAVAN Variant of **Kevin**. Irish, "Handsome." **Caven, Kavan**

CECIL Latin. "Blind one." **Cecilio, Cecilius, Celio**

CEDRIC Old English. "Battle leader." **Cad, Caddaric, Ced, Cedrick, Cerdic, Ceredic, Rick**

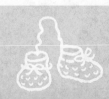

CELERINO Italian from Latin. "Speed up."

CEPHAS Hebrew. "Rock."

CHAD Old English. "Warrior." Also short form of **Chadwick**.
Ceadda, Chadd, Chaddie, Chaddy

CHADWICK Old English. "Warrior's camp." **Chad**

CHAIM Hebrew. "Life." **Chayim, Chayyim, Chayym, Hyman**
et al.

CHAL English Gypsy. "Boy."

CHANCE Middle English. "Good fortune."

CHANCELLOR Middle English. "Chief secretary." **Chance,**
Chaunce, Chauncey

CHANDLER Old French. "Candle maker." **Chan**

CHANEY Old French. "Oak tree." **Cheney**

CHANG Chinese. "Prosperity."

CHANNING Old French. "Official of the church." **Canning,**
Cannon, Canon, Chan, Chane

CHAPMAN Old English. "Peddler." **Chap, Chappy, Manny**

CHARLEMAGNE Old French. "Charles the Great."
Charlemagne I, emperor of the West (800–814), Carolingian
king of the Franks (768–814).

CHARLES Old German. "Man." **Carl, Carlie, Carling, Carlo,**
Carlos, Carlus, Carly, Carroll et al., **Cathal, Cathaoir, Char,**
Charlet, Charley, Charlie, Charlot, Charls, Charly, Chas,
Chaz, Chick, Chip, Chipper, Chuck, Karl et al.

CHARLESTON Middle English. "Charles's town." **Chariton**

CHAS English variant of **Charles**. **Chaz**

CHASE Old French. "Hunter."

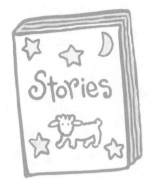

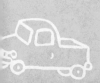

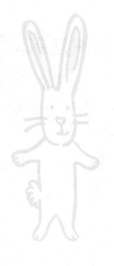

CHAUNCEY Middle English. "Church official." **Chance, Chancey, Chaune**

CHEN Chinese. "Great" or "fast."

CHESTER Old English, from Latin. "Camp." Also short form of **Rochester.**

CHET English. Nickname, usually for **Chester** or **Rochester.** Also Thai, "brother." Chet (Chester Burton) Atkins, 1924–2001, American finger-picking guitar player, creator of the "Nashville Sound" of country music. Chet (Chesney Henry) Baker, 1928–1988, American jazz trumpet player and singer.

CHETWIN Old English. "Little house on the lane." **Chetwyn, Chetwynd**

CHEVALIER French. "Knight." **Chevy**

CHEVY English. Nickname, usually for **Chevalier.** Chevy (Cornelius Crane) Chase, contemporary American comedian, an original cast member of the television show *Saturday Night Live.*

CHICK English. Nickname, usually for **Charles.** Chick Corea, contemporary American jazz pianist.

CHICO Spanish. Diminutive of **Francisco;** also "small" or "boy."

CHIEL Scottish. "Boy." **Chield**

CHILTON Old English. "Cold town."

CHIP English. Nickname, usually for **Charles.**

CHRIS Short form of **Christian, Christopher. Kris**

CHRISTIAN Greek. "Christian." **Chretien, Chris, Chrissie, Chrissy, Christiaan, Christiano, Christie, Christo, Cristian, Cristo, Cristy, Karsten** et al., **Kit, Kris, Kristian** et al.

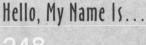 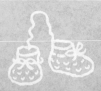

SON OF JESUS?

In the Ukraine and other Slavic countries, a person has three names, a given name such as *Ivan* or *Maria*, followed by a patronymic name—a name formed from the father's given name plus *ovich* ("son of") for men and *ovna* ("daughter of") for women—and then the surname.

This naming practice created an interesting situation in the Ukraine when the parents of a newborn son showed up at the local marriage registry and announced that they wanted to name their son *Khrystos,* or "Jesus Christ." Officials tried to convince the parents that the name would sound absurd, for two reasons. First, the child, whose father's first name is *Vladimir,* would be named *Khrystos Vladimirovich,* or "Jesus Christ, the son of Vladimir." Second, and even worse, if this boy grew up and had a son of his own, that offspring's patronymic name would be *Khrystosovich,* or "son of Jesus Christ." Officials added that the Orthodox Church would probably take a dim view of all this. Under Ukrainian law, however, parents can name babies whatever they want, so *Khrystos Vladimirovich* it is.

CHRISTMAS English. "Christ's mass," mid-winter holiday.

CHRISTO Bulgarian variant of **Christian.** Greek, "Christian." Cristo Javacheff, contemporary artist of enormous projects involving cloth. **Cristo**

CHRISTOPHER Greek. "Carrier of Christ." **Chris, Christie, Christof, Christoffer, Christoforo, Christoph, Christophe, Christophoros, Christos, Cris, Cristobal, Cristoforo, Kit, Kris, Kristofer** et al.

CHUCK Nickname for **Charles.** Old German, "man."

CHURCHILL Old English. "Church hill." Some parents have named their boys *Churchill* after Sir Winston Churchill, 1874–1947, British prime minister and author.

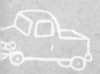

CIARAN Irish. "Black." **Ciaren, Kiaran, Kiaren, Kiraren, Kyran**

CICERO Latin. "Scholar." Roman orator, first century B.C. **Cicerone, Ciceroni**

CID Spanish, from Arabic. "Lord." El Cid, or Cid Campeador, a soldier romanticized in literature who fought first for the Christians, then for the Moors, and later against both. **Cyd**

CILAS Greek. "Wood." **Cilus**

CLANCY Irish. "Family." **Claney**

CLARENCE Latin. "Bright." **Clair, Clarance, Clarrance, Clarrence**

CLARK Old French. "Cleric, scholar." **Clarke, Clerc, Clerk**

CLAUDE Latin. "Lame." **Claud, Claudan, Claudell, Claudian, Claudianus, Claudien, Claudio, Claudius**

CLAUS Short form of **Nicholas.** Greek, "people of victory." **Claas, Claes, Clause, Klaus** et al.

CLAY Old English "Clay."

CLETIS Greek or Latin. "Illustrious." **Cletus**

CLAYBORNE Old English. "Stream near clay deposits." **Claiborn, Claiborne, Clay, Claybourne, Clayburn, Clayburne**

CLAYLAND Old English. "Clay land."

CLAYTON Old English. "Town near clay deposits."

CLEARY Irish. "Learned one."

CLEMENT Latin. "Granting mercy." St. Clement. **Clem, Clemens, Clemente, Clementius, Clemmie, Clemmy, Klemens, Klement, Kliment**

CLEON Greek. "Renowned." **Kleon**

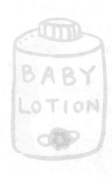

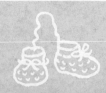

CLEVELAND Old English. "Hilly area." **Cleavland, Cleavon, Cleve, Clevon**

CLIFF Old English. "Steep slope." **Cliffie, Clyff**

CLIFFORD Old English. "Water crossing near a cliff." **Cliff, Cliffie, Clyff, Clyfford**

CLIFTON Old English. "Town near a cliff." **Cliff, Clift, Clyfton**

CLINT Old English "Headland." Clint Eastwood, contemporary American actor. **Klint**

CLINTON Old English. "Settlement near the headland." **Clint**

CLIVE Old English. "Cliff." **Cleve, Clyve**

CLOVIS Old German. "Renowned fighter." Clovis I, Frankish king, 481–511.

CLOYCE Middle English. "To hamper." **Cloy, Cloyd**

CLUNY Irish. "Meadow."

CLYDE Scottish. A river in Scotland. **Cly, Clydell, Clywd**

COBURN Old English. "Confluence." **Coby, Cockburn**

CODY Old English. "Pillow." Also a town in Wyoming. **Codee, Codey, Codie, Kody**

COLBERT Old English. "Renowned mariner." **Cole, Colt, Colvert, Culbert**

COLBY Old Norse. "Dark farmstead." **Collby**

COLE Middle English. "Coal."

COLEMAN English. "Coal man." **Colman**

COLIN Irish, Scottish. "Young creature." **Cailean, Colan, Cole, Collie, Collin, Colyn**

COLLEY Old English. "Dark-haired." **Collie**

Who represents the 'hood, Puff Daddy or Sean Combs?

Rap stars, those sometime bad boys and girls of music, turn out to have real names that mostly sound downright normal, if not a bit nerdy.

B-Real—Louis Freeze

Big Boi—Antoine Patton

Big Daddy Kane—Antonio Hardy

Big Punisher—Christopher Carlos Rios

Black Rob—Robert Ross

Bushwick Bill—Richard Steven Shaw

Canibus—Germaine Williams

Cappadonna—Darly Hill

Chuck D—Carlton Ridenhour

Coolio—Artis Ivey, Jr.

Da Brat—Shawntae Harris

DMX—Earl Simmons

Dr. Dre—Andre Brown

Eazy-E—Eric Wright

Eminem—Marshall Mathers

Funkmaster Flex—Aston Taylor

Ginuwine—Elgin Lumpkin

Heavy D.—Dwight Myers

Ice Cube—O'Shea Jackson

Ice-T—Tracy Marrow

J. Z.—Shawn Carter

Ja Rule—Jeffery Atkins

L. L. Cool J—James Todd Smith

Lil' Kim—Kimberly Denise Jones

M. C. Hammer—Stanley Kirk Burrell

Missy Elliott—Melissa Arnette

Mos Def—Dante Smith

Mystikal—Michael Tyler

Notorious B.I.G.—Christopher Wallace

Pharaohe Monch—Troy Jameson

Puffy/Puff Daddy—Sean Combs

Queen Latifah—Dana Owens

Redman—Reggie Noble

Scarface—Brad Jordan

Sisqo—Mark Andrews

Snoop Doggy Dogg—Cordazer Calvin Broadus

Timbaland—Tim Mosley

Vanilla Ice—Robert van Winkle

2Pac—Lesane Parish Crooks

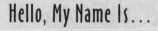

COLLIER Old English. "Coal miner." **Colier, Colis, Collayer, Collis, Collyer**

COLLINS Irish. "Holly."

COLTER Old English. "Colt herder."

COLTON Old English. "Dark town." **Collton, Colston**

COLUMBO Latin. "Dove." **Colón, Colum, Columb, Colombo, Columbus**

COLVILLE Old French. "Coal town." **Colvile, Colvill**

COLWYN Welsh. A river in Wales. **Collwyn, Colwin, Colwynn**

CONAN Irish. "High, lifted up." **Con, Conant, Conn, Conney, Connie, Conny**

CONLAN Irish. "Hero." **Conlen, Conley, Conlin, Conlon, Connlyn**

CONNOR Irish. "Desire." **Conor**

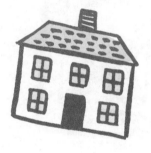

CONRAD Old German. "Wise counselor." **Con, Conn, Connie, Conny, Conrade, Conrado, Curt, Konrad** et al., **Kurt**

CONROY Irish. "Wise man."

CONSTANTINE Latin. "Steadfast." The name of Roman and Byzantine emperors. **Con, Conney, Connie, Considine, Consta, Constans, Constant, Constantin, Constantinius, Constantino, Costa, Costain, Costea** et al., **Custance, Konstantin** et al.

CONWAY Welsh. "Holy river." Conway Twitty, American singer and guitar player. **Conwy**

COOK English. "Cook." **Cooke**

COOPER Old English. "Barrel maker." **Coop**

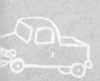

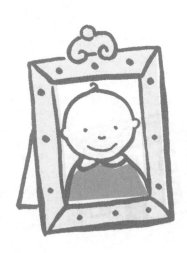

CORBETT Latin. "Raven." **Corb, Corbet, Corbie, Corbin, Corbit, Corbitt, Cory**

CORCORAN Irish. "Ruddy." **Cork**

CORDELL Old French. "Rope maker." **Cord, Cordas**

COREY Irish. "A hollow." **Correy, Corrie, Corry, Cory, Currie, Curry**

CORLISS Old English. "Benevolent." **Corley**

CORMICK Irish. "Chariot driver." **Cormac, Cormack**

CORNELIUS Latin. "Like a horn." **Con, Conney, Connie, Cornelious, Cornell** et al., **Cornelus, Corney, Cornie, Cornilius, Kornelisz, Neel, Neilus, Neely**

CORNELL French variant of **Cornelius. Cornall, Cornel, Corney, Kornel**

CORNWALLIS Old English. "Man from Cornwall." **Cornwall**

CORT Old German. "Brave." Also variant of **Court, Curt. Cortie, Corty, Kort**

CORWIN Old English. "Close companion." **Corwan, Corwyn, Corwynn, Cory**

CORYDON Greek. "Battle-ready." **Coridon, Coryden, Coryell**

COSGROVE Irish. "Champion." **Cosgrave**

COSMO Greek. "Organization." **Cosimo, Cosmas, Cosmé, Kosmé, Kosmo**

COSTEA Hungarian. "Constant." **Costin, Costine**

COUNT Old French. "Nobleman." **Counte**

COURT Old French. "Court." Also variant of **Curt. Cort**

COURTLAND Old English. "Land owned by the court." **Cortland, Cortlandt, Courtlandt**

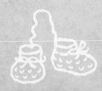

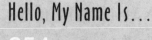

COURTNEY Old English. "Man of the court." **Cortney, Courtenay**

COVELL Old English. "Hill with a cave."

COVINGTON Old English. "Town on a cove."

COWAN Middle English. "Twin." **Coe, Cowen, Cowie**

COY Old French. "Modest." **Coye**

COYLE Irish. "Follows the battle."

CRADDOCK Variant of **Caradoc.** Welsh, "good-natured." **Caradoc, Caradog**

CRAIG Irish. "Rocky outcrop."

CRAMER Old German. "One who sells from a stall." **Cram, Kramer**

CRANDALL Old English. "Valley of cranes." **Crandal, Crandell**

CRANE Old English. "To stretch."

CRANLEY Old English. "Meadow with the cranes." **Cranlee, Cranleigh, Cranly**

CRANSTON Old English. "Town of cranes."

CRAWFORD Old English. "Crossing of the crows." **Craw, Crow**

CREIGHTON Old English. "Rocky town." **Crayton, Creight, Crichton, Crighton, Crite**

CRESSWELL Old English. "Well where watercress grows." **Carswell**

CRISPIN Latin. "Curly-haired." **Crepin, Crispian, Crispianus, Crispinian, Crispinianus, Crispino, Crispo, Crispus**

CROFTON Old English. "Small field." **Croft**

CROMWELL Old English. "Winding spring."

CROSBY Middle English. "At the cross." **Crosbey, Crosbie**

CROSLEY Old English. "Meadow of the cross." **Croslea, Crosleigh, Crosly, Crosslee, Crossley, Crosslie**

CROWTHER Old English. "Fiddler."

CUALGNE Irish. A district of ancient Ireland. **Cooley**

CULLEN Irish. "Handsome." **Cull, Cullan, Culley, Cullie, Cullin**

CULLEY Irish. "Woods." **Cully**

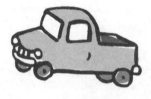

CULVER Old English. "Dove." **Colver, Cully**

CUNNINGHAM Irish. "Village of the milk pail." **Conyngham**

CURLEY English. "Curly-haired." **Curly**

CURRAN Irish. "Champion." **Curr, Currey, Currie, Curry**

CURTIS Old French. "Polite." **Cort, Cortie, Corty, Court, Courts, Curcio, Curt, Curtell, Curtice, Curtiss, Kurt, Kurtis**

CUTHBERT Old English. "Famous, brilliant." **Cudbert, Cudbright, Cuddie, Cuddy, Cumbert, Cuthbrid**

CUTLER Old English. "Knife maker."

CYPRIAN Greek. "From Cyprus." **Cipriano, Ciprien, Cyprien**

CYRANO Greek. "From Cyrene." Cyrano de Bergerac, the huge-nosed hero of a drama by the same name by Edmond Rostand.

CYRIL Greek. "Lord." **Ciril, Cirilio, Cirillo, Cirilo, Cyrill, Cyrille, Cyrillus, Kiril, Kirillos, Kyril**

CYRUS Persian. "Sun" or "throne." **Ciro, Cy, Cyrie**

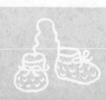
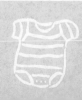

DACEY Latin. "From Dacia." **Dacian, Dacy, Daicey, Daicy**

DAEDALUS Greek. In myth, the architect who built the Labyrinth to confine the Minotaur, and the father of Icarus. **Dedalus**

DAG Scandinavian. "Day." Dag Hammarskjöld, secretary general of the United Nations from 1953 to 1961. **Dagny**

DAGAN Hebrew. "Grain." **Dagon**

DAGWOOD Old English. "Shining forest." The main character in the comic strip *Blondie*.

DAHI Welsh. "Agile." **Dathi**

DAKAR Capital of Senegal.

DAKOTA Sioux. "Friend." **Tadoka**

DALBERT Old English. "Bright-shining one." **Bert**

DALE Old Norse "Wide valley." **Dael, Dail, Dal, Daley, Dali, Dallan, Dallin, Dalt, Dayle, Delles**

DALLAS Scottish. "Skilled." A village in Scotland, and a city in Texas. **Dal, Dallis**

DALTON Old Norse. "Town in a valley." **Dallton, Dalten**

DALY Irish. "Assembly." **Daily, Daley, Dawley**

DALZIEL Scottish. "Small field."

DAMAN Irish. "To tame." **Damen, Damon** Damon Runyan, 1884–1946, American journalist and writer of fictional stories about New York City's underground.

IRISH NAMES

Irish names have come down from the many invaders who have swept through the Emerald Isle: the Vikings, the French, and the English, not to mention the Celts. For centuries, most people in Ireland spoke Irish (or "Gaelic" or "Irish Gaelic"), and gave their children names such as *Padraic* or *Maire*. However, in 1695, England imposed a series of penal laws aimed at eliminating Catholicism and otherwise subjugating the Irish. The Irish language was outlawed, and this brought about a shift in names to their English equivalents. *Padraic* became *Patrick*. *Maire* became *Mary*. *Sean* was transformed into *John,* and *Caitlin* became *Kathleen.* As the years wore on, Irish came to be spoken only in rural areas.

In 1893, the Gaelic League was founded with the purpose of keeping the Irish language alive. Chapters sprang up in the United States as well as in Ireland. During the twentieth century, Irish culture gradually became respectable and even fashionable. Along with celebrations of Irish music and dance came a new appreciation for the old Irish names. Now American schools have their Liams and Fionas, even from families who have no Irish background at all.

Following are some Irish names for boys:

Baird	"poet"
Barra ("bear-rah")	"fair-headed"
Carlus	Irish variant of *Charles*
Cualgne ("COO-al-ny")	district of ancient Ireland
Curran	"champion"
Daman ("DAY-mun")	"to tame"
Fergus	"best" or "strength"
Finn, Fynn	"fair"
Gaibrial ("gabe-ree-all")	Irish variant of *Gabriel*
Keir ("keer")	"dark-haired"
Miach ("MEE-ah")	"healer"
Murchadh ("MUR-cah")	"sea warrior"
Piaras ("PEE-ah-russ")	Irish variant of *Peter*
Ronan	"little seal"
Sean, Cian	Irish variant of *John*
Uilliam ("OOL-yum")	Irish variant of *William*

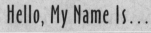
 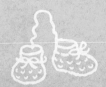

And here are some Irish names for girls:

Aife, Aoife ("EE-feh")	a legendary female warrior	
Ashling	"dream"	
Boenn ("BO-in")	unknown	
Cairenn ("KAY-ren")	"keel"	
Deirdre ("DEE-druh")	a legendary heroine	
Fiall ("FEE-all")	unknown	
Iseult ("EE-solt")	a legendary princess	

Jana ("JAH-nah")	feminine form of *John*
Maurya ("MAR-yah")	variant of *Mary*
Meath ("MEE-ath")	county in eastern Ireland
Morrigan	battle goddess
Noirin ("nor-EEN")	honor
Sinead ("shi-NADE")	variant of *Jane*
Sinann ("SHIN-on")	the river Shannon
Siobhan ("zhuh-VON")	variant of *Joan*

MOST POPULAR NAMES IN IRELAND

In a time when Irish names such as *Erin, Megan,* and *Maura* are popular, it's interesting to see what Irish people in Ireland name their babies. Here is a list of favorites from 2002, the most recent available.

Boys	**Girls**
Aaron	Amy
Adam	Aoife
Cian	Chloe
Conor	Ciara
Daniel	Emma
David	Hannah
Dylan	Katie
Jack	Lauren
James	Leah
John	Megan
Luke	Niamh
Michael	Rachel
Patrick	Rebecca
Ryan	Sarah
Sean	Sophie

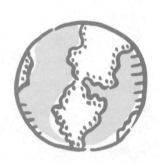

DAMIAN Greek. "Fate." **Daemon, Daimen, Daimon, Dame, Dameon, Damian, Damián, Damiano, Damien, Damion, Damlan, Damlano, Damyan, Damyen, Damyon, Darmon, Day, Dayman, Daymond, Demian**

DAN Short form of **Daniel.** Hebrew, "God is my judge."

DANE Old Norse. "From Denmark." **Dainard, Dana, Danie**

DANESH Arabic. "Wisdom," "learning," or "science." **Daanish**

DANIEL Hebrew. "God is my judge." **Dan, Dana, Danal, Dane, Daneal, Danel, Dani, Danial, Daniele, Danil, Danilo, Dannel, Dannet, Dannie, Danny, Danyal, Danyel, Deiniol, Dennel**

DANTE Latin. "Lasting." Dante Aligheri, 1265–1321, author of the *Divine Comedy.*

DARBY Old English. "Park with deer." **Dar, Darb, Darbie, Derby**

DARCY Irish. "Dark." **Dar, Darce, Darcey, Darsey, Darsy**

DARDANOS Greek. In myth, the founder of the Trojan race. **Dard**

DARIUS Greek. "Great." **Daare, Dar, Daria, Darian, Darien, Dario, Darrel** et al., **Darren** et al.

DARNELL Old English. "Hidden spot." **Darnall**

DARREL French variant of **Darius.** Greek, "great." **Dar, Dare, Darell, Darol, Darold, Darral, Darrell, Darrill, Darrol, Darryl, Daryl, Derril, Deryl, Deryll, Dorrel**

DARREN Variant of **Darius.** Greek, "great." **Dar, Dare, Daren, Darin, Daron, Darran, Darrin, Darron, Darryn, Deron, Derron**

DARROW Old English. "Spear." **Daro**

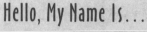

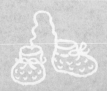

DARTON Old English. "Settlement of the deer."

DARWIN Old English. "Dear friend." **Darwyn, Derwin, Derwyn, Derwynn, Durwin**

DASHIELL Unknown origin. Dashiell Hammett, 1884–1961, American writer of detective novels. **Dashiel**

DAVID Hebrew. "Beloved by God." **Dab, Dabbey, Dabby, Dabko, Dabney, Daffy, Dafyd, Dafydd, Dahi, Dai, Dakin, Dako, Dathi, Daud, Daue, Dav, Dave, Daveed, Daven, Davey, Davi, Davidde, Davide, Davidyne, Davie, Davin, Daviot, Davit, Davon, Davy, Davyd, Daw, Dawe, Dawes, Dawood, Dawoodji, Dawud, Deakin, Deio, Devi**

DAVIS Old English. "David's son." **Dave, Davidson, Davies, Davison, Davy**

DAWSON Old English. "David's son."

DEAN Old English, "valley." Middle English, from Latin, "leader of ten." **Deane, Dee, Deen, Dene, Deno, Deyn, Dino, Dinu**

DEARBORN Old English. "Brook of the deer." **Dearborne, Dearbourn, Dearburne, Deerborn, Deerborne, Deerbourn, Deerbourne**

DECIMUS Latin. "Tenth."

DECLAN Irish. A fifth-century bishop.

DEDRICK English variant of **Theodoric.** Old German, "people's ruler." **Dedric, Diederick, Dietrick**

DEEMS Old English. "Judge's child."

DEEN Arabic. "Religious."

DELANEY Irish. "Offspring of the challenger." **Delaine, Delainey, Delainy, Delane, Delany**

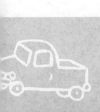

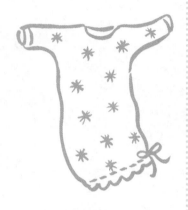

DELANO Old French. "Nut-tree forest."

DELBERT Old English. "Light as day." **Bert**

DELLING Old Norse. "Shining."

DELMORE Latin. "Of the sea." **Del, Delmar, Delmer, Delmor**

DELOS Greek. "Ring." **Deli, Delius**

DELROY French. "Of the king." **Delroi**

DELVIN Greek. "Dolphin." **Del, Delvinn**

DELWIN Old English. "Proud friend." **Dalwin, Dalwyn, Del, Delavan, Delevan, Dellwin, Delwyn, Delwynn**

DEMETRIUS Greek. Masculine form of **Demeter,** goddess of fertility. **Demetri, Demetrio, Demetris, Dhimitrios, Dimetre, Dimitri, Dimitrie, Dimitrios, Dimitry, Dimitru, Dmitri, Dmitrios, Dmitry**

DEMOS Greek. "The people." **Demas**

DEMPSEY Irish. "Proud." **Demp, Dempsy**

DEMPSTER Old English. "One who judges."

DENBY Scandinavian. "Danish village." **Danby, Den, Denbey, Denbigh, Denney, Dennie, Denny**

DENHAM Old English. "Village in a valley."

DENHOLM Swedish. "Home of the Danes."

DENLEY Old English. "Meadow in a valley." **Denlie, Denly**

DENMAN Old English. "Dane."

DENNIS Variant of **Dionysus,** Greek god of the vine. **Deenys, Den, Denies, Denis, Dennes, Dennet, Denney, Dennie, Denny, Dennys, Denys**

DENNISON Old English. "Son of Dennis." **Den, Denison, Dennyson, Tennyson**

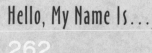

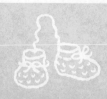

DENTON Old English. "Village in the valley." **Denny, Dent, Denten, Dentin**

DENVER Old English. "Forest valley." Capital of Colorado.

DENZIL Irish, Scottish. "Stronghold." **Denzel, Denzell, Denziel, Denzill.** Denzel Washington, contemporary film actor, winner of a 2002 Oscar.

DEODATUS Latin. "Gift of the gods." **Deodaonatus, Deodat, Dieudonné**

DERBY Old English. "Deer farm." **Darby** et al.

DEREK Variant of **Theodoric.** Old German, "people's ruler." **Darek, Darrick, Dereck, Deric, Derick, Derik, Derk, Derreck, Derrek, Derrick, Derrik, Derryck, Derryk, Deryk, Deryke, Dirk** et al.

DERMOT Variant of **Diarmuid.** Irish, "without envy." **Dermott**

DEROR Hebrew. "Freedom." **Derori, Dror**

DERRY Irish. Short form of *Londonderry,* the name of a city in Northern Ireland. **Derrie**

DERWARD Old English. "Gatehouse keeper." **Durward**

DERWIN Old English. "Dear friend." **Darwin, Darwyn, Derwyn, Derwynn, Durwin**

DESIDERIO Latin. "Desired." **Desi, Desideratus, Desiderius, Diderot** et al., **Didot, Dizier.** Desi Arnaz, twentieth-century musician, composer, actor, and husband of Lucille Ball.

DESMOND Irish. "From South Munster." **Des, Desi, Desmund, Dezi**

DEVERELL Old English. "River bank."

DEVEREUX French variant of **Eberhard.** Old German, "strength of a boar."

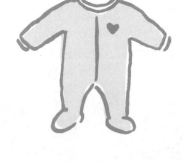

DEVIN Irish. "Bard." **Dev, Devon**

DEVINE Irish. "Ox."

DEVLIN Irish. "Fierce courage." **Devland, Devlen, Devlyn**

DEVON English. A county in England. **Devin, Devonn, Devyn**

DEWITT Flemish. "Blond." **Dewitt, Dwight, Wit, Witt**

DEXTER Latin. "Right-handed." **Decca, Deck, Dex**

DIAMOND Middle English. "Diamond" or, figuratively, "person of brilliant attainments."

DIARMUID Irish. "Without envy." In myth, a warrior for Finn mac Cumaill. Finn's fiancée forced Diarmuid to elope with her. **Dermot, Dermott, Diarmid, Diarmuit**

DICK Nickname for **Richard.** Old German, "great ruler."

DIEGO Spanish variant of **James.** Hebrew, "he who supplants."

DIETER Old German. "Army of the people."

DIETRICH Variant of **Theodoric.** Old German, "people's ruler." **Dedrick** et al., **Deke, Derek** et al., **Dierk, Dirk** et al., **Dtrik, Dytrych**

DIDIER French variant of **Desiderio.** "Desired."

DIGBY Old Norse. "Town by the canal."

DILBERT Frustrated office worker in the contemporary comic strip of the same name.

DILLON Irish. "Loyal." **Dilian, Dilon, Dyllon, Dylon**

DINO Italian variant of **Dean.** Latin, "leader of ten."

DINSMORE Irish. "Hill fortress." **Dinnie, Dinny, Dinse**

DINU Portuguese variant of **Dean.** Latin, "leader of ten."

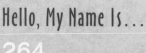

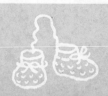

DIOMEDES Greek. In myth, a heroic fighter for Greece in the siege of Troy. **Diomed, Diomede**

DIONYSUS Greek. "God of the Nysa," a lovely, hidden valley. The god of the vine. **Dion, Dionisio, Dionysios, Dionysos, Dionysus**

DIRK Variant of **Theodoric.** Old German, "people's ruler." **Dirck, Dirke, Dyrk**

DIXON Old English. "Son of Dick." **Dickson, Diksin**

DOANE Old English. "Rolling hills."

DODGE Variant of **Roger.** Old German, "renowned spearman." **Dodger**

DOHERTY Irish. "Harmful." **Daugherty, Docherty, Dougherty, Douherty**

DOLAN Irish. "Black-haired."

DOMINIC Latin. "Lord." **Dom, Domenic, Domenico, Domenikos, Domingo, Domini, Dominick, Dominie, Dominik, Dominique, Nick**

DONAHUE Irish. "Dark fighter." **Donohoe, Donohue**

DONALD Scottish. "World mighty." **Donal, Donall, Donalt, Donaugh, Donny**

DONATO Latin. "Given." **Don, Donary, Donatus, Donny**

DONNEL Irish. "Hill." **Domhnall, Donn, Donnell, Donnelly, Donny, Doon, Dun**

DONOVAN Irish. "Dark." **Donavon, Donevin, Donevon, Donoven, Donovon**

DOOLEY Irish. "Dark hero."

DORAN Irish. "Fist." **Dore et al., Doron, Dorran, Dorren**

Keeping it short on the canvas

The Spanish painter known to the world as El Greco, which means "The Greek," was given this much longer name at birth: *Domenikos Theotokiopoulos.* That mouthful of a name would have taken up considerable space on his paintings, hence the shortened moniker.

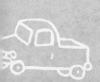

Tour de France winners

This famous bicycle race was canceled during both World War I and World War II, but otherwise it has taken place every year beginning in 1902. Here are the names and home countries of the winners.

Lance Armstrong *(United States, 1999–2004)*
Marco Pantani *(Italy, 1998)*
Jan Ullrich *(Germany, 1997)*
Bjarne Riis *(Denmark, 1996)*
Miguel Indurain *(Spain, 1991–1995)*
Greg LeMond *(United States, 1989, 1990)*
Pedro Delgado *(Spain, 1988)*
Stephen Roche *(Ireland, 1987)*
Greg LeMond *(United States, 1986)*
Bernard Hinault *(France, 1985)*
Laurent Fignon *(France, 1983, 1984)*
Bernard Hinault *(France, 1978, 1979, 1981, 1982)*
Joop Zoetemelk *(Netherlands, 1980)*
Bernard Thévenet *(France, 1975, 1977)*
Lucien Van Impe *(Belgium, 1976)*
Eddie Merckx *(Belgium, 1969–1972, 1974)*
Luis Ocana *(Spain, 1973)*
Jan Jansen *(Netherlands, 1968)*
Roger Pingeon *(France, 1967)*
Lucian Almar *(France, 1966)*
Felice Gimondi *(Italy, 1965)*

Jacques Anquetil *(France, 1961–1964)*
Gastone Nencini *(Italy, 1960)*
Federico Bahamontes *(Spain, 1959)*
Charly Gaul *(Luxembourg, 1958)*
Jacques Anquetil *(France, 1957)*
Roger Walkowiak *(France, 1956)*
Louison Bobet *(France, 1953–1955)*
Fausto Coppi *(Italy, 1949, 1952)*
Hugo Koblet *(Switzerland, 1951)*
Ferdinand Kubler *(Switzerland, 1950)*
Gino Bartali *(Italy, 1948)*
Jean Robic *(France, 1947)*
Sylvere Maes *(Belgium, 1936, 1939)*
Gino Bartali *(Italy, 1938)*
Roger Lapeble *(France, 1937)*
Romain Maes *(Belgium, 1935)*
Antonin Magne *(France, 1934)*
Georges Speicher *(France, 1933)*
André Leducq *(France, 1930, 1932)*
Antonin Magne *(France, 1931)*
Maurice Dewsele *(Belgium, 1929)*
Nicholas Frantz *(Luxembourg, 1927, 1928)*
Lucian Bruysee *(Belgium, 1926)*
Ottavio Bottecchia *(Italy, 1924, 1925)*
Henri Pellissier *(France, 1923)*
Firmin Lambot *(Belgium, 1919, 1922)*
Leon Scieur *(France, 1921)*
Phillipe Thys *(Belgium, 1913, 1914, 1920)*
Odile Defraye *(Belgium, 1912)*

Gustave Farrigou *(France, 1911)*
Octave Lapize *(France, 1910)*
François Faber *(Luxembourg, 1909)*
Lucien Petit-Breton *(France, 1907, 1908)*

René Pottier *(France, 1906)*
Louis Trousseller *(France, 1905)*
Henri Cornet *(France, 1904)*
Maurice Garin *(France, 1903)*

DORE Short form of **Isidore, Doran. Dorey, Dorie, Dory**

DORIAN Greek. "From Doris," a region of ancient Greece. **Dorien, Dorrian, Dorryen**

DOUGAL Celtic. "Dark stranger." **Doug, Dougall, Dougie, Doyle, Dug, Dugal, Dugald, Dugall, Duggy, Dugie**

DOUGLAS Scottish. "Dark water." **Doug, Dougie, Douglass, Dougy, Dugaid, Dugald, Duggie**

DOV Hebrew. "Bear."

DOW Irish. "Dark-haired." **Dowe**

DOYLE Varian of **Dougal.** Irish, "dark stranger."

DRACO Latin. "Dragon" or "serpent." Draco Malfoy, Harry Potter's antagonist at Hogwarts.

DRAKE Middle English. "Dragon."

DREW Welsh. "Wise." **Drewe, Dru**

DRISCOLL Irish. "Interpreter." **Driscol**

DRUMMOND Celtic. Unknown meaning.

DRURY Old French. "Loved one."

DRYDEN Old English. "Dry valley."

DUANE Irish. "Swarthy." **Dewain, Dewayne, Duwain, Duwayne, Dwain, Dwayne**

Naming by note

Herb Alpert, trumpet player and co-founder of A & M Records, named his son *Dore* for the first two notes of the musical scale.

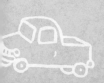

Would "Dylan" be as famous if Dylan Thomas had been an accountant?

When Dylan Thomas, the Welsh bard famous almost as much for his drunkenness as his poetry, was given his first name back in 1914, few people had heard of it, even in Wales. They pronounced it "dullan," and it was only later that the poet himself decided that he preferred that pronunciation to the one we use today.

Flash forward to a young folk singer named Robert Zimmerman, who began billing himself as Bob Dillon. He took the name from the main character, Matt Dillon, on the television show *Gunsmoke*. When Bob Dillon got to Greenwich Village, however, he decided that *Dylan* was far more hip.

So, apparently, have a lot of other people. In 1986, *Dylan* was the 86th most popular name for American boys. By 2003, it was number 19. A few girls have the name as well; in 1993 it was the 824th most popular girl's name, and in 2003 it had zoomed up to number 501.

DUDLEY Old English. "People's field."

DUFF Irish. "Swarthy." **Duffey, Duffy**

DUGAN Irish. "Swarthy." **Doogan, Dougan, Douggan, Dougie, Duggan, Dugie**

DUKE Middle English, from Old French. "Leader."

DUNCAN Scottish. "Brown fighter." **Dunn**

DUNHAM Irish, Scottish. "Brown one."

DUNLEY Old English. "Hill meadow."

DUNLOP Scottish. "Muddy hill."

DUNMORE Scottish. "Castle on a hill."

DUNN Irish, Scottish. "Brown." **Dunne**

DUNSTAN Old English. "Hill with boulders."

DUNTON Old English. "Hill town."

DURANT French, from Latin. "Lasting." **Durand, Durante, Duryea**

DURWARD Old English. "Gatehouse guard." **Derward**

DURWIN Old English. "Dear friend." **Derwin** et al., **Durwyn**

DUSTIN Old German. "Brave warrior." **Dustan, Dustie, Duston, Dusty, Dustyn**

DWIGHT Flemish. "Light-colored." **Dewitt, DeWitt, Diot, Doyt, Wit, Wittie, Witty**

DYER Old English. "Cloth dyer."

DYLAN Welsh. "Son of the sea." **Dill, Dillie, Dillon, Dilly**

DYSON Old English. "Son of a dyer."

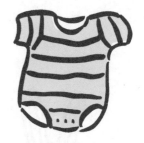

EAMON Irish variant of **Edmund.** Old English, "wealthy protector." **Eamonn**

EARL Old English. "Nobleman." **Earle, Earlie, Early, Erl, Erle**

EATON Old English. "Settlement on the river." **Eton, Eyton**

EBENEZER Hebrew. "Stone of help." Ebenezer Scrooge, the greedy misanthrope of Charles Dickens's *Christmas Carol.* **Eb, Ebbaneza, Eben, Ebeneezer, Ebeneser, Ebenezar, Eveneser**

EBERHARD Old German. "Strength of a boar." **Eberhardt, Everard** et al., **Everhardt**

EDBERT Old English. "Wealthy and bright."

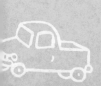

EDEL Old German. "Noble." **Adel**

EDEN Hebrew. "Pleasure." **Eaden, Eadin, Edin, Edyn**

EDGAR Old English. "Wealthy spearman." **Eadger, Ed, Eddie, Eddy, Edgard, Edgardo, Ned, Neddie, Neddy, Ted, Teddie, Teddy**

EDISON Old English. "Son of Edward." **Eddison, Eddy, Edson**

EDMUND Old English. "Wealthy protector." **Eadmund, Eamon, Eamonn, Ed, Eddie, Edmon, Edmond, Edmonde, Edmondo, Ned, Neddie, Ted, Teddy**

EDRIC Old English. "Wealthy ruler." **Edrick**

EDSEL Old English. "Wealthy man's house."

EDWARD Old English. "Wealthy defender." **Ed, Eddie, Eddy, Edik, Edouard, Eduard, Eduardo, Edvard, Ewart, Ned, Neddie, Ted, Teddie**

EDWIN Old English. "Wealthy friend." **Eadwinn, Ed, Eddy, Edlin, Eduino, Edwyn, Ned, Neddy, Ted**

EFRON Hebrew. "Singing bird."

EGAN Irish. "Burning." **Egann, Egen, Egon**

EGBERT Old English. "Shining sword." **Bert, Bertie, Berty**

EGERTON Old English. Place name. **Edgerton**

EGIDIO Italian, from Greek. "Young goat." St. Egidio, thirteenth-century Italian religious figure. **Egide, Egidius, Giles** et al.

EGINHARD German. "Sword power." **Eginhardt, Egon, Einhard, Einhardt**

EGOR Russian variant of **Ingemar**. Scandinavian, "Ing's soldier." **Igor**

EINAR Old Norse. "Leader." **Ejnar, Inar**

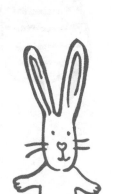

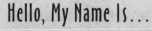

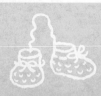

ELBERT Old German. "Illustrious." **Elbie, Ethelbert**

ELCHANAN Hebrew. "God is gracious." **Elhanan, Elhannan**

ELDEN Old English. "Old friend." **Alden** et al., **Aldwin** et al., **Eldwin** et al.

ELDER Old English. "Elder tree."

ELDON Old English. "Sacred hill."

ELDRED Old English. "Old counsel." **Aldred, Alldred, Eldrid, Elldred**

ELDRIDGE German. "Sage ruler." Eldridge Cleaver, activist for African-American rights. **Eldredge, Eldrege, Eldrige, Eldrich, Eldritch**

ELDWIN Old English. "Old friend." **Alden** et al., **Aldwin** et al., **Eldwyn, Eldwynn**

ELEAZER Variant of **Lazarus.** Hebrew, "the Lord will help." **Elazar, Eleasar, Eleazaro, Eli, Elie, Eliezer, Ely**

ELGAR Old English. "Noble spear." **Algar, Alger, Elger**

ELGIN English. "Noble" or "white."

ELI Hebrew. "On high." Also short form of **Eleazer, Elihu, Elijah. Elie, Eloi, Eloy, Ely**

ELIAS Hebrew. "The Lord is my God." **Elice, Ellice, Ellis, Elyas, Elys, Ilias**

ELIHU Hebrew. "The Lord." **Eli**

ELIJAH Hebrew. "The Lord is my God." **Eli, Elia, Elias, Elie, Eligio, Elio, Eliyahu, Ella, Elliot** et al., **Ilie, Ilija, Ilya**

ELISHA Hebrew. "The Lord is my help." **Elis, Elisee, Eliseo, Elizur, Ellas, Elly, Ely**

ELKANAH Hebrew. "God has made." **Elkan, Elkana**

ELLARD Old German. "Noble and valorous."

ELLERY Old English. "Island with elder trees." Ellery Queen, twentieth-century mystery writer. **Ellary, Ellerey**

ELLIOT English variant of **Elijah.** Hebrew, "the Lord is my God." **Eliot, Eliott, Elliott, Elyot, Elyott**

ELLIS English variant of **Elias.** Hebrew, "the Lord is my God." **Elys**

ELLISON Old English. "Son of Ellis." **Elison, Ellson, Ellyson, Elson**

ELLSWORTH Old English. "Nobleman's estate." **Ellswerth, Elsworth**

ELMER Old English. "Highborn and renowned." **Aylmer** et al., **Ellmer, Elmir, Eylmer**

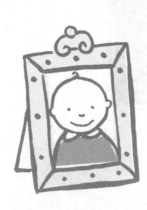

ELMO Variant of **Erasmus.** Greek, "desired." Saint Elmo.

ELMORE Old English. "Moor with elm trees."

ELROY Middle English, from Old French. "The king." **Elrad, Elrod**

ELSDON Old English. "Nobleman's hill."

ELSTON Old English. "Nobleman's town." **Ellston, Elsden, Elsdon**

ELTON Old English. "Old village." Elton John, a flamboyant pop singer with many hits in the 1970s and early 1980s. **Alton, Eldon, Ellton**

ELVIN Old English. "Of the elves." **Alvin** et al., **El, Elva**

ELVIS Scandinavian. "All-wise." Elvis Presley, rock-and-roll star. **Alvis, Alvys, Elvys**

ELWELL Old English. "Old well."

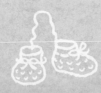

ELWOOD Old English. "Old forest." **Ellwood, Woody**

ELWYN Welsh. "Fair brow." Also variant of **Alwin. Elwin, Elwynn**

ELY Variant of **Eli.** Hebrew, "on high."

EMERSON Old German. "Emery's son."

EMERY Old German. "Home ruler." **Amerigo, Amory** et al., **Emeri, Emerich, Emmerich, Emmery, Emory**

EMIL Latin. "Eager to please." **Almericus, Almery, Amalrich, Aymil, Eemil, Emelen, Emile, Emilian, Emiliano, Emilio, Emillon, Emilyan, Emlen, Emlin**

EMLYN Welsh. Place name.

EMMANUEL Hebrew. "God is among us." **Eman, Emanual, Emanuel, Emanuele, Immanuel, Immanuele, Manny, Manuel** et al.

EMMETT Old German. "Universal." **Emmet, Emmit, Emmot, Emmott**

ENGELBERT Old German. "Angel-bright." **Bert, Berty, Ingelbert, Inglebert**

ENNIS Variant of **Angus.** Irish, "sole choice."

ENOCH Hebrew. "Dedicated." **Enock**

ENOS Hebrew. "Man." **Enosh**

ENRICO Italian variant of **Henry.** Old German, "estate ruler."

ENRIQUE Spanish variant of **Henry.** Old German, "estate ruler."

ENZO Italian variant of **Henry.** Old German, "estate ruler." Also short form of **Vincenzo, Lorenzo. Enzio**

EPHRAIM Hebrew. "Fertile." **Efraim, Efrain, Efrayim, Efrem, Efren, Ephream, Ephrem, Ephrim**

ERASMUS Greek. "Desired." **Elmo, Erasme, Erasmo, Eraste, Erastus, Ras, Rasmus**

ERASTUS Greek. "Beloved." **Eraste, Rastus**

ERCOLE Italian variant of **Hercules.** Greek, "splendid gift."

ERHARD Old German. "Strong resolve." **Erhardt, Erhart**

ERIC Scandinavian. "All-ruler." **Aric** et al., **Ehren, Erek, Erich, Erick, Erico, Erik, Erric, Errick, Eryk, Euric, Rick** et al.

ERIN Irish. "Of the island to the west," that is, Ireland.

ERLAND Old English. "Noble's land."

ERLING Old English. "Noble's son."

ERNEST Old English. "Sincere." **Earnest, Ern, Erneirs, Erneste, Ernesto, Ernestus, Ernie, Ernis, Erno, Ernst, Erny**

ERROL Scottish. "Wanderer." Errol Flynn, a Hollywood actor very popular in the 1930s and 1940s. **Erroll, Erryl, Rollo, Rolly**

ERSKINE Scottish. "High cliff." **Erskin, Kin, Kinney, Kinny**

ERVIN Scottish variant of **Irving.** Old English, "sea friend." **Earvin, Erv, Ervine, Ervyn**

ESAU Hebrew. "Hairy." In the Bible, a son of Rebekah and Isaac. Esau sold his birthright to his twin brother Jacob.

ESHAN Arabic. "Worthy."

ESMÉ French. "Esteemed."

ESMOND Old English. "Divine protector." **Esmand, Esmund**

ESTÉBAN Spanish variant of **Stephen.** Greek, "crowned." **Estaban, Estavan, Estéfan**

ESTES Spanish. "East."

ETHAN Hebrew. "Steadfastness." **Etan, Ethe**

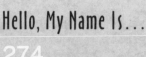

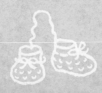

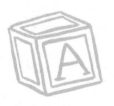
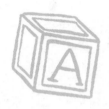
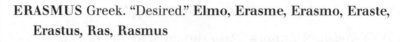

ETHELBERT Old English. "Illustrious." **Elbert, Elbie**

ETHELRED Old English. "Strong noble." **Aethelraed, Ailred, Alret, Edred**

ETHELWIN Old English. "Noble friend." **Ethelwyn, Ethelwynne**

ETIENNE French variant of **Stephen**. Greek, "crowned."

ETTORE Italian variant of **Hector**. "Loyal." **Ectore**

EUBIE English. Nickname, usually for **Eubule**. Eubie (James Herbert) Blake, twentieth-century composer and lyricist of ragtime, jazz, and pop music.

EUBULE Greek. "Good advice." **Euball, Eubie, Ewball**

EUDO Greek. "Well-being." **Eudes, Eudon, Udo, Udona**

EUGENE Greek. "Well-born." **Eugen, Eugeni, Eugenio, Eugenius, Evgeny, Gene, Yevgeny**

EUSEBIUS Greek. "Pious." **Eusebio, Eusebios.** St. Eusebio.

EUSTACE Greek. "Fertile." **Eustache, Eustachius, Eustachy, Eustashe, Eustasius, Eustatius, Eustazio, Eustis, Eustiss**

EVALD Old English. "Battle boar." **Evaldo, Ewald, Ewaldo, Ival, Ivol**

EVAN Welsh. "Young warrior." **Euan, Euen, Evans, Even, Evin, Evon, Evyn**

EVERARD Old English variant of **Eberhard**. "Strength of a boar." **Averitt, Devereux, Everardo, Everett** et al., **Evrard, Evraud, Eward, Ewart, Yves**

EVERETT Variant of **Everard**. Old English, "strength of a boar." **Averitt, Evered, Everet, Evertt**

EVERLEY Old English. "Boar meadow." **Everly**

EVERTON Old English. "Boar village."

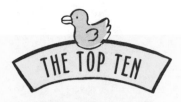

EWALD Old English. "Law-powerful." **Evald**

EWAN Celtic. Disputed meaning; "well-born" or "youth." **Euan, Euen, Ewen, Owen** et al.

EWERT Old English. "Shepherd."

EWING Old English. "Law-friend." **Ewin, Ewynn**

EZEKIEL Hebrew. "Strength of God." **Esequil, Ezechial, Ezechiel, Ezell, Eziechiele, Eziequel, Yehezekel, Zeke**

EZRA Hebrew. "Helper." **Azuriah** et al., **Esdras, Esra, Ezar, Ezer, Ezri, Ezzard, Ezzret**

FABIAN Latin. "Bean." **Fabe, Fabek, Faber, Fabert, Fabianno, Fabiano, Fabien, Fabio, Fabius, Fabiyus, Fabyan, Fabyen, Faybian, Faybien, Favian**

FABRICE French. "Works with the hands." **Fabricius, Fabrizio, Fabrizius**

FABRON French. "Young blacksmith." **Fabre, Fabroni**

FADEYKA Russian. "Courageous." **Fadey, Fadeushka, Fedeushka**

FAGAN Irish. "Fiery one." **Fagin.** In Charles Dickens's *Oliver Twist*, Fagin is the receiver of stolen goods and mentor of young thieves.

FAIRFAX Old English. "Blond."

FAISAL Arabic. "Resolute." The name of kings of Iraq and Saudi Arabia. **Faysal, Feisal**

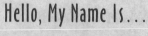

FALKNER Old English. "Falcon trainer." **Falconer, Falconner, Faulconer, Faulconner, Faulkner**

FANE Old English. "Joyous."

FARAMOND Old German. "Protected traveler." **Fara, Farman, Farmannus, Farrimond, Phareman**

FARLEY Old English. "Beautiful meadow." **Fairlay, Fairlee, Fairleigh, Fairlie, Farlay, Farlee, Farleigh, Farlie, Farly, Lee, Leigh**

FARNELL Old English. "Fern hill." **Farnall, Fernald, Furnald**

FARNHAM Old English. "Home with ferns." **Farnam, Farnum, Fernham**

FARNLEY Old English. "Meadow with ferns." **Farnlea, Farnlee, Farnleigh, Farnly, Fernleigh, Fernley**

FAROLD Old English. "Mighty voyager."

FARON Middle English. "Traveler." **Faren, Farren**

FAROUK Arabic. "Judge truth." The Egyptian king deposed for corruption in 1952. **Faruq, Faruqh**

FARQUHAR Scottish. "Very dear one." **Farquar**

FARQUHERSON Scottish. "Son of Farquhar." **Farquarson**

FARR Old English. "Voyager."

FARRELL Irish. "Valorous one." **Farrel, Farrill, Farryll, Ferrel, Ferrell, Ferryl**

FATE Latin. "Fate." **Fait, Faye**

FATEH Persian. "Victorious."

FAUST Latin. "Of good fortune." In legend, literature, and opera, a German magician and astrologer who sold his soul to the devil. **Faustino, Fausto, Faustus**

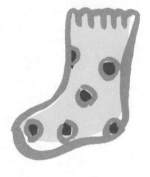

FAVIAN French variant of **Fabian**. Latin, "bean."

FAY Irish. "Raven." **Fayette**

FAZIO Short form of **Bonifacio**. Italian, from Latin. "Do-gooder."

FEDOR Variant of **Theodore**. Greek, "gift from God." **Feodor, Fyodor.** Feodor Dostoyevsky, 1828–1881, Russian novelist.

FÉLICIEN French. "Happiness."

FELIPE Spanish variant of **Philip**. Greek, "lover of horses." **Felippe, Filip, Filippo, Fillip, Flip, Lippo, Pepe, Pip, Pippo**

FELIX Latin. "Happy." **Fee, Felic, Felice, Felicio, Felike, Feliks, Felizio, Felyx**

FELTON Old English. "Village in the field." **Fell, Felt, Felten, Feltin**

FENTON Old English. "Village in the marsh." **Fen, Fennie, Fenny**

FERD German. "Horse." **Ferde, Ferdie, Ferdy**

FERDINAND Old German. "Explorer." **Ferd, Ferdie, Ferdinando, Ferdo, Ferdynand, Fernand, Fernando, Hernán, Hernando, Nando**

FERGUS Irish. "Best" or "strength." **Fearghas, Fearghus, Feargus, Fergie**

FERGUSON English. "Son of Fergus." **Fergusson**

FERMÍN Spanish. "Firm, strong." St. Fermín. **Firmín**

FERNLEY Old English. "Fern meadow." **Farnlea, Farnlee, Farnleigh, Farnley, Fernlea, Fernlee, Fernleigh, Lee, Leigh**

FERRANT Old French. "Farrier." **Farand, Farrand, Farrant, Ferrand, Ferrant**

FERRIS Irish. Disputed meaning. **Farris, Farrish, Ferriss**

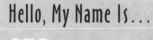

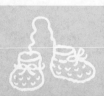

FIDEL Latin. "Faithful." **Fidele, Fidelio, Fidelis, Fido**

FIELDING Old English. "The field." **Felding**

FILBERT Middle English. "Bright loving" or "hazelnut" (because the feast day of St. Philibert occurs at about the time hazelnuts ripen). **Bert, Filberte, Filberto, Philbert, Philibert**

FILMORE Old English. "Very famous." **Fillmore, Fylmer**

FINIAN Irish. "Fair." **Finn, Finnian, Fionan, Fynn, Phinean, Phinian**

FINLAY Irish. "Fair-haired courageous one." **Findlay, Findley, Finlea, Finlee, Finley, Finn, Finnlea, Finnley, Lee, Leigh**

FINN Irish, "fair." Old Norse, "Finnish." Finn mac Cumaill, in myth the leader of a band of military men. **Eifion, Fin, Finan, Finbar, Finbarr, Finegan, Finian** et al., **Finnegan, Fion, Fionn**

FINNEGAN Irish. "Fair." *Finnegans Wake,* a novel by James Joyce, published in 1939. **Finegan**

FIORELLO Italian. "Little flower."

FIRMIN Latin. "Firm, strong." **Fermín**

FISK Middle English. "Fish." **Fish, Fiske**

FITCH Middle English, from Old French. "Fix."

FITZ Old French. "Son of."

FITZGERALD Old German. "Son of Gerald."

FITZHUGH Old German. "Son of Hugh."

FITZPATRICK Old French. "Son of Patrick."

FITZROY Old French. "Son of the king."

FLAMINIO Spanish. "Roman priest."

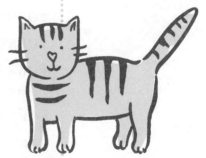

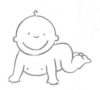

FLANN Irish. "Ruddy, red-haired." **Flannery**

FLAVIAN Latin. "Blond hair." **Flavel, Flavelle, Flavien, Flavio, Flaviu, Flavius, Flawiusz**

FLEMING Old English. "Flemish." **Flemming, Flemmyng, Flemyng**

FLETCHER Middle English. "Arrow maker." **Flecher, Fletch**

FLINT Old English. "Hard stone." **Flynt**

FLORENT Old French. "Blooming." **Florentin, Florentino, Florenz, Florinio, Florino**

FLORIAN Latin. "Blooming." **Florien, Florrian, Floryan**

FLOYD Welsh. "Gray-haired." **Lloyd, Loyd**

FLYNN Irish. "Son of the ruddy man." **Flin, Flinn, Flyn**

FOLKE Scandinavian. "Guardian of the people." **Folke, Folker, Volker, Vollker**

FORBES Scottish. "Field."

FORD Old English. "Water crossing."

FOREST Middle English, from Old French. "Woods." **Forrest**

FORESTER Middle English, from Old French. "Forester." **Forrester, Forster, Foster**

FORTNEY French. "Stronghold." **Fort, Fortnum**

FORTUNE Old French. "Lucky." **Fortunato, Fortunatus, Fortune, Fortunto**

FOWLER Old English. "Bird catcher."

FRANCIS Latin. "Frenchman." **Chico, Fran, Francesco, Franchot, Francisco, Franciskus, Franck, Franco, François, Frank, Frankie, Franko, Frann, Frannie, Frans, Fransisco,**

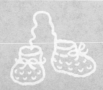

Keeping it short and sweet

Many famous people choose to ignore their given names and just go by initials. For a time, television shows and movies about hard-nosed executives often featured men who used their initials. J. R. Ewing of the TV show *Dallas* was a classic example of this.

P. T. Barnum, hoaxer and founder of a circus

J. M. Barrie, author of *Peter Pan*

L. L. Bean, outfitter of WASPs

e. e. cummings, poet

W. E. B. DuBois, intellectual and civil-rights leader

T. S. Eliot, cat fancier

M. C. Escher, illustrator of dormitory posters

W. C. Field, actor and curmudgeon

M. C. Hammer, pre-rap star

W. C. Handy, father of the blues

B. B. King, blues giant

k. d. lang, musician

D. H. Lawrence, author

T. E. Lawrence, Arabist

A. A. Milne, creator of Winnie the Pooh

I. M. Pei, architect

S. J. Perelman, *New Yorker* humorist

J. K. Rowling, creator of Harry Potter

J. D. Salinger, recluse

O. J. Simpson, running reprobate

B. F. Skinner, student of pigeons

J. R. R. Tolkien, hobbit fancier

H. G. Wells, futurist

E. B. White, author of *Charlotte's Web*

P. G. Wodehouse, creator of Jeeves

Frants, Franz, Franzel, Franzen, Franzin, Frasco, Frascuelo, Frasquito

FRANK Short form of **Francis, Franklin. Frankie**

FRANKLIN Middle English. "Free landholder." **Francklin, Francklyn, Frank, Franklinn, Franklyn, Franklynn**

FRAYNE Middle English. "Foreign." **Fraine, Frayn, Frean, Freen, Freyne**

FRAZER Disputed origin. **Fraser, Frasier, Frazier**

FREDERICK Old German. "Peaceful ruler." **Federico, Federigo, Fred, Fredd, Freddie, Fredek, Frederic, Frederich, Frédéric, Frederico, Frederigo, Frederik, Fredi, Fredric, Fredrick, Fredrik, Fridrich, Fridrick, Friedel, Friedrich, Friedrick, Fritz, Fritzchen, Fritzi, Fritzl, Fryderyk, Rick** et al.

FREEBORN Old English. "Freeborn."

FREEDMAN Old English. "Freed man." **Friedman, Friedmann**

FREEDOM English. "Freedom."

FREELAND Old English. "Free land." **Frieland**

FREEMAN Old English. "Free man." **Freemon**

FREMONT Old German. "Protector of freedom."

FREWIN Old English. "Free friend." **Frewen**

FRICK Old English. "Brave man."

FRIDOLF Old English. "Peaceful wolf." **Freydolf, Freydulf, Fridulf**

FRITZ German. "Peaceful ruler."

FULBRIGHT English. "Very bright."

FULLER Old English. "Cloth treader or beater."

FULTON Old English. "Village of the fowl."

FYFE Scottish. A county in Scotland. **Fife, Fyffe, Phyfe**

GABRIEL Hebrew. "Hero of God." **Gab, Gabbie, Gabby, Gabe, Gabi, Gabie, Gabirel, Gable, Gabriele, Gabrielli, Gabriello, Gabrielo, Gaby, Gaibrial, Gavriel, Gavril, Gavrilo**

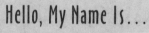

GADIEL Arabic. "God is my fortune."

GAETAN Italian. "From Gaeta," a city on Italy's west coast. **Gaetano**

GAGE Old French. "Oath."

GAIR Irish. "Short one." **Gaer, Geir**

GALBRAITH Irish. "Scottish." **Galbrait, Galbreath**

GALE Irish, "Irish." Scottish, "Scottish Highlander" or "Celt." **Gael, Gail, Gaile, Gayle**

GALEN Greek. "Calm one." A second-century Roman physician and writer. **Gaelan, Galeno, Galin, Gaylen, Gaylin, Gaylinn, Gaylon**

GALLAGHER Irish. "Foreign helper."

GALLOWAY Irish. **Gallway, Galway.** Galway, a city in western Ireland.

GALTON Old English. "Landleaser." **Gallton**

GALVIN Irish. "Sparrow." **Gal, Gallven, Galivin, Galvan, Galven**

GAMAL Arabic. "Camel." **Gamali, Gamli, Gamul**

GAMALIEL Hebrew. "Recompense of God."

GAMMEL Old Norse. "Old." **Gamel, Gemmel**

GARDNER Middle English. "Gardener." **Gar, Gard, Garden, Gardener, Gardie, Gardiner, Gardy**

GARETH Welsh. "Gentle." **Garith, Garreth, Garyth**

GARFIELD Old English. "Battlefield." **Gar**

GARLAND Old French. "Wreath." **Garlan, Garlen, Garllan**

GARMAN Old English. "Spearman." **Garmann, Garrman**

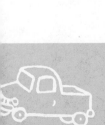

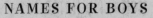

GARNER Middle English. "To gather grain." **Garnier**

GARNETT Old English. "Lance." **Garner, Garnet, Garm**

GARNOCK Old Welsh. "River of alder trees."

GARRETT English variant of **Gerard.** Old French, "Strong spear." **Garrat, Garratt, Garret, Garritt, Garrot, Garrott**

GARRICK Old English. "Warrior" or "ruler." **Garek, Garreck, Garrik, Garryck, Garryk**

GARROWAY Old English. "Spear-fighter." **Garraway**

GARSON Old French. "To protect." **Garrison**

GARTH Scandinavian. "Gardener." **Garton**

GARTON Old English. "Fenced farm." Also variant of **Garth.**

GARVEY Irish. "Rough peace." **Garrvey, Garrvie, Garvie, Garvy**

GARVIN Old English. "Spear-friend." **Garvan, Garven, Garvyn, Garwen, Garwin, Garwyn, Garwynn**

GARWOOD Old English. "Wood with pine trees." **Garrwood, Woody**

GARY Old English. "Spear." Also short form of **Gerald. Garey, Gari, Garrie, Garry**

GASPAR Variant of **Casper.** Persian, "guard." **Gaspard, Gasparo, Gasper, Jasper** et al., **Kaspar** et al.

GASTON French. "From Gascony." **Gascon, Gastone**

GAUTHIER Teutonic. "Ruler of the people." **Galtero, Gualteero, Gualterio, Gualtiero**

GAVIN Variant of **Gawain.** Welsh, "white falcon." **Gauen, Gauvin, Gav, Gavan, Gaven, Gavyn, Gavynn**

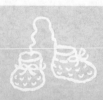

GAWAIN Welsh. "White falcon." In Arthurian and earlier legend, a heroic knight. **Gauen, Gavin** et al., **Gawain, Gawaine, Gawayn, Gawayne, Gawen, Gwaine, Gwayn**

GAYLORD Old French. "Active." **Gaillard, Gallard, Gay, Gayelor, Gayelord, Gayler, Gaylor**

GAYNOR Irish. "Son of the fair-skinned one." **Gainer, Gainor, Gay, Gayner, Gaynnor**

GEARY Middle English. "Changing." **Gearey, Gery**

GEDALIA Hebrew. "God is great." **Gedaliah, Gedaliahu, Gedelio**

GEFANIA Hebrew. "Vineyard of God." **Gefaniah, Gephania, Gephaniah**

GEIRR Norwegian. "Spear."

GENE Short form of **Eugene**. Greek, "well-born." **Genio, Geno, Jeno**

GEOFFREY Variant of **Jeffrey**. Old German, "district." **Geoff, Geoffery, Geoffroy, Geoffry, Geofrey**

GEORGE Greek. "Farmer." **Egor, Geo, Georas, Geordie, Georg, Georges, Georgi, Georgie, Georgios, Georgy, Gheorghe, Giorgio, Giorgos, Goran, Gyorgy, Gyuri, Jarge, Jiri, Jorge, Jorgen** et al., **Jurek, Juri** et al., **Jurik, Youri, Yuri, Yurik**

GERAINT Old English. "Old."

GERALD Old German. "Spear ruler." **Garald, Garold, Gary, Gearalt, Geralde, Geraldo, Gerard, Geraud, Gerek, Gerhard, Gerik, Gerold, Gerrald, Gerri, Gerrild, Gerrold, Gerry, Geryld, Giraldo, Giraud, Girauld**

GERARD Old French. "Strong spear." **Garrard, Garret** et al., **Gearard, Gerardo, Geraud, Gerhard** et al., **Gerrard, Gerri, Gerry, Gherardo**

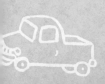

GEREMIA Italian variant of **Jeremiah.** Hebrew, "the Lord exalts."

GERHARD Old German. "Strong spear." **Gerard** et al., **Gerhardt, Gerhart**

GERMAIN French. "From Germany." St. Germain. **Germaine, Germán, Germane, Germano, Germayn, Germayne, Jermaine** et al.

GERONIMO Italian variant of **Jerome.** Greek, "sacred name." Geronimo, c. 1829–1909, leader of the Chirichahua Apaches. He battled white authorities for ten years before his final capture. **Hieronymos** et al., **Jeronimo**

GERSHOM Hebrew. "Exile." **Gersham, Gershon, Gerson**

GERVASE Old German. "Honorable." **Gervais, Gervaise, Gervase, Gervaso, Gervayse, Gervise, Gerwazy, Jarvis** et al.

GIACOMO Italian variant of **Jacob.** Hebrew, "he who supplants."

GIBSON Old English. "Son of Gilbert." **Gibb, Gibbons, Gibbs, Gillson, Gilson**

GIDEON Hebrew. "Feller of trees." In the Bible, Gideon led the Israelites in raids against the Midianites. **Gideone, Gidi, Hedeon**

GIFFORD Old English. Disputed derivation. **Giferd, Giff, Giffard, Gifferd, Giffie, Giffy, Gilford**

GIL Hebrew. "Joy."

GILAD Arabic. "Hump of a camel." **Gil, Gilead**

GILBERT Old German. "Shining pledge." **Bert, Bertie, Burt, Gib, Gibb, Gil, Gilberto, Gilburt, Gill, Gillett** et al., **Giselbert, Giselberto, Giselbertus, Guilbert**

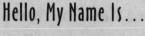

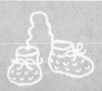

GILBY Irish. "Blond." **Gilbey, Gillbey, Gillbie, Gillby**

GILCHRIST Irish. "Christ's servant."

GILES English variant of **Egidio.** Italian, from Greek, "young goat." **Gide, Gil, Gilles, Gyles**

GILLEAN Irish. "John's servant." **Gillan, Gillen, Gillian**

GILLESPIE Irish. "Bishop's servant." **Gillis**

GILLETT Old French. "Young Gilbert." **Gelett, Gelette, Gillette**

GILMER Old English. "Renowned person." **Gil, Gill, Gillie**

GILMORE Old English "Root." **Gil, Gill, Gillie, Gillmore, Gillmour, Gilmour**

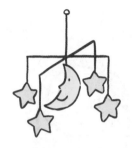

GILROY Irish. "Servant of the redhead." **Gilderoy, Gildray, Gildroy, Gillroy, Roy**

GIOVANNI Italian variant of **John.** Hebrew, "the Lord is gracious." **Gian, Giannes, Gianni, Giannino, Gianninos, Gio**

GIRVIN Irish. "Small feisty one." **Girvan, Girven, Girvon**

GIULIO Italian variant of **Julius.** Latin, "youthful." **Giuliano**

GLADWYN Old English. "Lighthearted friend." **Gladwinn, Gladwyn, Gladwynne**

GLEN Irish. "Glen." **Glanard, Gleann, Glenn, Glennie, Glenny, Glin, Glyn, Glynn**

GLENDON Scottish. "Town in the glen." **Glenden, Glendin, Glenton**

GLENVILLE Middle English. "Village in the glen." **Glanville**

GODDARD Old English. "Strong God." **Godard, Godart, Goddart, Godhard, Godhardt, Godhart, Gotthard, Gotthardt, Gotthart**

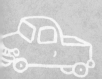

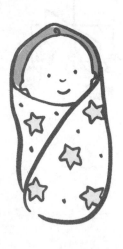

GODFREY Old German. "God's peace." **Godefroi, Godfry, Godofredo, Goffredo, Gotffrid, Gottfried**

GODRIC Old English. "Good ruler." **Godrich, Goodrich**

GODWIN Old English. "Friend of God" or "good friend." **Godewyn, Godwinn, Godwyn, Goodwin, Goodwyn, Goodwynn, Goodwynne, Win, Winny, Wyn**

GOLDING Old English. "Little golden one." **Golden**

GOLDMAN English, German. "Goldsmith" or "gold merchant." **Goldmann**

GOLDSMITH English. "Goldsmith."

GOLDWIN Old English. "Golden friend." **Goldewin, Goldewyn, Goldwinn, Goldwyn, Goldwynn**

GOLIATH Hebrew. "Exile." In the Bible, the giant Philistine slain by David. **Golliath**

GOMER Old English. "Famous battle." Gomer Pyle, 1960s television character played by Jim Nabors.

GONZALO Spanish. "Safety through battle." St. Gonzalo. **Gonçalve, Gonsalve, Gonzales**

GORDON Old English. Disputed meaning; possibly "triangular hill." **Goran, Gordan, Gorden, Gordie, Gordius, Gordy, Gore, Gorrell**

GORE Old English. Disputed meaning; "spear" or "triangular piece of land."

GORHAM Old English. "Village on the gore."

GORMAN Irish. "Small blue-eyed one."

GORO Japanese. "Fifth son."

GORTON Old English. "Town on the gore."

  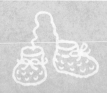

GOWER Old Welsh. "Pure." **Gowall**

GRADY Irish. "Renowned." **Gradea, Gradee, Gradey, Graidey, Graidy**

GRAHAM Old English. "Gray homestead." **Graeham, Graeme, Grahame**

GRANGER Middle French. "Farmer." **Grainger, Grange**

GRANT French. "Tall."

GRANTHAM Middle English. "Large home."

GRANTLAND Middle English. "Large fields."

GRANTLEY Middle English. "Large meadow." **Grantleigh, Grantly**

GRANVILLE Old French. "Big town." **Granvil, Granvile, Granvill, Grenville**

GRAY Old English "Gray-haired." **Grey**

GRAYDON Old English. "Gray hill."

GRAYSON Old English. "Grey's son." **Greyson**

GREELEY Scottish. "Watchful." **Greelea, Greeleigh, Greely**

GREENWOOD Old English. "Green forest."

GREGORY Greek. "Vigilant." **Graig, Greg, Greger, Gregg, Greggory, Gregoire, Gregoor, Gregor, Gregorio, Gregorius, Gregos, Grigor, Grigorios, Grischa**

GRESHAM Old English. "Village surrounded by pasture."

GREVILLE Old French. "Gray town." **Grevill**

GRIFFIN English, from French. "Griffin," an imaginary animal with the head of an eagle and the body of a lion. **Griff, Griffon, Gruffydd, Gryphon**

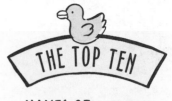

THE TOP TEN

NAMES OF 1987

The Year Madonna Won the MTV Video Music Award for Best Female Video, *Papa Don't Preach*

BOYS

Michael
Christopher
Matthew
Joshua
Andrew
Daniel
David
Justin
James
Robert

GIRLS

Jessica
Ashley
Amanda
Jennifer
Sarah
Stephanie
Nicole
Brittany
Elizabeth
Heather

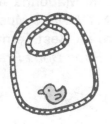

GRIFFITH Welsh. "Strong chief." **Griff**

GRIMBALD Old German. "Fierce." **Grimbel, Grimbold, Grimm**

GRIMSHAW Old English. "Dark woods."

GRISWOLD Old French, German. "Gray woods." **Gris, Griswald, Gritz, Griz**

GROSVENOR Old French. "Great hunter."

GROVER Old English. "One who lives in a grove." **Grove**

GUILDFORD Old English. "Ford with yellow flowers." **Gilford, Guilford**

GUILLAUME French variant of **William.** Old German, "will-helmet." **Guglielmo, Guilherme, Guillermo, Gwillym, Gwilym, Ulleam**

GUNDULF Old Norse. "War." **Gunn**

GUNTHER Scandinavian. "Warrior." **Guenter, Guenther, Gun, Gunnar, Gunner, Guntar, Günter, Guntero, Gunthar, Guntur**

GURION Hebrew. "Lion." **Gur, Guri, Guriel**

GURNEY Latin. "Grunt." **Gornus, Gourney**

GUS Short form of **Angus, Augustus, Gustave. Guss, Gussie**

GUSTAVE Scandinavian. "Staff of the gods." **Gus** et al., **Gustaf, Gustaff, Gustaof, Gustav, Gustavo, Gustavus, Gustof, Gustus, Gusztav**

GUTHRIE Celtic. "Hero." **Guthry**

GUY Middle English. "Guide." **Guido, Guyon, Wido**

GWYNN Old Welsh. "Fair." **Gwin, Gwyn, Gwynne**

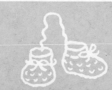

HABIB Arabic. "Loved one."

HACKETT Old French, German. "Little woodcutter." **Hacket, Hackit, Hackitt**

HACKMAN Old French, German. "Woodcutter."

HADDEN Old English. "Hill of heather." **Had, Haddan, Haddon, Haden, Hadon**

HADI Persian. "Leader."

HADLEY Old English. "Heather meadow." **Hadlea, Hadlee, Hadleigh, Hadly, Lee, Leigh**

HADRIAN Variant of **Adrian.** Latin, "from Adria," a city in northern Italy. **Hadrien**

HADWIN Old English. "Friend in war." **Hadwinn, Hadwyn, Hadwynne**

HAGEN Irish. "Youthful one." **Hagan, Hagen, Haggan**

HAGLEY Old English. "Enclosed meadow." **Haglea, Haglee, Hagleigh, Hagly, Lee, Leigh**

HAIG Old English. "Enclosed with bushes."

HAKIM Arabic. "Wise." **Hakeem**

HAKON Scandinavian. "Of the highest race." **Haaken, Haakin, Haakon, Hacon, Hak, Hakan, Hako**

HAL English. Nickname for **Henry,** variant of **Hale.**

HALBERT Old English. "Shining hero." **Halburt**

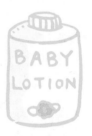

HALDAN Scandinavian. "Half-Danish." **Haldane, Halden, Halfdan, Halvdan**

HALE Old English. "Hall." **Hal, Hayle**

HALEY Old English. "Hay meadow." **Hailey, Haily, Haleigh, Hayleigh, Hayley, Lee, Leigh**

HALFORD Old English. "Valley ford." **Halfford**

HALL Old English. "Hall."

HALLAM Old English. "Valley."

HALLEY Old English. "Meadow near the hall."

HALLIWELL Old English. "Holy well." **Hallewell, Hellewell, Helliwell, Holliwell, Hollwell, Holwell**

HALLWARD Old English. "Guardian of the hall." **Halward**

HALSEY Old English. "Hal's island." **Hallsey, Hallsy, Halsy**

HALSTEAD Old English. "Manor grounds." **Halsted**

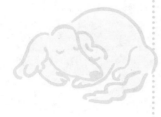

HAM Hebrew. "Heat." In the bible, the son of Noah cursed by his father to be a servant to his brothers. **Hammie**

HAMAL Arabic. "Lamb."

HAMAR Old Norse. "Hammer."

HAMILL Old French. "Home." **Hamel, Hamell, , Hamil, Hammill**

HAMILTON Middle English. "Home town." **Hamelton**

HAMISH Scottish variant of **James.** Hebrew, "he who supplants."

HAMLET Old French. "Home." Hamlet, the prince in Shakespeare's tragedy of the same name. Hamnet, Shakespeare's son, who died in childhood. **Amleth, Amothi, Haimes, Ham, Hames, Hamil, Hammet, Hammett, Hamnet, Hamnett**

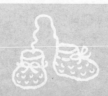

Adopting new names and new children

Ellen DeVilbiss lives in Louisville, Colorado.

"We adopted four children, two when they were infants and two when they were six and five years old. Adoptive children often become available on very short notice, so you have to have your names ready. For our first son, John Kenneth, we had one and a half hours' notice, but we were ready; we chose *John* for my husband's father and *Kenneth* for my husband.

"For our second child, we had signed up for a girl and had several girls' names picked out, but the agency called and asked if we would take a boy. We said yes, and then we had twelve hours to come up with a boy's name. Since we already had John, I looked for a *J* name so that the monogrammed hand-me-downs would match. I wanted a name with a good meaning, so we chose *Jason,* which means 'healer.' *William* came from my father.

"We still wanted to adopt a girl, and when the agency called about one year later, they told us that she came with a brother. So we happily took him as well. She was five years old and he was six, so they already had names—*Kayleen* and *Michael.* It would not have been a good idea to change these names. The children did not know their middle names, however, so we got to choose those. Their maternal birth-grandparents had been so helpful during the adoption that we decided to honor them by using their names.

"For Kayleen, we chose *Rose* for her maternal grandmother, and for Michael we chose *Gene,* the name of his maternal grandfather. *Kayleen* is a version of *Katherine,* which means 'pure,' and *Rose* means 'rose.' So we had *Pure Rose*—a perfect name for a red-headed girl."

HAMLIN Old German. "Little home-lover." **Hamblin, Hamelin, Hamlen, Hamlyn**

HANFORD Old English. "High ford."

HANK English. Nickname for **Henry.**

HANLEY Old English. "High meadow." **Handlea, Handleigh, Handley, Hanlea, Hanlee, Hanleigh, Hanly, Henley** et al.

HANNIBAL Carthaginian general. **Annibal, Annibale, Hanniball, Honeyball**

HANS Scandinavian variant of **John.** Hebrew, "the Lord is gracious." **Hanan, Hanes, Hannes, Hanns, Hansel, Hanshen, Haynes, Heinz**

HANSEN Scandinavian. "Han's son." **Hanson**

HARBIN Old French, German. "Little bright warrior."

HARCOURT Old French. "Fortified farm." **Harcort, Harry**

HARDEN Old English. "Valley of the hares." **Hardin**

HARDING Old English. "Son of the courageous one."

HARDWIN Old English. "Courageous friend." **Harding, Hardwinn, Hardwyn, Hardwynn**

HARDY English. "Courageous."

HARFORD Old English. "Ford of the hares."

HARGROVE Old English. "Grove of the hares." **Hargrave, Hargreaves**

HARKIN Irish. "Dark red." **Harkan, Harken**

HARLAN Old English. "Army land." **Harland, Harlen, Harlenn, Harlin, Harlyn, Harlynn**

HARLEY Old English. "Meadow of the hares." **Arley** et al., **Harlea, Harlee, Harleigh, Harly, Lee, Leigh**

HARLOW Old English. "Army hill."

HARMON Variant of **Herman.** Old German, "soldier." **Harman**

HAROLD Scandinavian. "Army ruler." **Araldo, Aralt, Arold, Aroldo, Arry, Garald, Garold, Hal, Harald, Haralds, Haroldas, Harry, Herold, Herrold**

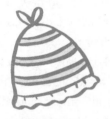

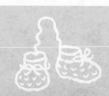

HAROUN Arabic. "Exalted."

HARPER Old English. "Harp player."

HARRISON Old English. "Son of Harry." **Harris, Harriss**

HARRY Diminutive of **Harcourt, Henry.**

HART Old English. "Stag." **Harte**

HARTFORD Old English. "Stag ford."

HARTLEY Old English. "Stag meadow." **Hartlea, Hartlee, Hartleigh, Hartly**

HARTMAN Old German. "Strong man."

HARTWELL Old English. "Well of the stags." **Harwell, Harwill**

HARVESON Middle English. "Harvey's son."

HARVEY Old French. "Burning for battle." **Erve, Harv, Harve, Harveson, Harvie, Hervey, Hervie**

HARWOOD Old English. "Forest of the hares."

HASHIM Arabic. "Crusher of evil." **Hasheem**

HASKEL Hebrew. "Intellect." **Haskell, Hassal, Hassel**

HASLETT Old English. "Point with the hazel trees." **Hazel, Hazlett, Hazlitt**

HASSAN Arabic. "Handsome." **Asan, Assan, Hasan**

HASTINGS Old English. "Swift one." **Hastie, Hasting, Hasty**

HAVELOCK Scandinavian. "Sea competition."

HAVEN Old English. "Sanctuary." **Havin**

HAWLEY Old English. "Hedged meadow." **Hawleigh, Hawly**

HAWTHORN Old English. "Hawthorn tree." **Hawthorne**

HAYDEN Old French. "Hedged valley." **Haden, Haydn, Haydon**

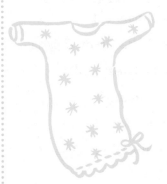

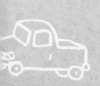

The Greats

Muhammad Ali may be known as "The Greatest," but a lot of people have proudly worn the title "The Great":

Alexander the Great, Greece

Catherine the Great, Russia

Charles the Great, a.k.a. **Charlemagne,** France

Frederick the Great, Prussia

Herod the Great, Judea

Ivan the Great, Russia

Peter the Great, Russia

Ramses the Great, Egypt

HAYES Old English. "Hedged area." **Hays**

HAYWARD Old English. "Gardener."

HAYWOOD Old English. "Hedged forest." **Heywood, Woody**

HEATH Middle English. "Heath."

HEATHCLIFF Middle English. "Cliff with heath."

HEBER Hebrew. "Togetherness." **Hebor**

HECTOR Greek. "Loyal." In myth, a Trojan hero in the Trojan War. **Ectore, Ettore**

HEDLEY Old English. "Heathered meadow." **Headley, Headly, Hedly, Lee, Leigh**

HEINRICH Old German. "Estate ruler." **Heike, Heindrick, Heiner, Heinrick, Heinrik, Heinz, Hendrick, Hendrik, Hernerik, Henri, Henrik, Henrique, Henry** et al., **Henryk, Hinrich**

HELI Greek. "Sun." **Helios**

HELMUT German. "Helmet." **Hellmut, Helm**

HENDERSON Old English. "Son of Henry." **Hendricksen, Hendrickson, Hendrie, Hendries, Hendriksen, Hendron, Henriksen, Henryson**

HENLEY Variant of **Hanley.** Old English, "high meadow." **Henlea, Henleigh**

HENRY Old German. "Estate ruler." **Arrigo, Enrico, Enrikos, Enrique, Enzio, Hal, Hank, Harry, Heinrich** et al., **Henning, Henri**

HERBERT Old German. "Shining warrior." **Bert, Bertie, Erberto, Harbert, Hebert, Herb, Herbie, Heribert, Heriberto**

HERCULES Greek. "Splendid gift." In myth, an exceptionally strong hero. **Ercole, Herakles, Herc, Herculano, Hercule, Herculie**

HERMAN Old German. "Soldier." **Armand** et al., **Ermanno, Ermano, Ermin, Harman, Harmon, Hermann, Hermie, Hermon**

HERN Middle English. "Heron." **Herne, Heron**

HERNANDO Spanish variant of **Ferdinand.** Old German, "explorer." **Hernán**

HEROD Greek. "Protector." Herod the Great, King of Judea, 37–4 B.C.

HERRICK Old German. "War ruler." **Herrik, Herryck**

HERSHEL Hebrew. "Deer." **Hersch, Herschel, Herschell, Hertz, Herzl, Heshel, Hirsch, Hirschel, Hirsh, Hirshel, Hischel**

HESKETH Hebrew. "God's strength." **Hezeki, Hezekiah**

HESPEROS Greek. "Evening." **Hespero**

HEWSON Old English. "Hugh's son."

HEZEKIAH Hebrew. "God gives strength."

HIEREMIAS Greek variant of **Jeremiah.** Hebrew, "the Lord exhalts."

HIERONYMOS Greek variant of **Jerome.** Hebrew, "sacred name." **Heironymous, Hierome, Hieronim, Hieronimos, Hieronymo, Hieronymus**

HILAL Arabic. "New moon." **Hilel**

HILARY Greek. "Joyful." **Alair, Alaire, Helier, Hilaire, Hilarie, Hilario, Hilarion, Hilarius, Hillary, Hillery, Hilliary, Ilario, Larie, Lary**

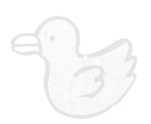

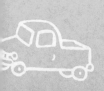

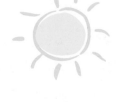

HILDEBRAND Old German. "Battle sword." **Hildabrand, Hildreth**

HILLARD Old German. "Hard warrior." **Hillier, Hillyer**

HILL Old English. "Hill."

HILLEL Hebrew. "Praised."

HILLIARD Old German. "Battle guard." **Hiller, Hillierd, Hillyard, Hillyer, Hillyerd**

HILMER Old English. "Hill by the sea."

HILTON Old English. "Hill settlement." **Hylton**

HIPPOLYTUS Greek. "Freeing the horses." In myth, Hippolytus, falsely accused of killing his stepmother, lost his horses when they were frightened by a sea monster. They broke away from his chariot, mortally wounding him. **Hippolit, Hippolitus, Hippolyte, Ippolito, Ippolitus, Ypolit, Ypolitus**

HIRAM Hebrew. "Noble brother." **Hi, Hirom, Hy, Hyrum**

HIROSHI Japanese. "Generous."

HISOKA Japanese. "Secretive."

HITOSHI Japanese. "One."

HO Chinese. "Good."

HOBSON Old English. "Son of Robert." **Hob, Hobs, Hopson**

HODGSON Old English. "Son of Roger."

HOGAN Irish. "Youth."

HOLBROOK Old English. "Stream near the hollow." **Brook, Holbrooke**

HOLCOMB Old English. "Deep valley."

HOLDEN Old English. "Hollow valley."

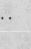
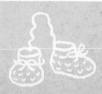
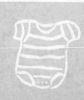

HOLLEB Polish. "Like a dove." **Hollub, Holub**

HOLLIS Old English. "Holly-tree grove."

HOLM Old Norse. "Islet in a stream." **Hume**

HOLMES Middle English. "Coarse cloth from Ulm (Germany)."

HOLT Old English. "Wood."

HOMER Greek. "Pledge." Ancient Greek author of the *Iliad* and the *Odyssey*. **Homere, Homeros, Homerus, Omero**

HONORÉ Latin. "Honored one." **Honoratus, Honorius**

HORACE Latin. Clan name. Roman poet, 65–8 B.C. **Horacio, Horatio, Horatiu, Horatius, Horaz, Oratio, Orazio**

HORST Old German. "Thicket."

HORTON Old English. "Gray town." **Horten, Orton**

HOSA Arapaho. "Young crow."

HOSEA Hebrew. "Salvation." **Hoseia, Hoshal, Hoshayah, Osee, Osia, Osias**

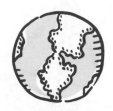

HOUGHTON Old English. "Settlement on the point."

HOUSTON Old English. "Settlement on the hill." Also a city in Texas. **Huston**

HUTCHINSON English. "Houston's son." **Hutcheson**

HOWARD Teutonic. "Guardian of the home." **Howey, Howie, Ward**

HOWELL Welsh. "Worthy of respect." **Hoel, Hough, Howe, Howel, Howey, Hywel**

HOWLAND Old English. "Hilly land." **Howlan, Howlen**

HUBERT Old German. "Shining intellect." **Bert, Hobard, Hobart, Hubbard, Hube, Huberto, Hubie**

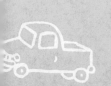

HUDSON Old English. "Hugh's son." **Hughes, Hugues**

HUGH Old German. "Intellect." **Hew, Hewe, Huey, Hughie, Hugo, Huw, Ugo**

HULBERT Old German. "Grace." **Bert, Hulbard, Hulberd, Hulburd, Hulburt**

HUMBERT Old German. "Famous warrior." **Hum, Humberto, Umberto**

HUMPHREY Old German. "Protector of the peace." **Humfrey, Humfrid, Humfried, Humfry, Humph, Humphery, Humphry, Hunfredo, Onfre, Onfroi, Onofredo, Onofrio, Umphrey**

HUNTER Old English. "Hunter."

HUNTINGTON Old English. "Hunter's town." **Huntingdon**

HUNTLEY Old English. "Meadow of the hunt." **Huntlea, Huntlee, Huntleigh, Huntly**

HURLBERT Old English. "Victorious army." **Hurlburt, Hurlbutt**

HURLEY Irish. "Sea tide." **Hurlee, Hurleigh, Hurly**

HURST Middle English. "Thicket of trees." **Hearst, Hirst**

HUSSEIN Arabic. "Small handsome one." **Hosein, Hossein, Husain, Husein, Hussain**

HUTTON Old English. "Settlement on the bluff." **Hutten**

HUXFORD Old English. "Hugh's ford."

HUXLEY Old English. "Hugh's meadow." **Hux, Huxlea, Huxlee, Huxleigh, Huxly**

HYACINTHE French. "Hyacinth."

HYAM Hebrew. "Life." **Chaim**

HYATT Old English. "Lofty gate."

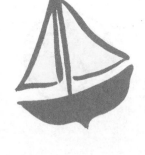

HYDE Old English. An old measure of land. **Hyder**

HYLAND Old English. "High land." **Highland, Hy**

HYMAN Variant of **Chaim.** Hebrew, "life." **Hayim, Hayvim, Hayyim, Hymie, Mannie**

HYMEN Greek. God of the wedding feast.

IAGO Spanish variant of **James.** Hebrew, "the Lord supplants." **Jago**

IAN Scottish variant of **John.** Hebrew, "the Lord is gracious." **Ean, Eann, Iain**

IB Danish. "Baal's pledge."

IBRAHIM Arabic. "Father of many."

ICHABOD Hebrew. "The glory is gone." Ichabod Crane, the credulous schoolmaster in Washington Irving's *Legend of Sleepy Hollow.*

ICHIRO Japanese. "First son."

IDRIS Welsh. "Eager lord."

IGNATIUS Greek. "Fire." **Eneco, Iggie, Iggy, Ignac, Ignace, Ignacio, Ignacius, Ignatious, Ignatz, Ignaz, Ignazio, Iñigo, Iñigue**

IGOR Russian variant of **Ingemar.** Scandinavian, "Ing's soldier." **Egor**

ILARIO Italian variant of **Hilary.** Greek, "cheerful."

ILIAS Greek variant of **Elijah.** Hebrew, "the Lord is my God."

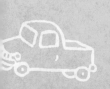

JAPANESE NAMES

Since the Japanese have no middle names, parents get to select only one name. In selecting this name, however, the parents can decide how it will be written in Japanese characters, and here another dimension of creativity emerges. Japanese mothers and fathers can choose from over two thousand *kanji* (characters) with which to write a baby's name. Some names can be written forty or more different ways. All this variation vanishes, however, when a Japanese name is written with roman letters.

Here are some Japanese names for boys:

Akihiko	"bright"
Goro	"fifth son"
Hiroshi	"generous"
Hitoshi	"one"
Ichiro	"first son"
Kenji	"second son"
Kenta	"healthy"
Masao ("mah-sah-o")	"holy"
Nori	"rule"
Osamu	"law-abiding

Rokuro	"sixth son"
Seiji	"lawful"
Taizo ("tah-ee-zo")	"third son"
Taro ("tah-ro")	"strong first son"
Yukio	"snow boy"

And some Japanese names for girls:

Asako	"child of sunrise"
Aumi ("ah-you-me")	"peace"
Etsu	"delight"
Haruko	"spring child"
Kiku	"chrysanthemum branch"
Kinu	"silk"
Koneko ("ko-neh-ko")	"kitten"
Nariko	"gentle child"
Riku	"land"
Sachiko	"child of bliss"
Shinako	"faithful child"
Tamiko	"people child"
Tomako ("to-mah-ko")	"jewel child"
Yoko	"positive"
Yukiko ("yu-kee-ko")	"snow child"

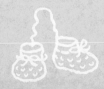

MOST POPULAR NAMES IN JAPAN

Here is the list from 2002, the most recent available.

Boys	Girls
Shun	Misaki
Takumi, Shou (tie)	Aoi
Ren	Nanami
Shouta, Souta (tie)	Miu
Kaito	Riko
Kenta	Miyu
Daiki	Moe ("mo-ay")
Yuu	Mitsuki, Yuuka ("yoo-ooh-ka"), Rin ("ren"), Ai (tie)

IMAD Arabic. "Support, mainstay."

IMRI Hebrew. "Tall." **Imray, Imre, Imric, Imrie**

INCE Hungarian. "Innocent."

ING Old Norse. God of fertility. **Inge**

INGEMAR Scandinavian. "Ing's son." **Ingamar, Ingemur, Ingmar, Ingevar, Ingvar**

INGELBERT Variant of **Engelbert**. Old English, "angel-bright." **Inglebert**

INGRAM Old English. "Ing's raven." **Ingraham, Ingrim**

INGVAR Scandinavian. "Ing's soldier." **Ingevar**

IÑIGO Spanish variant of **Ignatius**. Greek, "fire."

INNIS Scottish, Irish. "Island." **Innes, Inness, Inniss**

INNOCENZIO Italian. "Innocent." **Innocenty, Inocencio**

IOAKIM Russian variant of **Joachim**. Hebrew, "God will judge." **Ioachime**

IRA Hebrew. "Watchful."

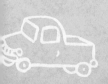

How about a boy named iTunes?

In 2001, a company named Internet Underground Music Archive, or IUMA, offered $5,000 to any couple willing to name their child *Iuma*. Two parents in Hutchinson, Kansas, thought this was a great idea, so they named their firstborn son *Iuma Dylan-Lucas Thornhill*. Iuma's father is a bass player in a band called Opus, which describes itself on the IUMA website as "hardcore/industrial, electronic, hard rock, heavy metal."

IRVING Old English. "Sea friend." **Ervin** et al., **Irv, Irvin, Irvine**

IRWIN Old English. "Boar friend." **Erwin** et al., **Irwinn, Irwyn**

ISAAC Hebrew. "Laughter." **Eisig, Ike, Ikey, Ikie, Isaak, Isac, Isacco, Isak, Itzak, Izaak, Izak, Izik, Izsak, Yitzchak, Yitzhak, Zack, Zak**

ISAIAH Hebrew. "The Lord helps me." In the Bible, a prophet. **Esaias, Ikaia, Ikaika, Is, Isa, Isaia, Isia, Isiah, Issiah**

ISHAM Old English. "Home of the iron one."

ISHMAEL Hebrew. "The Lord will hear." **Ismail**

ISIDORE Greek. "Gift of Isis." **Dore, Dory, Isador, Isadore, Isidor, Isidoro, Isidro, Issy, Izidor, Izydor, Izzy, Ysidro**

ISRAEL Hebrew. "Let God contend." The ancient Hebrews descended from Jacob, Jews past and present, and the modern Jewish state. **Yisrael**

ISTVAN Hungarian variant of **Stephen.** Greek, "crowned."

IUMA Contemporary name, acronym for the Internet Underground Music Archive (see sidebar).

IVAN Russian variant of **John.** Hebrew, "God is gracious." **Evo, Evon, Ivann, Ivon, Yvan, Yvon**

IVAR Old Norse. "Archer." **Ifor, Ivair, Ive, Iver, Ivor, Yvon, Yvor**

IVO Old German. "Yew wood." **Yvo**

JABEZ Hebrew. "Born in pain." **Jabes, Jabesh**

JABIR Arabic. "Consolation."

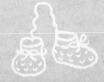

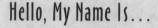

JACINTO Spanish. "Hyacinth." **Giacintho, Giacinto, Jacindo**

JACK English variant of **John.** Hebrew, "The Lord is gracious." **Jackie, Jacko, Jacky**

JACKSON Old English. "Son of Jack." **Jack, Jackie, Jacky, Jakson**

JACOB Hebrew. "He who supplants." **Akevy, Akiba, Akiva, Akkoobjee, Akkub, Cob, Cobb, Cobby, Como, Coppo, Diego, Geemes, Giacamo, Giacobo, Giacomo, Giacopo, Hamish, Iacopo, Iacovo, Iago, Iakob, Iakobos, Iakov, Jack** et al., **Jaco, Jacobo, Jacques, Jacquet, Jago, Jake, Jakie, Jakob, Jakov, Jakub, James** et al., **Jay, Kivi, Kub, Kubaa, Lapo, Santiago, Seamus** et al., **Yaakov** et al., **Yuki**

JACQUES French variant of **Jacob.** Hebrew, "he who supplants." **Jacque**

JAEL Hebrew. "Mountain goat." **Yael**

JAIME Spanish variant of **James.** Hebrew, "he who supplants." **Jaimie, Jammey, Jayme, Jaymie**

JAKE Short form of **Jacob.** Hebrew, "he who supplants." **Jackie**

JAMAL Arabic. "Handsome." **Jamaal, Jamahl, Jamall, Jameel, Jamell, Jamil, Jamill, Jammal**

JAMES Variant of **Jacob.** Hebrew, "he who supplants." **Diego, Giamo, Hamish, Jaime** et al., **Jaimes, Jamesie, Jamesy, Jamie** et al., **Jaymes, Jim** et al.. **Seamus** et al.

JAMESON Old English. "Son of James." **Jamieson, Jamison**

JAMIE Diminutive of **James. Jaime, Jaimey, Jaimie, Jamey, Jayme**

JAN Dutch, Scandinavian variant of **John.** Hebrew, "the Lord is gracious." **Janek, Janos**

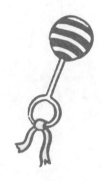

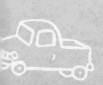

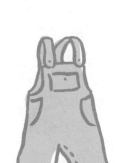

JANSON Scandinavian. "Jan's son." **Jansen, Jantzen, Janzen, Jensen, Jenson**

JANUS Latin. "Passage." In myth, the god of good beginnings, for whom the month of January is named. **Janis, Janiusz, Januarius**

JAPHETH Hebrew. "Comely." **Japhet, Yafet, Yaphet**

JAREB Hebrew. "He will struggle." **Jarib**

JARED Hebrew. "He descends." **Jarad, Jarid, Jarrad, Jarred, Jarrid, Jarrod, Jerad, Jerrad**

JAREK Slavic. "January," the month of Janus.

JARMAN Variant of **Germaine.** Old German, "German." **Jerman**

JAROSLAV Slavic. "Beauty of spring."

JARRETT Contemporary variant of **Gareth, Garrett,** or **Jared. Jarret, Jarrot, Jarrott**

JARVIS Variant of **Gervase.** Old German, "spear servant." **Gervais, Jary, Jarvey, Jerve, Jervey, Jervis**

JASON Hebrew. "The Lord is salvation." **Jaeson, Jaisen, Jaison, Jase, Jasen, Jasin, Jasun, Jay, Jayson**

JASPER English variant of **Casper.** Persian, "guard." **Jaspar, Josper**

JAVIER Variant of **Xavier.** Basque, "new house."

JAY Latin. "Jaybird." Also a variant of **Jason. Gaius, Jae, Jaye**

JEAN French variant of **John.** Hebrew, "the Lord is gracious." **Jeannot**

JEDEDIAH Hebrew. "Beloved of the Lord." **Didi, Jed, Jedd, Yehial**

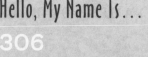
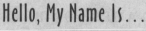

JEFFERSON Old English. "Son of Jeffrey." Many parents have named their sons *Jefferson* after Thomas Jefferson, third president of the United States. **Jeff, Jeffer, Jeffers, Jeffey, Jeffie**

JEFFREY Old German. "District." **Geoffrey** et al., **Jefery, Jeff, Jefferies, Jeffery, Jeffey, Jeffie, Jeffree, Jeffries, Jeffry, Jeffy, Jefry, Jeoffroi**

JEHOVAH Hebrew. "Eternal one."

JENKIN Flemish. "Little John." **Jenkins, Jenkyn, Jenkyns, Jennings**

JENS Scandinavian variant of **John.** Hebrew, "the Lord is gracious."

JENSEN Scandinavian. "Son of John." **Janson** et al., **Jenson**

JEPHTHAH Hebrew. "He will open." **Jephtah, Yiftach, Yiftah**

JERALD Variant of **Gerald.** Old German, "battle ruler." **Jerold, Jerrold, Jerry**

JEREMIAH Hebrew. "The Lord exalts." **Geremia, Jem, Jemmie, Jeremia, Jeremias, Jeremija, Jeremiya, Jeremy** et al., **Jerry**

JEREMY English variant of **Jeremiah. Jem, Jemmie, Jemmy, Jeramee, Jeramey, Jeramie, Jere, Jereme, Jeremie, Jeromy, Jerry**

JERMAINE Variant of **Germaine.** Old German, "German." **Jarman, Jerman, Jermane, Jermayn, Jermayne**

JEROME Greek. "Sacred name." St. Jerome, early Christian scholar. **Gerome, Geronimo, Gerrie, Gerry, Hieronymos** et al., **Jeroen, Jeromo, Jeronimo, Jerrome**

JERRY Diminutive of **Gerald, Jeremiah, Jerome.**

JESSE Hebrew. "The Lord exists." **Jess, Jessamine, Jessie**

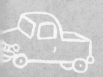

JESUS Hebrew. "The Lord is salvation."

JETHRO Hebrew. "Preeminence." **Jeth, Jett**

JIBBEN Romany. "Life." **Jivvil**

JIM Short form of **James.** Hebrew, "he who supplants." **Jimmie, Jimmy**

JÍMEN Spanish variant of **Simon.** Hebrew, "one who listened." **Gímen, Xímen**

JIN Chinese. "Gold."

JOAB Hebrew. "Praise Jehovah."

JOACHIM Hebrew. "God will judge." **Akim, Giachimo, Ioakim, Joacheim, Joakim, Joaquim, Joaquin**

JOB Hebrew. "The afflicted." **Jobe**

JODY Variant of **Joseph.** Hebrew, "Jehovah increases." **Jodi, Jodie**

JOEL Hebrew. "Jehovah is the Lord."

JOHANN German variant of **John.** Hebrew, "the Lord is gracious." **Johan, Johannes**

JOHN Hebrew. "The Lord is gracious." **Anno, Evan** et al., **Giovanni** et al., **Hanno, Hans** et al., **Honus, Ian** et al., **Ioannes, Ioannis, Ivan** et al., **Jack** et al., **Jan** et al., **Jancsi, Janko, Janne, Jean, Jeannot, Jehan, Jens, Joao, Jock, Jocko, Johann** et al, **Johnie, Johnnie, Johnny, Jon, Jona, Jonnie, Juan, Juanito, Sean** et al., **Shane** et al., **Vanek, Vanko, Vanya** et al., **Yannis** et al., **Zane**

JOHNSON Old English. "Son of John." **Johnston, Jonson**

JONAH Hebrew. "Dove." **Jo, Jonas, Jonás, Yona, Yonah**

JONATHAN Hebrew. "Gift of Jehovah." **Johnathan, Johnathon, Jon, Jonathon**

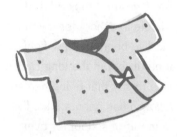

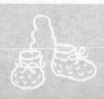

JORAH Variant of **Yora.** Hebrew, "teach."

JORDAN Hebrew. "Descend." **Giordano, Jordaan, Jordao, Jordon, Jori, Jory, Jourdain, Jourdan, Yarden**

JORGE Spanish variant of **George.** Greek, "farmer."

JORGEN Danish variant of **George.** Greek, "farmer." **Jeorg, Jerzy, Jorg, Jori, Joris, Jurgen**

JOSÉ Spanish variant of **Joseph. Joselito, Pepe, Pepito**

JOSEPH Hebrew. "Jehovah increases." **Ché, Giuseppe, Giuseppino, Iosep, Jo, Jodi, Jodie, Jody, Joe, Joey, JoJo, Jo Jo, Joop, Joos, José** et al.**, Josef, Josephe, Josephus, Josif, Josip, Joszef, Jozef, Osip, Pino, Pipo, Sepp, Seppi, Yousef, Yusuf, Yusup, Yuszef**

JOSHUA Hebrew. "The Lord is salvation." **Giosuè, Josh, Joshuah, Josua, Josue, Jozua**

JOSIAH Hebrew. "The Lord supports." **Josia, Josias**

JUAN Spanish variant of **John.** Hebrew. "The Lord is gracious." **Juanito**

JUDAH Hebrew. "Praise." **Jud, Judas, Judd, Jude, Yehudi** et al.

JUDAS Hebrew. "Praise." Judas Iscariot, disciple and betrayer of Jesus.

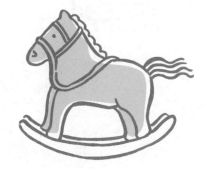

JUDE English variant of **Judas.** St. Jude, or St. Judas, a disciple of Jesus. He is called *Jude* in English to distinguish him from Judas Iscariot.

JULES French variant of **Julius.** Latin clan name. **Jule**

JULIAN Variant of **Julius.** Latin clan name. **Jolyon, Julien**

JULIUS Latin. Clan name. Julius Caesar, c. 102–44 B.C., Roman statesman and general. **Giulio, Jolyon, Jule, Jules, Julio, Yuli**

NAMES FOR BOYS

JURI Slavic variant of **George. Jaris, Yuri**

JUSTIN Latin. "Just." **Giustino, Giusto, Justen, Justinas, Justinian, Justinius, Justino, Justinus, Justis, Justo, Justus, Justyn**

JUVENTINO Spanish. "Young."

KAHIL Turkish. "Inexperienced." **Cahil**

KAHLIL Arabic. "Friend." Kahlil Gibran, 1883–1931, Lebanese mystic poet and novelist. **Kaleel, Kalil, Khaleel, Khalil**

KAIKANE Hawaiian. "Ocean." **Kai**

KAISER German. "Ruler."

KALOOSH Armenian. "Blessed coming."

KAMAL Arabic. "Perfection." **Kameel, Kamil**

KAMALI Zimbabwean. "Spirit."

KANE Irish. "Tribute." **Cahan, Cain, Kahan, Kain, Kaine, Kayne**

KARIM Arabic. "Generous noble." **Kareem**

KARL Old German. "Man." **Carl, Karlan, Karlens, Karli**

KARMEL Variant of **Carmel.** Hebrew, "orchid." **Karmeli, Karmi, Karmiel**

KARSTEN Old German. "Christian." **Carsten, Kerstan, Kerston**

KASEY Irish variant of **Casey.** "Alert."

KASPAR Persian. "Guard." **Casper** et al., **Gaspar** et al., **Kasper**

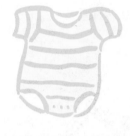

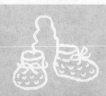

People known by first initial and middle name

America claims to be a classless society, but one of the tip-offs that someone is upper-class—or aspires to be—is the practice of using the initial of the first name followed by the middle name. There's a whiff of pretension around people who do this, but here are a few who have managed to pull it off.

F. Murray Abraham, actor

L. Frank Baum, author of *The Wizard of Oz*

E. Power Biggs, organist extraordinaire

H. Rider Haggard, English adventure author

J. Edgar Hoover, head of the FBI

L. Ron Hubbard, science fiction writer

E. Howard Hunt, Republican burglar

G. Gordon Liddy, Republican burglar

F. Scott Fitzgerald, author of *The Great Gatsby*

W. Somerset Maugham, English novelist

H. Ross Perot, entrepreneur and presidential candidate

J. Paul Getty, American, then British, oil man

J. Alfred Prufrock, famed for love song

J. Pierpont Morgan, financier

KAVAN Variant of **Kevin.** Irish, "handsome." **Cavan**

KAVANAGH Irish. "Follower of Kevin." **Cavanagh, Cavanaugh, Kavanaugh**

KAY Old Welsh. "Rejoicing."

KAZIMIERZ Variant of **Casimir.** Slavic, "bringing peace." **Kaz, Kazimir, Kazmer**

KEANE Old English. "Keen, fast-thinking." **Kane, Kani, Kayne, Kean, Keen, Keene**

KEARNEY Irish. "Winner." **Carney, Carny, Karney, Karny, Kearny**

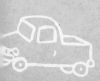

KEDAR Arabic. "Powerful." **Kadar**

KEEFE Irish. "Handsome."

KEEGAN Irish. "Little and ardent."

KEELAN Irish. "Little and thin."

KEELEY Irish. "Handsome." **Kealey, Kealy, Keelie, Keely**

KEENAN Irish. "Ancient and little." **Keen, Keenen, Kienan, Kienen**

KEISHON Contemporary American. **Keishaun, Keshon, Keyshaun, Keyshawn, Keyshon**

KEITH Scottish. "Forest."

KELBY Old Norse. "Farm near a spring." **Kelbey, Kelbie, Kellby**

KELL Old Norse. "Spring."

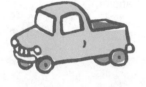

KELLY Irish. "Warrior." **Kelley, Kellie**

KELSEY Middle English. "Keel." **Kelcey, Kelsie, Kelsy**

KELSON Middle English. "A line of timber placed inside a ship along the floor timbers and parallel with the keel."

KELTON Old English. "Port." **Keldon, Kelten, Keltonn**

KELVIN Disputed origin. **Kelvan, Kelven, Kelvyn, Kelwin, Kelwyn**

KEMEN Basque. "Strong."

KEMP Middle English. "Victorious warrior."

KEMPTON Middle English. "Camp town."

KEN Short form of **Kenneth.** Irish, "handsome."

KENDALL Old English. "The valley of the Kent River." **Kendal, Kendell, Kenny**

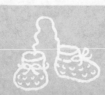

KENDRICK Old English. "Royal ruler." **Kendricks, Kendrik, Kendryck, Kenric, Kenrick, Kenricks, Kenrik**

KENELM Old English. "Brave helmet."

KENJI Japanese. "Second son."

KENLEY Old English. "King's meadow." **Kenlea, Kenlee, Kenleigh, Kenlie, Kenly**

KENN Welsh. "Bright water."

KENNARD Old English. "Brave and strong." **Kennaird**

KENNEDY Irish. Disputed meaning. **Canaday, Canady, Kennedey**

KENNETH Irish. "Handsome." **Ken, Kennet, Kennett, Kenney, Kennie, Kennith, Kenny**

KENT Old English. A county in England.

KENTA Japanese. "Healthy."

KENTON Old English. "Royal camp."

KENWARD Old English. "Royal guard."

KENWAY Old English. "Royal fighter."

KENYON Irish. "Blond."

KEREY Romany. "Home-bound."

KERMIT Irish. "Without envy." On the children's television show *Sesame Street*, a frog puppet.

KERN Irish. "Small swarthy one."

KERNAGHAN Irish. "Victorious." **Carnahan, Kernohan**

KERR Scandinavian. "Swampy place." **Carr, Karr**

KERRY Irish. "Dark one." Also a county in Ireland. **Kearie, Keary, Kerrey, Kerrie**

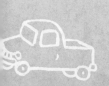

Kiefer Sutherland by any other name

The actor known to the world as Kiefer Sutherland actually has a much longer name: *Kiefer William Frederick Dempsey George Rufus Sutherland.* This blockbuster of a name was given to him by his parents, actors Donald Sutherland and Shirley Douglas.

KERWIN Irish. "Little dark one." **Kervyn, Kerwinn**

KEVIN Irish. "Handsome." **Cavan, Cavin, Kavan, Kavin, Kevan, Keven, Kevon, Kevyn**

KEY Middle English. "Key." **Keyes**

KHALID Arabic. "Never-ending."

KIDD Middle English. "Young goat."

KIEFER German. "Barrel-maker." Kiefer Sutherland, contemporary actor and director in television and film. **Keefer, Keifer, Keiffer, Kieffer**

KIERAN Irish. "Dark, swarthy." **Keir, Keiran, Keiron, Kernan, Kiernan, Kieron, Kiraren, Kyran**

KILLIAN Irish. "Small and fierce."

KIMBALL Old English. "Bold war leader." **Kimbal, Kimbell, Kimble**

KIMBERLY Old English. "Chief." Also a town in South Africa made famous during the Boer War. **Kim, Kimba, Kimber, Kimberlee, Kimberleigh, Kimberley, Kimberlie, Kimbli, Kimbly, Kimmie, Kimmy, Kym, Kymberlee, Kymberley, Kymberly**

KIN Japanese. "Golden."

KINCAID Irish. "Battle leader."

KINCHEN Old Norse. "Family."

KING Old English. "King."

KINGMAN Old English. "King's man." **Kingsman**

KINGSLEY Old English. "King's meadow." **Kingslea, Kingslie, Kingsly, Kinslea, Kinslee, Kinsley, Kinslie, Kinsly**

KINGSTON Old English. "King's town."

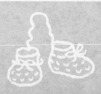

KINGSWELL Old English. "King's well."

KINNARD Irish. "Tall hill." **Kinnaird**

KINNELL Irish. "Top of the cliff."

KINTA Choctaw. "Beaver."

KIPP Old English. "Pointed hill." **Kip**

KIRBY Old English. "Church village." **Kerbey, Kerbie, Kirbey, Kirbie, Kirkby**

KIRIL Greek. "The Lord." **Cyril** et al., **Kirillos, Kyril**

KIRK Old Norse. "Church." **Kerk**

KIRKLEY Old English. "Church meadow." **Kirklea, Kirklee, Kirklie, Kirkly**

KIRKWELL Old English. "Church spring."

KIRKWOOD Old English. "Church forest."

KIT Short form of **Christopher.** Greek, "carrier of Christ." Kit Carson, 1809–1868, Union general, frontier guide and hunter, and Indian agent.

KIYOSHI Japanese. "Quiet."

KLEIN German. "Small." **Kline**

KLEMENS Variant of **Clement.** Latin, "giving mercy." **Klemenis, Klement, Kliment**

KOHANA Sioux. "Swift."

KONG Chinese. "Glorious."

KONRAD Variant of **Conrad.** Old German, "courageous advisor." **Koenrad, Kord**

KONSTANTIN Variant of **Constantine.** Latin, "steadfast." **Konstant, Konstantio, Konstanty, Konstanz, Kostas**

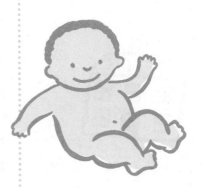

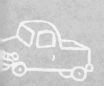

KORAH Hebrew. "Bald." **Korach**

KORNEL Variant of **Cornell.** Latin, "like a horn."

KNOX Old English. "Hills."

KNUTE Scandinavian. "Knot." **Canute, Cnut, Knud, Knut**

KRISPIN Variant of **Crispin.** Latin, "curly-haired."

KRISTIAN Variant of **Christian.** Greek, "Christian." **Krist, Kristo, Kristos, Krystian, Khrystos**

KRISTOFER Variant of **Christopher.** Greek, "carrier of Christ." **Kristoffer, Kristofor, Kristopher, Kristophor, Krzysztof**

KUN Chinese. "Mountain range."

KURT Variant of **Konrad.** Old German, "courageous advisor." **Curt**

KYLE Scottish. "Narrow spit of land." **Kile, Ky**

KYLOE Old English. "Grazing meadow."

LABAN Hebrew. "White."

LACHLAN Scottish. "Fighting spirit."

LADD Middle English. "Manservant" or "young man," "lad." **Lad, Laddey, Laddie, Laddy**

LAFFIT Old French. "The faith." **Lafitte**

LAIRD Scottish. "Lord of the land."

LAMAR Spanish. "The sea." **Lamarr, Lemarr**

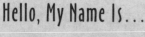

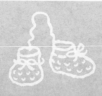

LAMBERT Old German. "Brilliant land." **Bert, Lamberto, Lambirt, Landbert**

LAMONT Old French. "The mountain." **Lammond, Lamond, Lemond**

LANCE Variant of **Lancelot.** Old French, "servant." **Lantz, Lanz, Launce**

LANCELOT Old French. "Servant." **Lance** et al., **Launcelot**

LANDER Middle English."Lion-man." **Landers, Landor**

LANDON Old English. "Plains." **Landan, Landen, Landin**

LANE Middle English. "Narrow road." **Laine, Layne**

LANG Old Norse. "Long." **Lange**

LANGDON Old English. "Long hill." **Landon, Langden**

LANGFORD Old English. "Long ford."

LANGLEY Old English. "Long meadow." **Langlea, Langlee, Langleigh, Langly**

LANGSTON Old English. "Long town." (James) Langston Hughes, 1902–1967, African-American poet and major figure in the Harlem Renaissance. **Langsden, Langsdon**

LANGWARD Old English. "Tall guard."

LANGWORTH Old English. "Long paddock."

LARKIN Irish. "Fierce." **Larkins**

LARRIMORE Old French. "The armorer." **Larimore, Larmor**

LARRON Old French. "Thief." **Laront, Larront, Latheron, Lathron**

LARS Scandinavian variant of **Lawrence.** Latin, "from Laurentium."

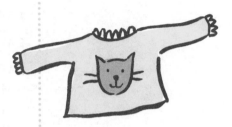

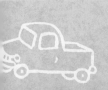

LARSON Scandinavian. "Son of Lars." **Larsen, Larssen, Larsson**

LASZLO Hungarian. "Famous ruler." **Laslo, Lazlo**

LATHAM Old English. "District."

LATHROP Old English. "District with barns."

LATIMER Middle English. "Interpreter." **Latymer**

LAVERN French. "The spring." **Laverne, Lavrans**

LAWFORD Old English. "Hill ford."

LAWLER Irish. "Mutterer." **Lawlor, Lollar, Loller**

LAWRENCE Latin. "From Laurentium." **Larrance, Larrey, Larry, Lars, Laurance, Lauren, Laurence, Laurens, Laurent, Laurentios, Laurentius, Laurenz, Laurie, Laurindo, Laurits, Lauritz, Lawrance, Lawrey, Lawrie, Lawry, Lenci, Lon, Lonny, Lorant, Loren, Lorenc, Lorencz, Lorens, Lorenzo, Lorin, Loritz, Lorry, Lowrance**

LAWSON Old English. "Son of Lawrence."

LAWTON Old English. "Town on a hill." **Laughton**

LAXTON Old English. "Salmon town." **Lexton**

LAZARUS Hebrew. "The Lord will help." **Eleazer** et al., **Lazar, Lazare, Lázaro, Lazzaro**

LEANDER Greek. "Lion man." **Ander, Leandre, Leandro, Leandros, Lee, Leo**

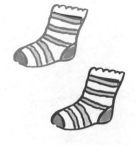

LEBEN Yiddish. "Life." **Lieben**

LEBRON Contemporary American. **Labron**

LEE Old English. "Meadow." **Leigh**

LEGGETT Old French. "Emissary." **Legate, Leggitt, Liggett**

LEI Chinese "Thunder."

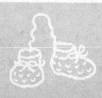

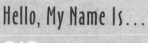

LEIF Scandinavian. "Loved." **Lief**

LEIGHTON Old English. "Meadow town." **Layton, Leyton**

LEITH Scottish. "Broad river."

LELAND Old English. "Meadow land." **Leeland, Leighland, Leyland**

LEMUEL Hebrew. "Devoted to God." **Lem, Lemmie**

LENIS Latin. "Gentle."

LENNON Irish. "Cape."

LENNOR Romany. "Summer."

LENNOX Scottish. "Grove of elm trees." **Lenox**

LEO Latin. "Lion." **Lee, Leon, Leontios, Lion, Lyon**

LEOFRIC Old English. "Loved ruler."

LEON Spanish variant of **Leo.** Latin, "lion." **León**

LEONARD Old German. "Lion strength." **Lee, Len, Lenard, Lennard, Lennerd, Lennie, Lenny, Leo** et al., **Leon, Leonardo, Leonerd, Leonhard, Leonid, Leonidas, Leonides, Lonnard, Lonny**

LEOPOLD Old German. "Brave as a lion." **Leo, Leupold**

LERON Old French. "The king." **Lerone, Lerin, Lerrin**

LEROY Old French. "The king." **Elroi, Elroy, Lee, Leeroy, Leroi, Roy**

LESHEM Hebrew. "Precious stone."

LESLIE Scottish. "Meadowlands." **Leslea, Leslee, Lesley, Lesly, Lezly**

LESTER Old English. "Leicester," a city in England. Also short form of **Alastair. Les**

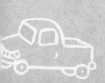

How about Lex Luthor?

Sara Lindenger and Johan Leisten of Sweden wanted to name their baby boy *David Rune Staalman Leisten*, but when they tried to register the child with the local tax authority, *Staalman,* which means "Superman" in Swedish, was turned down. The nameless officials, evidently not fans of the Man of Steel, claimed that the name "might lead to discomfort for the person who uses it."

LEV Hebrew. "Lion."

LEVERETT Old French. "Baby rabbit." **Leveret, Leverit, Leveritt**

LEVERTON Old English. "Lord's estate."

LEVI Hebrew. "Attached." **Levey, Levin, Levon, Levy**

LEWIS English variant of **Aloysius.** Old German, "renowned warrior." **Lew, Lewes, Louis** et al.

LEX Short form of **Alexander.** Greek, "man's protector."

LIAM Irish. "Determined protector."

LIANG Chinese. "Good."

LIBERIO Portuguese. "Freedom."

LIBERTY American. "Liberty."

LIDIO Portuguese. "From Lydia," an ancient country in Asia Minor.

LIN Chinese. "Forest."

LINCOLN Old English. "Village by the water." **Linc, Link**

LINDBERG Old German. "Linden-tree mountain." **Lindbergh, Lindburg, Lindy**

LINDELL Old English. "Linden-tree valley." **Lindall, Lindel, Lyndall, Lyndell**

LINDLEY Old English. "Linden-tree meadow." **Lindlea, Lindlee, Lindleigh, Lindly**

LINDSAY Old English. "Linden-tree island." **Lind, Lindsee, Lindsey, Lindsy, Linsay, Linsey, Lyndsay, Lyndsey, Lyndsie**

LINFORD Old English. "Flax ford." **Lynford**

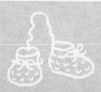

LINGREL Old English. "Hill." **Linc, Link**

LINLEY Old English. "Flax meadow." **Linlea, Linlee, Linleigh, Linly**

LINTON Old English. "Flax settlement." **Lintonn, Lynton, Lyntonn**

LINUS Greek. "Flax."

LIONEL Latin. "Young lion." **Lionello**

LIPMAN German. "Dear man." **Lieberman, Liebermann**

LISTER Short form of **Alastair.** Scottish, from Greek, "man's defender."

LITTON Old English. "Town on the hill." **Lytton**

LIVINGSTON Old English. "Leif's settlement." **Livingstone**

LLEWELLYN Welsh. "Resembling a lion." **Fluellen, Lew, Llewellen**

LLOYD Welsh. "Grey-haired." **Floyd, Loyd**

LOCADIO Latin. "Peace."

LOCKE Old English. "Fortified place." **Lock**

LOCKWOOD Old English. "Enclosed wood."

LODGE Old French. "Cottage."

LOGAN Irish. "Small hollow."

LOK Chinese. "Happy."

LOMBARD Latin. "Long-bearded." **Lombardo, Bard, Bardo**

LONG Chinese. "Dragon."

LORAL Old German. "To instruct."

LOREDO Italian. "From Loreo," a town in northern Italy. **Lorado**

LORENZO Italian. "Crowned with laurels."

LORIMER Latin. "Harness maker." **Lorrie, Lorrimer**

LORING Old German. "Son of the famous warrior." **Lorring**

LOT Hebrew. "Covering." **Lotan**

LOUIS Variant of **Aloysius.** Old German, "renowned warrior." **Lewis** et al., **Lou, Louie, Luis**

LOWELL Old English. "Praise." **Lovel, Lovell, Lowe, Lowel, Loyte**

LUBOMIR Polish. "Loves peace."

LUCIAN Latin. "Light." **Luciano, Lucianus, Lucien, Lucjan, Lukianos, Lukyan**

LUCIUS Latin. "Light." **Luca, Lucas, Luce, Lucias, Lucio, Lukas, Luke**

LUDLOW Old English. "Nobleman's hill." **Ludlowe**

LUDOVICUS Latin variant of **Aloysius.** Old German, "renowned warrior." **Lodowick, Ludovick, Ludovico**

LUDWIG Variant of **Aloysius.** Old German, "renowned warrior." **Ludvig, Ludvik**

LUIGI Italian variant of **Aloysius.** Old German, "renowned warrior."

LUKE Greek. "From Lucanus," a place in southern Italy. **Loukas, Luc, Lucas, Lucian, Lucien, Lucio, Lucius, Luck, Lucky, Lukacs, Lukas**

LUMUMBA Congolese. "Gifted."

LUNDY Scottish. "Grove near the island."

LUNN Irish." Strong." **Lon, Lonn**

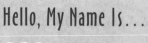
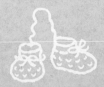

LUTHER Old German. "Soldier." **Lotario, Lothair, Lothar, Lothario, Lutero**

LUTHERUM Romany. "Deep sleep."

LUZERNE Latin. "Lamp." **Luc, Lucerne, Luz**

LYDE Old English. "Hill." **Lydell**

LYLE Old French. "The island." **Lisle, Lyall, Lyell, Lysle**

LYMAN Old English. "Meadow dweller." **Leaman, Leyman**

LYNCH Irish. "Mariner."

LYNDON Old English. "Linden-tree hill." **Lin, Linden, Lindon, Lindy, Lyn, Lynden**

LYNN Old English. "Bubbling brook." **Lyn, Lynne**

LYSANDER Greek. "Liberator."

LYULF Old English. "Burning wolf." **Ligulf, Liulf, Lyolf**

MAC Irish, Scottish. "Son of." **Mack, Mackey, Mackie**

MACABEE Hebrew. "Hammer." **Maccabee**

MACADAM Scottish. "Son of Adam." **MacAdam, McAdam**

MACALLISTER Irish. "Son of Alistair." **MacAlister, McAlister, McAllister**

MACARDLE Irish. "Son of great courage." **MacArdell, McCardell**

MACBRIDE Irish. "Son of a follower of Saint Brigid." **Macbryde, McBride**

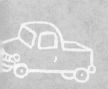

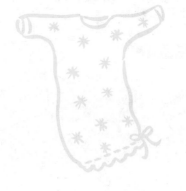

MACCREA Irish. "Son of grace." **MacCrae, MacCray, MacCrea, Macrae, McCrea**

MACDONALD Scottish. "Son of Donald." **McDonald**

MACDOUGAL Scottish. "Son of Dougal." **MacDowell, McDougal, McDowell**

MACE Old French. "Club." **Maceo, Macey, Macy**

MACGOWAN Irish. "Son of the blacksmith." **Magowan, McGowan**

MACKENZIE Irish. "Son of the wise ruler." **McKenzie**

MACKINLEY Irish. "Learned ruler." **McKinley**

MACMAHON Irish. "Son of the bear." **McMahon**

MACMURRAY Irish. "Son of the sailor." **McMurray**

MACON Old English. "To create."

MACY Old French. "Matthew's estate." **Macey**

MADDOX Anglo-Welsh. "Benefactor's son." **Madox**

MADISON Old English. "Son of the mighty warrior." **Maddison, Maddy, Madisson**

MADOC Old Welsh. "Fortunate." **Maddock, Madock, Madog**

MAGEE Irish. "Son of Hugh." **MacGee, MacGhee, McGee**

MAGEN Hebrew. "Protector."

MAGNUS Latin. "Great." **Magnes, Manus**

MAGUIRE Irish. "Son of the beige one." **MacGuire, McGuire, McGwire**

MAHIR Arabic. "Productive worker."

MAJOR Latin. "Greater." **Mager, Majer, Mayer, Mayor**

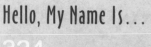

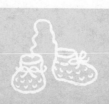

MAKARIOS Greek. "Blessed." **Macario, Macarios, Maccario, Maccarios**

MALACHAI Hebrew. "Messenger." **Malachie, Malachy, Malechy**

MALCOLM Scottish. "Devotee of St. Columba." **Malcolum, Malkolm**

MALDON Old English. "Council." **Malden, Malton**

MALIK Arabic. "Master." **Maliq**

MALIN Old English. "Little strong warrior." **Mallin, Mallon**

MALLORY Old French. "Of bad fortune." **Mallery, Mallorle, Malory**

MALONEY Irish. "Pious." **Malone, Malony**

MALVIN Variant of **Melvin.** Disputed meaning. **Malvinn, Malvyn**

MAMO Hawaiian. "Saffron flower."

MANCE Short form of **Emancipation.** English, "freedom." Mance Lipscombe, blues singer and guitarist.

MANCHU Chinese. "Pure."

MANDEL German. "Almond." **Mandell**

MANDELA South African. Parents have named their sons *Mandela* after Nelson Mandela, South African freedom fighter and president.

MANFRED Old English. "Man of peace." **Manfrid, Manfried, Mannfred, Mannfryd**

MANIPI Native American. "Amazing."

MANKATO Sioux. "Blue earth."

MANLEY Old English. "Man's meadow." **Manlea, Manleigh, Manly**

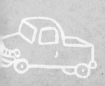

Novel names from a master storyteller

All novelists get to give their characters names, and Charles Dickens (1812–1870) created wonderful ones in his books and stories.

Arabella Allen, *The Pickwick Papers*

Bayham Badger, *Bleak House*

Tite Barnacle, *Little Dorrit*

Noddy Boffin, *Our Mutual Friend*

Rosa Bud, *The Mystery of Edwin Drood*

Hannibal Chollop, *Martin Chuzzlewit*

David Copperfield, *David Copperfield*

Bob Cratchit, *A Christmas Carol*

Volumnia Dedlock, *Bleak House*

Amy Dorrit, *Little Dorrit*

Edwin Drood, *The Mystery of Edwin Drood*

Bentley Drummle, *Great Expectations*

Affery Flintwinch, *Little Dorrit*

Augustus Folair, *Nicholas Nickleby*

Uriah Heep, *David Copperfield*

Gaffer Hexam, *Our Mutual Friend*

Jaggers, *Great Expectations*

Jarvis Lorry, *A Tale of Two Cities*

Abel Magwitch, *Great Expectations*

Jacob Marley, *A Christmas Carol*

Wilkins Micawber, *David Copperfield*

Nicholas Nickleby, *Nicholas Nickleby*

Newman Noggs, *Nicholas Nickleby*

Kit Nubbles, *The Old Curiosity Shop*

Dolge Orlick, *Great Expectations*

Seth Pecksniff, *Martin Chuzzlewit*

Ham Peggotty, *David Copperfield*

Phillip "Pip" Pirrip, *Great Expectations*

Barnaby Rudge, *Barnaby Rudge*

Zephaniah Scadder, *Martin Chuzzlewit*

Ebenezer Scrooge, *A Christmas Carol*

Cleopatra Skewton, *Dombey and Son*

Chevy Slyme, *Martin Chuzzlewit*

Dora Spenlow, *David Copperfield*

Wackford Squeers, *Nicholas Nickleby*

Montigue Tigg, *Martin Chuzzlewit*

Polly Toodle, *Dombey and Son*

Lucretia Tox, *Dombey and Son*

Gabriel Varden, *Barnaby Rudge*

Sophie Wackles, *The Old Curiosity Shop*

Silas Wegg, *Our Mutual Friend*

Bella Wilfer, *Our Mutual Friend*

Eugene Wrayburn, *Our Mutual Friend*

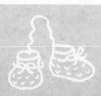

MANNING Old English. "Son of the man."

MANSEL Old English. "From the manse." **Mansell**

MANSFIELD Old English. "Field by the little river."

MANTON Old English. "Hero's town." **Manten, Mannton**

MANUEL Diminutive of **Emanuel.** Hebrew, "God be with us." **Mano, Manolo, Manual, Manuelo**

MANVILLE Old French. "Great town." **Mandeville, Manvile, Manvill**

MARCEL French. Latin. "Little warrior." Marcel Marceau, famous mime. **Marceau, Marcelin, Marcellin, Marcellino, Marcello, Marcellus, Marcelo, Marcely**

MARCUS Latin. "Warlike." **Marc, Marco, Marcos, Marko, Markus**

MARDEN Old English. "The Valley with the pool."

MARIO Italian variant of **Mark.** Latin, "warlike." **Marius**

MARION Masculine form of **Mary.** Hebrew, "bitter." **Marian, Mariano**

MARK Latin. "Warlike." **Marc, Marcus** et al., **Mario, Marius**

MARLAND Old English. "Land near the lake."

MARLEY Old English. "Meadow near the lake." **Marlea, Marleigh, Marly**

MARLON Old French. "Little hawk." **Marlin, Merlin** et al.

MARLOW Old English. "Hill near the lake." **Marlowe**

MARMION Old French. "Tiny one." **Marmyon**

MARNIN Hebrew. "Minstrel."

MARS Latin. In myth, the god of war. Also the fourth planet from the sun.

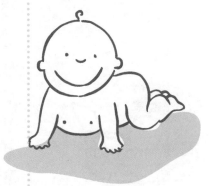

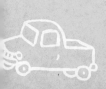

MARSDEN Old English. "Swampy valley." **Marsdon**

MARSH Old English. "Marsh."

MARSHALL Old French. "Horse keeper." **Marschal, Marshal, Marshell**

MARSTON Old English. "Town by the marsh."

MARTIN Latin. "Warlike." **Marinos, Mart, Martel, Martell, Marten, Martie, Martijn, Martinien, Martino, Martinos, Martinus, Marton, Marty, Martyn**

MARVELL Latin. "Extraordinary." **Marvel, Marvelle**

MARVIN Old English. "Friend of the sea." **Marve, Marven, Marwin, Marwynn**

MARWOOD Old English. "Lake near the woods."

MASAO Japanese. "Holy."

MASKIL Hebrew. "Learned."

MASLIN Old French. "Little Thomas." **Maslen, Masling**

MASON Old French. "Stoneworker."

MASUD Arabic. "Lucky."

MATHER Old English. "Powerful army."

MATO Sioux. "Bear."

MATTHEW Hebrew. "Gift of the Lord." **Mat, Mata, Mateo, Mateusz, Mathé, Matheu, Mathew, Mathian, Mathias, Mathieu, Matias, Mats, Matt, Mattaeus, Mattaus, Matteo, Matthaus, Mattheus, Matthias, Matthiew, Mattias, Mattie, Mattieu, Matty, Matvey, Matyas, Matz**

MAURICE Latin. "Moor." **Mauricio, Maurids, Maurie, Maurise, Maurits, Maurizio, Maury, Maurycy, Morey, Morice,**

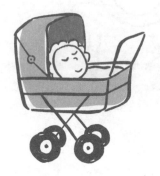

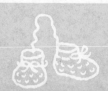

Moricz, Moris, Moritz, Moriz, Morrel, Morrey, Morrice, Morrill, Morris et al., **Moss**

MAXIMILIAN Latin. "Greatest." **Mac, Mack, Maks, Maksim, Maksym, Maksymilian, Massimiliano, Massimo, Max, Maxemilian, Maxemilion, Maxey, Maxie, Maxim, Maxime, Maximiliano, Maximilianus, Maximilien, Maximillian, Maximino, Maximo, Maximos, Maxy, Maxymilian, Maxymillian**

MAXWELL Scottish. "From the stream of Magnus."

MAYER Latin. "Greater." **Mayor**

MAYFELD Old English. "Strong one's field."

MAYNARD Old English. "Hard strength." **Mayne, Maynhard, Meinhard, Meinhardt, Menard**

MAYO Irish. "Yew tree plain." Also a county name in Ireland.

MCCOY Irish. "Son of Hugh." **MacCoy**

MEAD Old English. "Meadow." **Meade, Meed**

MEDRIC Old English. "Prospering meadow."

MEDWIN Old German. "Strong friend."

MEGED Hebrew. "Goodness."

MEINHARD German. "Hard strength." **Maynard, Meinhardt**

MEINRAD German. "Strong counsel."

MEIR Hebrew. "Shining." **Meier, Meyer**

MELBOURNE Old English. "Mill stream." Also a city in Australia. **Mel, Melborn, Melburn, Milbourn, Milbourne, Milburn, Millburn, Millburne**

MELCHIOR Polish. "King." In Christian folklore, one of the Magi. **Melker, Melldor**

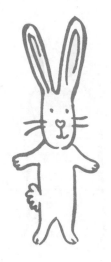

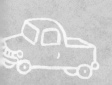

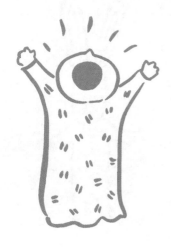

MELDON Old English. "Mill hill." **Melden**

MELDRICK Old English. "Mill ruler."

MELVILLE Old French. "Mill town."

MELVIN Old French. "Mill worker." **Malvin, Malvinn, Malvyn, Melvyn**

MENACHEM Hebrew. "Comforter." **Menahem, Nachman** et al.

MENDEL Arabic. "Learned individual." **Mendell, Mendeley**

MENELAUS Greek. In myth, King of Sparta and Helen's husband. **Mene**

MERCER Middle English. "Storekeeper." **Merce**

MERCURY Latin. Roman name for Hermes, Zeus's messenger. Mercury was the god of commerce, a master thief, and the guide of the dead to their last home.

MEREDITH Welsh. "Great ruler." **Meredyth, Merideth, Meridith**

MERLE French. "Blackbird." **Merl, Myrl, Myrle**

MERLIN Middle English. "Small falcon." In Arthurian legend, a great wizard. **Marlin, Marlon, Merlen, Merlinn, Merlyn, Merlynn**

MERRIPEN Romany. "Life," "death."

MERRITT Old English. "Little renowned one." **Merit, Meritt, Merrett**

MERTON Old English. "Town by the lake." **Murton**

MERVIN Old Welsh. "Friend of the sea." **Mervyn, Mervynn, Merwin, Merwinn, Merwyn, Murvin, Murvyn**

MESHACH Hebrew. Unknown meaning.

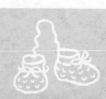

MEYER German. "Farmer." Meyer Lansky, gangster. **Mayeer, Mayer, Mayor, Meier, Meir, Myer**

MIACH Irish. "Healer."

MICAH Variant of **Michael.** Hebrew, "who is like the Lord?" **Mike, Mikey, Mycah**

MICHAEL Hebrew. "Who is like the Lord?" **Micael, Mical, Michail, Michal, Micheal, Michel, Michele, Michiel, Mick, Mickey, Micky, Miguel, Mihai, Mihail, Mihaly, Mikael, Mikal, Mike, Mikel, Mikey, Mikhail, Mikhalis, Mikhos, Mikkel, Mikol, Mischa, Misha, Mitchell** et al., **Mychal, Mykal, Mykell**

MICKEY Variant of **Michael.** Hebrew, "who is like the Lord?" Mickey Mantle, one of the greatest sluggers in baseball history, who played with the New York Yankees. Mickey Mouse, Disney character. **Mick, Micky**

MIDGARD Old Norse. "Middle place." In myth, the place where humans lived. **Midgarth, Midrag, Mithgarthr**

MIGUEL Spanish variant of **Michael.** Hebrew, "who is like the Lord?"

MILAN Czech. "Favored one."

MILES Latin. "Soldier." **Milo, Myles**

MILFORD Old English. "Mill crossing."

MILILEILANI Hawaiian. "To praise." **Mili**

MILLARD Old English. "Guardian of the mill." **Millward, Milward**

MILLER Old English. "Miller." **Millar, Myller**

MILTON Old English. "Mill town." **Milt, Mylton**

Royally flushing the last name

The royal family of England has not always been known as the House of Windsor. In the middle of World War I, when England was at war with Germany, the family became increasingly embarrassed at their Germanic surname, *Saxe-Coburg-Gotha.* King George V changed the family's last name to *Windsor.* This allegedly prompted Kaiser Wilhelm II, the king's cousin, known in happier days as Willy, to remark that he looked forward to seeing a production of Shakespeare's *Merry Wives of Saxe-Coburg-Gotha.*

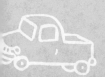

MING Chinese. "Shining" or "clear."

MINOR Latin. "Younger." **Mynor**

MINOS Greek. In myth, the son of Europa and Zeus.

MIROSLAV Slavic. "Great glory."

MISHA Russian variant of **Michael. Mischa**

MISU Miwok. "Water."

MITCHELL Middle English variant of **Michael.** Hebrew, "who is like the Lord?" **Mitch, Mitchel, Mytch**

MODESTUS Latin. "Moderate." The name of several saints. **Modesto**

MODRED Old English. "To consume." **Mordred**

MOHAMMED Arabic. "Highly praised." Founder of Islam. **Hamid, Hammad, Mahmoud, Mahmud, Mahomet, Mohamet, Mohammad, Muhamet, Muhammad, Muhammed**

MOHAN Hindi. "Pleasant."

MONAHAN Irish. "Monk." **Monaghan, Monoghan**

MONROE Irish. Place name. **Monro, Munro, Munroe**

MONTAGUE French. "Sharply pointed hilltop." **Montagu, Montigue**

MONTGOMERY Old English. "Mount of the rich man." **Montgomerie, Montie, Monty**

MOORE Old English. "Moor" (open, rolling land). **More**

MORDECAI Hebrew. In the Bible, the cousin and foster-father of Esther. By refusing to bow before King Haman, Mordecai provoked the king's wrath against all Jews. **Mordechai, Mordy, Mort**

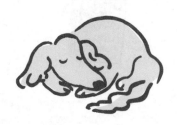

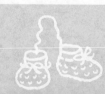

MORELAND Old English. "Moor land." **Moorland, Morland**

MORGAN Disputed origin. **Morgen, Morgun, Morrgan**

MORLEY Old English. "Meadow on the moor." **Moorley, Moorly, Morlee, Morleigh, Morly, Morrley, Morrly**

MORRIS English variant of **Maurice**. Latin, "Moor." **Morice, Moris, Moriss**

MORRISON Old English. "Son of Morris." **Morrisson, Morse**

MORTIMER Old French. "Still water." **Mort, Morty, Mortymer**

MORTON Old English. "Moor town." **Morten**

MORVEN Scottish. "Huge mountain." **Morfin, Morfinn, Morfyn, Morvyn**

MOSES In the Bible, a prophet and lawgiver who led the Jews out of Egypt. **Mo, Moe, Moise, Moises, Mose, Moshe, Mosheh, Mosie, Moss, Moyses, Mozes**

MUHAMMAD Variant of **Mohammad**. Arabic, "highly praised."

MUIR Scottish. "Moor."

MURACO Native American. "White moon."

MURCHADH Irish. "Sea warrior."

MURDOCK Scottish. "Sea warrior." **Murdo, Murdoch, Murtagh, Murtaugh**

MURIEL Irish. "Bright sea."

MURPHY Irish. "Sea fighter." **Murfey**

MURRAY Scottish. "Mariner." **Moray, Murrey, Murry**

MYRON Greek. "Fragrant oil."

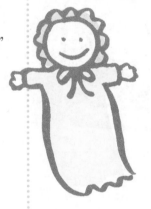

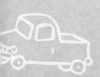

NABIL Arabic. "Prince." **Nabeel**

NABOTH Hebrew. "Prophecy."

NACHMAN Hebrew. "Comforter." **Menachem, Menahem, Nachum, Nahum**

NADIM Arabic. "Friend."

NAIRN Scottish. "River with alder trees." **Nairne**

NAJIB Arabic. "Noble." **Najeeb**

NAMIR Arabic. "Leopard."

NAPHTALI Hebrew. Ancient Israeli place name. **Nappie, Nappy**

NAPOLEON Greek. "New town." Napoleon Bonaparte, 1769–1821, French military commander and emperor. **Leon, Nap, Napoleone**

NARCISSE French variant of **Narcissus.**

NARCISSUS Latin, from Greek. In myth, a youth who fell in love with his own reflection. Also New Latin, from Greek, "daffodil." **Narcisse, Narkissos**

NASHOBA Chocktaw. "Wolf."

NASIR Arabic. "Helper" or "friend."

NASSER Arabic. "Victorious."

NATAL Spanish. "Of birth." **Natalino, Natalio**

NATALE Italian. "Birth" or "birthday." **Nataly**

NATHAN Hebrew. "Given." **Nat, Natan, Nate, Nathen**

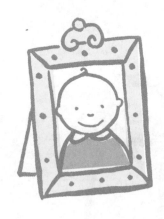

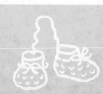

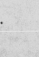

NATHANIEL Hebrew. "Given by God." **Nat, Natanael, Nataniel, Nate, Nathan, Nathaneal, Nathanial, Nathanyal, Nathanyel, Nethaniel, Nethanyel, Thaniel**

NAV Romanian. "Name." **Nev**

NAVAD Hebrew. "Giver."

NAVID Persian. "Good news."

NAYATI Native American. "Wrestler."

NEAL Variant of **Neil.** Irish, "champion." **Neale, Neall, Nealle, Neel**

NED Old English. "Guardian." **Neddie, Neddy**

NEGEV Hebrew. "To the south." A desert in southern Israel.

NEHEMIAH Hebrew. "The Lord's comfort." **Nechemya**

NEIL Irish. "Champion." **Neal** et al., **Neile, Neill, Neille, Nial, Niall, Niel, Nigel**

NELSON English. "Son of Neil." **Nealson, Neils, Nels, Niles, Nils, Nilson, Nilsson**

NEMESIO Spanish. "Justice."

NEPTUNE Latin. In myth, god of the sea.

NESBIT Old English. "River-bend shaped like a nose." **Naisbit, Naisbitt, Nesbitt, Nisbet, Nisbett**

NESTOR Greek. "Traveler."

NEVILLE Old French. "New town." **Nev, Nevil, Nevile, Nevyle**

NEVIN Irish. "Holy." **Nev, Nevan, Nevins, Niven**

NEWELL Old English. "New hall." **Newall, Newel, Newhall**

NEWLAND Old English. "New land."

NEWLIN Old Welsh. "New pond."

Letting the baby decide

Rabbi Zalman Schachter-Shalomi is the pioneering father of the Jewish Renewal movement, founder of the Spiritual Eldering Institute, and an active and original teacher of Jewish mysticism.

"I get concerned when I hear people say they have picked out a name for a baby without holding the child in their arms. People have ideas about names, but those names come from the head. It is important to consider the meaning of a name, and to choose one that will not have a troublesome nickname, but it is more important to let the child help make the decision.

"You can talk to babies when they are still in the womb. They can hear you. You can tell them what names you are considering and ask them to let you know which one they prefer. Sometimes they will come to you in a dream and tell you.

"When I named my son, I held him and recited the various names we had chosen. You might say I crooned them to him. When I felt an energy response from him, I knew what name he wanted. It was *Yotam*."

NEWMAN Old English. "Newcomer."

NEWTON Old English. "New town."

NIALL Variant of **Neil**. Irish, "champion." **Nial**

NICHOLAS Greek. "Victory of the people." **Claus** et al., **Colas, Cole, Colet, Klaus** et al., **Nic, Nicanor, Niccolo, Nichol, Nichole, Nicholl, Nichols, Nick** et al., **Nicklas, Nickolas, Nickolaus, Nicodema, Nicodemus, Nicol, Nicola, Nicolaas, Nicolae, Nicolai, Nicolao, Nicolas, Nicolis, Nicoll, Nicolls, Nicolo, Nicu, Niculaie, Nikita, Niklaas, Niklas, Nikodema, Nikolai, Nikolas, Nikolaus, Nikolay, Nikolos, Nikos, Nilos**

NICK Short form of **Dominic, Nicholas, Nicodemus**. **Nic, Nickey, Nickie, Nicky, Nik, Niki, Nikki, Nikky**

NICODEMUS Greek. "Victory of the people." **Nikodema**

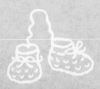

NIELS Danish variant of **Nelson**. English, "son of Neil." **Nils**

NIGEL Variant of **Neil**. Irish, "champion."

NILES Variant of **Nelson**. Irish, "son of Neil."

NIR Hebrew. "Cultivated field."

NISSIM Hebrew. "Wondrous things."

NITIS Native American. "Good friend."

NIV Arabic. "Speech."

NIWOT Arapaho. "Left hand."

NIXON Old English. "Son of Nicholas."

NOAH Hebrew. In the Bible, the boatbuilder who saved the animals from the flood. **Noach, Noak, Noé**

NOAM Hebrew. "Sweetness." Noam Chomsky, contemporary linguist and political commentator.

NOBLE Latin. "Aristocratic."

NOEL French. "Christmas." **Nowel, Nowell**

NOGA Hebrew. "Famous."

NOLAN Irish. "Renowned." **Noland, Nolen, Nolin, Nollan**

NORBERT Old German. "Renowned northerner." **Bert, Bertie, Berty, Norberto**

NORI Japanese. "Rule."

NORMAN Old French. "Northerner." **Norm, Normand, Normen, Normie**

NORRIS Old French. "Northerner."

NORTHCLIFF Old English. "Northern cliff." **Northcliffe, Northclyff, Northclyffe**

NORTHROP Old English. "Northern farm." **Northrup**

NORTON Old English. "Northern town."

NORVILLE Middle English. "Northern town." **Norval, Norvel, Norvell, Norvil, Norvill, Norvylle**

NORVIN Old English. "Northern friend." **Norvyn, Norwin, Norwinn, Norwyn, Norwynn**

NORWARD Old English. "Warden of the north." **Norwerd**

NORWELL Old English. "Northern well."

NORWOOD Old English. "Northern woods."

NUNCIO Italian. "Messenger." **Nunzio**

NURI Arabic. "Light." **Noori, Nur, Nuriel, Nuris**

NYE Middle English. "Island." **Nyle**

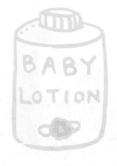

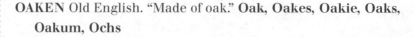

OAKEN Old English. "Made of oak." **Oak, Oakes, Oakie, Oaks, Oakum, Ochs**

OAKLEY Old English. "Oak-tree meadow." **Oaklee, Oakleigh, Oakly**

OBADIAH Hebrew. "Servant of God." **Abdias, Obadias, Oban, Obed, Obediah, Obie, Oby, Ovadiach, Ovadiah**

OBERON Old German. "Highborn and bear-like." **Auberon, Auberron, Oberron, Oeberon**

OBERT Old German. "Wealthy and bright."

OCTAVIUS Latin. "Eighth." **Octave, Octavian, Octavien, Octavio, Octavo, Octavus, Otavio, Otavus, Ottavio**

ODAM Middle English. "Son-in-law." **Odum**

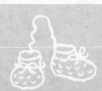

ODELL Disputed origin. **Del, Dell, Odall, Odd, Ode, Odey, Odie, Odile, Odo, Ody**

ODIN Old Norse. In myth, the ruler of the gods. **Ode, Odie, Ody**

ODO Old English. "Rich." **Aodh, Audo, Oddie, Oddo, Oddy, Odey, Odie, Ody**

ODOLF Old German. "Prosperous wolf." **Odolff, Odulf**

ODYSSEUS Greek. "Wrathful." In the *Odyssey,* the hero of many adventures on his way home from the siege of Troy.

OEDIPUS Greek. In myth, the hero who slew his father and married his mother.

OFER Hebrew. "Fawn." **Opher**

OGDEN Old English. "Oak-tree valley." **Ogdan, Ogdon**

OGIER Old German. "Wonderous spear." **Oger, Ogere**

OLAF Scandinavian. "Ancestor." **Olaff, Olav, Olave, Ole, Olen, Olie, Olif, Olin** et al., **Olle, Ollie, Olof, Olov**

OLEG Russian. "Holy." Oleg Cassini, contemporary fashion designer. **Ole**

OLIN English variant of **Olaf. Olen, Olney, Olyn**

OLIVER Latin. "Olive." **Alivar, Aliver, Alvar, Noll, Nollie, Nolly, Oliverio, Olivero, Olivier, Oliviero, Olivor, Olley, Ollie, Olliver, Ollivor, Olly, Olvan**

OMAR Arabic. "Highest." Omar Khayyam, twelfth-century Persian poet. Omar Sharif, contemporary actor.

OMRI Hebrew. In the Bible, a king of ancient Israel. Omri is the main character in Lynne Reid Banks' *Indian in the Cupboard.*

ONACONA Cherokee. "White owl."

ONAN Turkish. "Affluent."

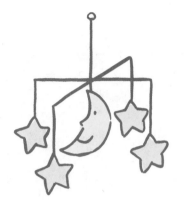

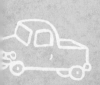

ONSLOW Old English. "Enthusiast's hill." **Enslo, Enslow, Ounslow**

OPAL Sanskrit. "Gem."

ORAN Irish. "Green." **Oren, Orin, Orran, Orren, Orrin**

ORAZIO Italian variant of **Horace, Horatio**. Latin clan name.

ORBAN Latin. "Globe."

OREN Hebrew, "tree." Irish, "pale-skinned." **Oran, Orin, Orren, Orrin**

ORESTES Greek. "Man of the mountain." In Aeschylus's tragedy *Oresteia*, Orestes murdered his mother to avenge his father's death. **Aresty, Orest, Oreste**

ORFORD Old English. "Ford of cattle."

ORION Greek. In myth, a giant and mighty hunter who became, after his death, a constellation. **Orie, Orien, Orin, Oron, Orrin**

ORLANDO Spanish variant of **Roland**. Old German, "famous land." **Arland, Arlando, Orlan, Orland, Orley, Orlin, Orlo**

ORMAN Old German. "Seaman." **Ormand**

ORMOND Disputed origin. **Orma, Orman, Ormand, Ormonde**

ORNETTE Contemporary American. Ornette Coleman, saxophone player and jazz composer.

ORO Spanish. "Gold."

ORPHEUS Greek. "Ear." In myth, a musician who followed his lover, Eurydice, to Hades, then lost her by failing to heed the gods' warning not to look at her until they reached the upper world.

ORRICK Old English. "Old oak tree." **Orick, Orric**

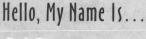

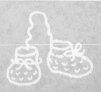

ORSON Latin. "Bear." Orson Welles, twentieth-century actor and director. **Orsen, Orsin, Orsini, Orsino, Sonnie, Sonny, Urson**

ORTON Old English. "Grey settlement."

ORVAL Old English. "Strong spear."

ORVILLE Old French. "Town of gold." **Orv, Orval, Orvell, Orvil**

ORVIN Old English. "Spear-friend." **Orwin, Orwynn**

OSAMA Arabic. "Like a lion." **Osamah, Usama, Usamah**

OSBERT Old English. "Divine and bright." **Osbrett**

OSBORN Old English. "Bear god." **Osborne, Osbourn, Osbourne, Osburn, Osburne, Ozzie**

OSCAR Scandinavian. "Divine spear." **Oke, Osber, Oskar, Ossie, Ossy, Ozzie, Ozzy**

OSGOOD Old English. "Divine Goth." **Osgoode**

OSIA Variant of **Hosea.** Hebrew, "salvation." **Osias**

OSIRIS Egyptian. God of the dead.

OSMAR Old English. "Divine and wonderful."

OSMOND Old English. "Divine protector." **Osman, Osmand, Osmande, Osmonde, Osmont, Osmund, Osmunde, Oswin, Oz**

OSRED Old English. "Divine counsel."

OSRIC Old English. "Divine ruler." **Osrick**

OSWALD Old English. "God's power." **Ossie, Osvald, Oswal, Oswaldo, Oswall, Oswell, Ozzie, Ozzy, Waldo**

OSWIN Old English. "Divine friend." **Osvin, Oswinn, Oswyn, Oswynn**

Need a name? Ask Jeeves.

P. G. Wodehouse chronicled and caricatured the British upper classes in a wonderful series of books centered on Bertie Wooster and his faithful manservant, Jeeves. Part of the charm of these books is the names of the other characters.

Madeline Bassett

Beech the Butler

Earl of Blandings

Lord Emsworth

Gussie Fink-Nottle

Barmy Fotheringay-Phipps

Agatha Gregson

Bin go Little

Psmith

Roderick Spode

Dahlia Travers

Oofy Wegg-Prosser

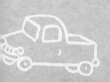

OTHELLO Italian. "Prosperous." Main character of the eponymous Shakespearean tragedy and of operas by Rossini and Verdi. A noble Moor who slew his devoted wife out of jealousy. **Otello, Otelo**

OTHMAN Old German. "Wealthy man." **Otheman, Otman, Ottman**

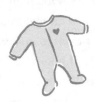

OTIS Old English. "Son of Otto." **Oates, Otes, Otess, Ottes**

OTTO Old German. "Prosperous." **Otho, Oto**

OURAY Ute. "Arrow."

OVED Hebrew. "Follower." **Ovedde**

OVERTON Middle English. "Upper town."

OVID Latin. "Egg." Roman poet, 43 B.C.–17 A.D.

OWEN Welsh variant of **Eugene.** Greek, "well-born." **Ewan** et al., **Owain, Owayne, Owin, Uwen**

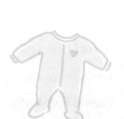

OXFORD Old English. "Crossing of the oxen."

OZ Hebrew. "Strength." **Ozzie, Ozzman, Ozzy**

PABLO Spanish variant of **Paul.** Latin. "Small."

PACO Spanish nickname for **Francis.** Latin, "Frenchman." **Pacorro, Paquito**

PADDY Irish variant of **Patrick.** "Upper class." In the nineteenth and twentieth centuries, an epithet for any Irishman. **Paddey, Paddie, Padraic, Padraig, Patti, Pattie, Patty**

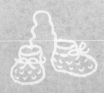

PAGE French. "Young messenger." **Padget, Padgett, Paget, Pagett, Paige, Payge**

PALL Variant of **Paul**. Latin, "small."

PALMER Middle English, from French. "One who wears a palm cross to show that has has made a pilgrimage to the Holy Land." **Pallmer, Palmar**

PAN Greek. God of shepherds, flocks, and fornication.

PANCHO Spanish. "Calm." Pancho Villa, c. 1877–1923, Mexican outlaw, revolutionary leader, and folk hero.

PARIS Old English. "From Paris." Also Greek. In myth, a Trojan prince who started the Trojan War by stealing away Helen, queen of Sparta, from her husband. **Parris**

PARKER Old English. "Park keeper." **Parke, Parkes, Parks**

PARKIN Old English. "Little Peter." **Perkin** et al.

PARNELL Old French. "Little Peter." **Parrnell, Parnell**

PARR Old English. "Castle park."

PARRISH Old French. "Parish." **Parish, Parrie, Parry**

PARRY Old Welsh. "Son of Harry." Also variant of **Parrish**. **Parrey, Parrie**

PARSA Persian. "Pious."

PARSON Middle English, from French. "Representative of the church parish."

PASCAL French. "Of Easter." **Pascale, Pascalle, Paschal, Paschalis, Pasco, Pascoe**

PASQUALE Italian. "Of Easter." **Pascal** et al., **Pascuale**

PATRICK Latin. "Upper class." **Pad, Paddey, Paddie, Paddy, Padhraig, Padraic, Padraig, Padriac, Padrig, Pat, Patric,**

Naming for artistic proclivities

Painter Charles Wilson Peale (1741–1827) wielded more than a brush. Although he is famous in art circles for his portraits of Benjamin Franklin, fourteen paintings of George Washington, and many paintings of children, he also fathered seventeen offspring from two sequential wives. His first four children, who bore unremarkable names, died in infancy. The rest were named for famous scientists and artists, among the latter *Raphaelle, Rembrandt, Rubens,* and *Titian.* Remarkably, all four lived up to their names by becoming artists themselves.

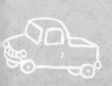

Patrice, Patricio, Patrik, Patrizio, Patrizius, Patryk, Pats, Patsy, Patti, Pattie, Patty

PATTON Old English. "Fighter's town." **Paten, Patin, Paton, Patten**

PAUL Latin. "Small." **Pablo, Pall, Paolo, Paulie, Paulin, Paulinus, Paullus, Paulus, Pauly, Pavel, Pawel, Pawley, Poll, Pollard et al., Poul**

PAXTON Latin. "Peace town." **Packston, Paxon, Paxtun, Payton**

PAYNE Latin. "Countryman." **Paine**

PELAGIUS Greek. "Sea." In myth, the grandson of the river god Inachus and founder of the Pelagic division of the Greek people. **Pelagiusto, Pelagyus**

PELL Middle English. "Parchment." **Pall**

PELLMAN Middle English. "Parchment man." **Pellton**

PEMBROKE Old English. "Broken hill." **Pembrook**

PENLEY Old English. "Enclosed meadow." **Penlea, Penleigh, Penly, Pennlea, Pennleigh, Pennley**

PENN Latin. "Writing instrument." **Pen, Pennie, Penny, Penrod**

PEPE Spanish. Nickname for **Felipe, José. Pepito**

PEPPER English. "Having pep, energy."

PEPPIN Old German. "One who petitions." **Pepin, Peppi, Peppie, Peppy, Pip, Pipin, Pippie, Pippin, Pippy**

PERCIVAL Old French. In Arthurian legend, Sir Percival sought the Holy Grail. **Parsafal, Parsefal, Parsifal, Perce, Perceval, Percevall, Percey, Percie, Percivall, Percy, Purcell**

PERCY French. Short form of **Percival. Pearcy, Percey, Percie**

PEREGRINE Latin. "Traveler." **Peregrin, Peregrino, Peregryn**

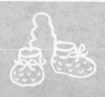

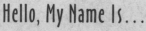
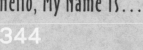

PERFECTO Spanish. "Perfect."

PERKIN Old English. "Little Peter." **Parkin, Perkins, Perkyn, Perrin**

PEROOZ Persian. "Victorious."

PERRY Old English. "Traveler."

PERSEUS Greek. In myth, the killer of Medusa. **Persius, Persi**

PERVIS Latin. "Passage."

PESACH Hebrew. "Spared." **Pessach**

PETER Greek. "Rock." **Peadar, Pearce, Peder, Pedro, Peerus, Per, Perkin** et al., **Pero, Perry, Petar, Pete, Peterus, Petey, Petr, Petros, Petrus, Petur, Piaras, Piero, Pierre, Piers** et al., **Piet, Pieter, Pietr, Pietrek, Pietro, Piotr, Pjotr, Pyotr**

PEVERELL Old French. "Piper." **Peveral, Peverall, Peverel, Peveril**

PEYTON Old English. "Warrior's lands." **Payton**

PHELAN Irish. "Wolf."

PHELPS Old English. "Son of Philip." **Phellps**

PHILEMON Greek. "Kiss." In myth, Baucis and Philemon were an old couple who treated Jupiter and Mercury hospitably when they visited Phrygia in disguise as wayfarers. The gods rewarded them with a temple and with life after death as two trees, an oak and a linden, growing from a single trunk. **Philo**

PHILIP Greek. "Lover of horses." **Felipe** et al., **Fyllip, Lipp, Lippo, Pepe, Phil, Philipp, Philippe, Phillip, Phillips, Phip, Phyllip, Pip, Pippo**

PHILMORE Greek. "Ocean lover."

PHILO Greek. "Loving." Also short form of **Philemon.**

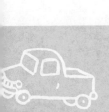

ROMANIAN NAMES

As with other eastern European countries, Romania has had many conquerors, and all of them—Roman, German, various Slavic neighbors, and Russia—shared their names with this country. Catholic saints' names show up here, sometimes with distinctive spellings. Romania was a source of many children adopted by American parents following the 1989 execution of Communist leader Nicolae Ceauşescu.

Here are some Romanian boys' names:

Adrian	"dark" or "from Adria"
Anatolie	"from the east"
Bodgan, Bogdan	"gift of God"
Catalin	"pure"
Costea, Costin, Costine	"constant"
Dimitrie, Dimitry, Dumitru	"follower of Demeter"
Emil	"excellent"
Flaviu, Flavius	"blond hair"
George, Gheorghe	"farmer"
Horatiu	"timekeeper"
Ivan	"God is gracious"

Marian	"bitter" or "rebellious"
Mihai	"who is like the Lord?"
Miroslav	"great glory"
Nic, Nicolae, Nicu, Niculaie	"victory of the people"
Radu	meaning unknown
Simu	"one who listened"
Stefan	"crowned"
Teo, Teodor, Teodosie	"gift of God"
Vlad, Vladimir	"renowned prince"

Here are some Romanian girls' names:

Adriana, Adrianna, Andreea	"dark" or "from Adria"
Amelia	"industrious"
Anica	"grace"
Aurelia	"gold"
Chesna	"peaceful"
Dorina	"brooding" or "gilded"
Ihrin, Irina	"peace"
Lenuta, Leunta	"mild"
Luba	"lover"
Marina, Marinela	"from the sea"
Melita	"honey"

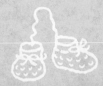

Mirela	"admirable"	Teofila	"divinely loved"
Nicoleta	"victory of the people"	Vanda	"wanderer"
Petronela	"rock"	Violeta	"purple"
Rodica, Rodika	"renowned ruler"	Viorela	meaning unknown
Simona	"one who listened"	Zora	"dawn"

PHINEAS Disputed origin. Possibly Hebrew, "oracle." **Fineas, Phinhas, Pincas, Pinchas, Pinchos, Pincus.** Pinchas Zuckerman, contemporary Israeli violinist and conductor.

PHOENIX Greek. "One who rises from fire." In myth, a magical bird that burned itself and was reborn in the ashes every 500 years. A symbol of death and rebirth. Also the capital of Arizona.

PIARAS Irish variant of **Peter.** Greek, "rock."

PICKFORD Old English. "Ford with pike fish."

PIERRE French variant of **Peter.** Greek, "rock."

PIERS Greek. "Rock." **Pearce, Pears, Peirce, Pierce, Pierson, Piersson**

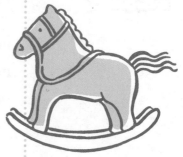

PIERSON English. "Son of Piers." **Pearson**

PIO Latin. "Pious." **Pius**

PITNEY Old English. "Island of the stubborn one." **Pittney**

PITT Old English. "Pit."

PLÁCIDO Spanish. "Serene." Plácido Domingo, contemporary musician. **Placid, Placidus, Placyd, Placydo**

PLATO Greek. "Broad-shouldered." Ancient Greek philosopher, pupil and friend of Socrates. **Platon**

PLATT Old French. "Flat land." **Platte**

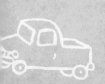

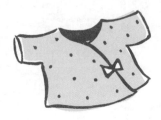

POCO Italian. "Little."

POLLARD English variant of **Paul**. Latin, "small." **Poll, Pollerd, Pollyrd**

POLLOCK Old English variant of **Pollux**. Greek, "crown." **Pollack, Polloch**

POLLUX Greek. "Crown."

POMEROY Old French. "Apple orchard." **Pom, Pommeray, Pommeroy, Pommie, Pommy**

PONTIUS Latin. "From Pontus," an ancient province in Asia Minor. Pontius Pilate, the Roman governor of Judea at the time of Jesus' death. **Ponce, Poncio**

POPE Greek. "Father."

PORFIRIO Greek. "Purple stone." **Porphirio, Porphirios, Prophyrios**

PORTER English from Latin. "Gatekeeper."

POWELL Old English. "Son of Howell." **Powel**

PRENTICE Middle English. "Apprentice." **Prentis, Prentiss**

PRESCOTT Old English. "Priest's cottage." **Prescot, Prestcot, Prestcott, Scott**

PRESLEY Old English. "Priest's meadow." **Presleigh, Presly, Presslee, Pressley, Prestley, Priestley, Priestly**

PRESTON Old English. "Priest's estate."

PREWITT Old French. "Brave little one." **Prewet, Prewett, Prewit, Pruitt**

PRIAM Greek. King of Troy during the Trojan War.

PRICE Welsh. "Prize." **Brice, Bryce, Pryce**

PRIMITIVO Spanish. "Primitive." St. Primitivo.

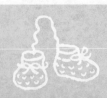

PRIMO Italian. "First." **Preemo, Premo, Prim, Prime**

PRINCE Latin. "Chief." **Prinz, Prinze**

PROCTOR Latin. "Administrator." **Prockter, Procter**

PROSPERO Latin. "Fortunate." In Shakespeare's *Tempest*, Prospero was the magician and exiled duke of Milan. **Prosper**

PRYOR Latin. "Monastic leader." **Prior**

PUCK English. "Mischievous sprite." **Puckeridge**

PURNAL Latin. "Pear."

PURVIS French. "To look after." **Purves, Purviss**

PUTNAM Latin. "Gardner." **Putnem, Putnum**

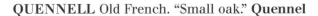

QUENNELL Old French. "Small oak." **Quennel**

QUENTIN Latin. "Fifth." **Quent, Quenten, Quenton, Quint, Quintin, Quinton, Quintus**

QUIGLEY Irish. Disputed meaning. **Quigly**

QUILLAN Irish. "Cub." **Quillen**

QUIMBY Old Norse. "Estate of the woman." **Quimby**

QUINCY Old French. "Estate of the fifth son." **Quince, Quincey**

QUINLAN Irish. "Strong." **Quindlen**

QUINN Irish. "Wise leader." **Quin**

QUIRINAL Latin. One of the seven hills of Rome.

QUIRINUS Latin. In myth, the deified Romulus, the founder of Rome.

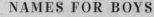

RABI Arabic. "Gentle wind." **Rabbi, Rabee**

RAD Old English. "Adviser."

RADAMA Madagascarian. A king of Madagascar.

RADBERT Old English. "Bright adviser." **Radburt**

RADBURN Old English. "Red brook." **Radborn, Radborne, Radbourn, Radbourne, Radburne**

RADCLIFF Old English. "Red cliff." **Radcliffe, Radclyffe**

RADFORD Old English. "Red ford." **Radferd, Radfurd**

RADLEY Old English. "Red meadow." **Radlea, Radlee, Radleigh, Radly**

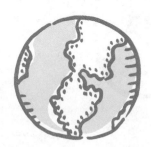

RADNOR Old English. "Red shore."

RADU Romanian. Unknown meaning.

RAFE English variant of **Raphael.**

RAFFERTY Irish. "Prosperity wielder." **Rafe, Raferty, Raff, Raffarty**

RAFI Arabic. "Holding high." **Rafee, Raff, Raffi, Raffy**

RAGNAR Norwegian. "Powerful army." **Ragnor, Rainer, Rainier, Rayner, Raynor**

RAJA Sanskrit. "King." **Raj**

RALEIGH Old English. "Meadow of deer." **Ralegh, Rawleigh, Rawley, Rawly**

RALPH Old English. "Wolf-counsel." **Raaf, Raff, Ralf, Raoul, Raoulin, Rauf, Rauffe, Raul**

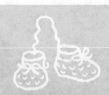

RALSTON Old English. "Ralph's town."

RAMIRO Portuguese. "Great judge." **Ramirez**

RAMÓN Spanish variant of **Raymond.** Old German, "guardian."

RAMSAY Old English. "Ram's island." **Ram, Ramsey**

RAMSDEN Old English. "Ram's valley."

RAMSES Egyptian. "Sun-born." Egyptian kings of the XIX and XX dynasties. **Rameses, Ramesses**

RANAN Hebrew. "Vibrant." **Raanan, Ranen, Ranon**

RAND Old English. "Fighter."

RANDALL Variant of **Randolph.** Old English, "shield-wolf." **Randal, Randel, Randell, Randie, Randl, Randle, Randy**

RANDOLPH Old English. "Shield-wolf." **Randall** et al., **Randolf**

RANGER Old French. "Forest guardian." **Rainger, Range**

RANKIN Old English. "Little shield."

RANSFORD Old English. "Raven's ford." **Rainsford**

RANSLEY Old English. "Raven's meadow." **Ransleigh, Ransly**

RANSOM Latin. "Release."

RAOUL French variant of **Ralph.** "Wolf-counsel." **Raul**

RAPHAEL Hebrew. "God has healed." **Falito, Rafal, Rafael, Rafaelle, Rafaello, Rafe, Rafel, Rafello, Raffael, Raffaello, Raffi, Rafi, Rafit, Raphaello, Raphello**

RASHID Turkish. "Righteous." **Rasheed, Rasheid, Rasheyd**

RAVEN Old English. "Raven."

RAVI Hindi. "Sun." **Ravee**

RAVID Hebrew. "Ornament."

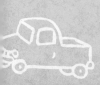

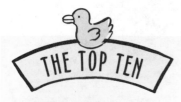

THE TOP TEN

NAMES OF 1997

The Year *Titanic* Won the
Oscar for Best Picture

BOYS

Michael
Jacob
Matthew
Christopher
Nicholas
Austin
Joshua
Andrew
Joseph
Brandon

GIRLS

Emily
Sarah
Taylor
Jessica
Ashley
Samantha
Madison
Hannah
Kayla
Alexis

RAWLINS Old French. "Son of a wise wolf." **Rawlens, Rawlinson, Rawson**

RAY Short form of **Raymond**. Old German, "guardian." Also variant of **Rey. Rae, Raye, Reigh, Reo**

RAYBURN Old English. "Brook with ray fish." **Burn, Raeborn, Raeborne, Raebourn, Raeburn, Raeburne, Rayborn, Raybourne, Rayburne**

RAYMOND Old German. "Guardian." **Raemond, Raemondo, Raimond, Raimondo, Raimund, Raimundo, Rajmund, Ramon, Ramond, Ramonde, Ramóne, Ray, Rayment, Raymondo, Raymund, Raymunde, Raymundo, Raynard, Redmond** et al.

RAYN Arabic. One of the gates of Heaven.

RAYNOR Norwegian. "Mighty army." **Ragnar, Rainer, Rainier, Rainor, Ranieri, Raynar, Rayner**

RAYYAN Arabic. "Full" or "pretty."

READ Old English. "Red-haired." **Reade, Red, Redd, Reed, Reid, Reidar, Reide, Reyd**

READING Old English. "Son of the red-haired one." **Raiding, Redding, Reeding**

RED English. "Red-haired." **Redd**

REDFORD Old English. "Quick ford." **Radford, Ford**

REDLEY Old English. "Red meadow." **Radley, Redlea, Redleigh, Redly**

REDMOND Irish variant of **Raymond**. Old German, "guardian." **Radmond, Radmund, Redmund**

REECE Welsh. "With zeal." **Rees, Reese, Rhys, Rice**

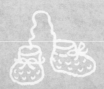

REED Old English. "Red-haired." **Read, Reade, Red, Redd, Reid, Reidar, Reyd**

REEVE Middle English. "Bailiff." **Reave, Reeves**

REGAN Irish. "Little king." **Reagan, Regen**

REGINALD Old English. "Powerful ruler." **Naldo, Ragnold, Reg, Reggie, Reginaldo, Reginalt, Reginauld, Reginault, Regnauld, Regnault, Reynard** et al., **Reynold** et al., **Ronald** et al.

REINART Old German. "Powerful ruler." **Rainart, Rainhard, Rainhardt, Reginhart, Reinhard, Reinhardt, Reinhart**

REMINGTON Old English. "Raven-family village." **Remi, Remy**

REMUS Latin. "Swift." In myth, the twin brother of Romulus. **Remer, Remi, Remis**

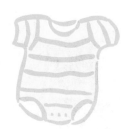

REMY French. "From Rheims." **Remee, Remi, Remie, Remmy**

RENALDO Spanish. "Powerful ruler." **Rinaldo, Ronaldo**

RENART French variant of **Reginhart.** Old German, "powerful ruler." The name of the fox in the medieval animal epic *Roman de Renart.* **Rainard, Ray, Raynard, Renard, Renaud, Renauld, Rey, Reynard, Reynart, Reynaud, Reyner**

RENATUS Latin. "Reborn." **Ren, Renat, Renato**

RENÉ French. "Reborn." **Renay**

RENFRED Old English. "Wise counsel for peace."

RENFREW Old Welsh. "Calm river."

RENNY Irish. "Small and mighty." **Renney, Renni**

RENSHAW Old English. "Raven woods." **Renishaw**

RENTON Old English. "Camp of the roe deer."

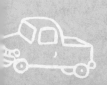

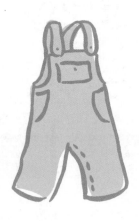

REUBEN Hebrew. "Behold, a child." **Reuban, Reubin, Reuven, Rouvin, Rube, Ruben, Rubens, Rubin, Ruby**

REX Latin. "King." **Regis**

REXFORD Old English. "King's crossing." **Rexer**

REY Spanish. "King." Also short form of **Reynard. Ray, Reyes**

REYNARD English variant of **Renart**, the name of the fox in the medieval animal epic *Roman de Renart*.

REYNOLD Variant of **Reginald.** Old English, "powerful ruler." **Rainalt, Rainhold, Raynold, Raynolt, Reinald, Reinaldo, Reinaldos, Reinhold, Reinold, Reinolt, Renado, Renaldo, Rinald**

RHETT Variant of **Rhys.** Welsh. "With zeal." Rhett Butler, Scarlett O'Hara's third husband in Margaret Mitchell's *Gone with the Wind*.

RHODES Greek. "Where roses grow." **Rhodas, Rodas**

RHODRIC German. "Renowned ruler." **Roderick, Rodrick, Rodrik**

RHYS Welsh. "With zeal." **Reece, Reese, Rey, Rhett, Rice, Rise**

RICH Short form of **Aldrich, Richard. Richie, Richy, Ritchey, Ritchie, Ritchy**

RICHARD Old German. "Great ruler." **Dic, Dick, Dickie, Dicky, Dix, Dixie, Dixy, Ric, Ricardo, Riccardo, Rich** et al., **Richardo, Richardon, Richart, Richerd, Rick** et al., **Rickard, Rickert, Rickey, Rico, Rikard, Riocard, Ritchard, Ritcherd, Ritchyrd, Ritshard, Ritsherd, Ryszard**

RICHMOND Old German. "Powerful protector." Also the name of cities in California, Virginia, New South Wales, New Zealand, and South Africa.

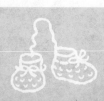

RICK Short form of **Aldrich, Cedric, Dietrich, Frederick, Heinrich, Richard. Ricci, Rici, Ricki, Rickie, Ricky, Riki, Rikki**

RICKWARD Old English. "Mighty guardian." **Rickwerd, Rickwood**

RIDER Old English. "Horseman." **Ridder, Ryder**

RIDGE Old English. "Ridge."

RIDGEWAY Old English. "Path on the ridge."

RIDGLEY Old English. "Ridge meadow." **Ridgeleigh, Ridgeley, Ridglea, Ridgleigh, Ridgley**

RIDLEY Old English. "Cleared meadow." **Riddley, Ridlea, Ridleigh, Ridly**

RILEY Irish. "Courageous." **Reilly, Ryley, Ryly**

RING Old English. "Ring."

RIORDAN Irish. "Minstrel." **Rearden, Reardon, Ri**

RIPLEY Old English. "Ripe meadow." **Rip, Ripleigh, Riply**

RISLEY Old English. "Meadow with shrubs." **Rislea, Rislee, Risleigh, Risly, Wrisley**

RISTON Old English. "Town near the shrubs." **Wriston**

RITTER German. "Knight." **Rit, Ritt**

RIVER English. "River." **Rivers**

ROALD Old German. "Famous and powerful." Roald Dahl, contemporary author of *Charlie and the Chocolate Factory* and other books.

ROARK Irish. "Mighty ruler." **Roarke, Rorke, Rourke, Ruark**

ROBERT Old English. "Bright fame." **Bert, Bertie, Bob, Bobbie, Bobby, Rab, Rabbie, Riobard, Rip, Rob, Robb,**

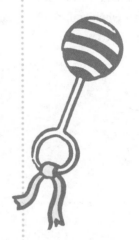

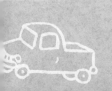

U. S. Chess Hall of Fame inductees

This strategic crowd, who attained their fame by hunching over chess boards, have some names worthy of consideration when you make your naming move.

Lev Alburt
Hans Berliner
Pal Benko
Arthur Bisguier
Walter Browne
Donald Byrne
Robert Byrne
John Collins
Arthur Dake
Arnold Denker
Ed Edmondson
Arpad Elo
Larry Evans
Reuben Fine
Robert (Bobby) Fischer
Benjamin Franklin
Gisela Gresser

Kenneth Harkness
Hermann Helms
I. A. Horowitz
Isaac Kashdan
Lubomir Kavalek
George Koltanowski
Sam Loyd
George Mackenzie
Frank Marshall
Edmar Mednis
Paul Morphy
Victor Palciauskas
Harry Pillsbury
Fred Reinfeld
Sammy Reshevsky
Wilhelm Steinitz
Milan Vukcevich

Robbie, Robby, Robers, Roberto, Roberts, Robi, Robin et al., **Rupert** et al.

ROBERTSON Old English. "Son of Robert."

ROBIN Old English variant of **Robert. Robben, Robbin, Robbins, Robyn**

ROBINSON Old English. "Son of Robert." **Robbinson, Robeson, Robynson, Robson**

ROCCO Italian. "Rock."

ROCHE Old French. "Rock." **Roc, Roch, Roque**

ROCHESTER Old English. "Stone fortress." Also cities in England, Canada, Australia, Minnesota, New Hampshire, and New York. **Chester, Chet, Rocco, Rock**

ROCKY English. "Rocky." **Rock**

ROCKLEY Old English. "Rock meadow." **Rocklee, Rockleigh, Rockly**

ROCKWELL Old English. "Rock spring."

ROKURO Japanese. "Sixth son."

ROD Short form of **Roderick**. Old German, "renowned ruler."

RODERICK Old German. "Renowned ruler." **Rod, Rodd, Rodderick, Roddie, Roddrick, Roddy, Roderic, Roderich, Roderyck, Rodrick, Rodrigo** et al., **Rodrik, Rodryck, Rodryk, Rory, Rurik, Ruy**

RODMAN Old German. "Renowned man." **Rodmen**

RODNEY Old English. "Island near the clearing." **Rod, Rodnee, Rodnie**

RODRIGO Spanish variant of **Roderick**. Old German, "renowned ruler." **Roderigo, Rodrigue, Rodrigues, Rodrique**

ROE Middle English. "Roe deer." **Row, Rowe**

ROGAN Irish. "Red-haired."

ROGER Old German. "Renowned spearman." **Dodge, Dodger, Rodge, Rodger, Rodgers, Rog, Rogelio, Rogerio, Rogers, Rogiero, Roj, Ruger, Rugero, Ruggiero, Rutger, Ruttger**

ROLAND Old German. "Famous." **Lannie, Lanny, Orlando, Roeland, Rolan, Rolando, Roldan, Roley, Rollan, Rolland, Rollen, Rollie, Rollin, Rollins, Rolly, Rowe, Rowland**

ROLF Old German. "Cunning wolf." **Rolfe, Rolph, Rolphe, Roulf**

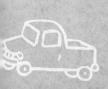

ROLLO Old French. "Famed land." **Rolle, Rolli, Rollie, Rolo**

ROMAN Latin. "From Rome." **Rome, Romain, Romano, Romanos, Romanus**

ROMEO Italian. "Pilgrim to Rome." **Rommey, Rommy, Romo, Romolo**

ROMNEY Old Welsh. "Winding river."

ROMULUS Latin. In myth, the founder of Rome. **Romallus, Romalus**

RONALD Old English. "Powerful ruler." **Ranald, Ron, Roneld, Roni, Ronnie, Ronny**

RONAN Irish. "Little seal." **Ronen**

RONSON Old English. "Son of Ronald."

ROONEY Irish. "Red-haired." **Rowney**

ROOSEVELT Old Dutch. "Rose field." Many boys have been named *Roosevelt* after Theodore Roosevelt and, especially, Franklin Delano Roosevelt, both U.S. presidents.

ROPER Old English. "Rope maker."

RORY Irish. "Red." **Rorey, Rorie, Rorrey, Rorrie, Rorry**

ROSARIO Portuguese. "Rosary." **Rosarius**

ROSCOE Scandinavian. "Deer woods." **Rosco**

ROSS Scottish. "Woody meadow." **Rosse, Rossie, Rossy**

ROSSO Italian. "Red."

ROSWELL Old English. "Rose spring."

ROTH Old German. "Red."

ROTHWELL Old Norse. "Red spring."

ROVER Middle English. "Wanderer."

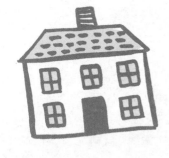

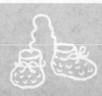

ROWAN Old English. "Rowan tree." **Roan, Rowe, Rowen, Rowney**

ROWELL Old English. "Roe-deer well." **Rowel**

ROWLEY Old English. "Roughly cleared meadow." **Rowlea, Rowlee, Rowleigh, Rowly**

ROXBURY Old English. "Rook's village." **Roxburshe**

ROY Scottish, "red." French, "king." **Roi, Roye, Ruy**

ROYAL Old French. "Royal." **Royall, Royle**

ROYCE Old English. Disputed meaning. **Roice**

ROYDEN Old English. "Rye hill." **Roydan, Roydon**

ROYSTON Old English. A city in England.

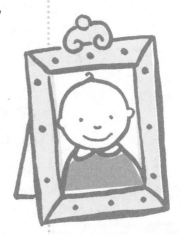

RUDOLPH Old German. "Famous wolf." **Dolph, Rodolfo, Rodolph, Rodolphe, Rodolpho, Rodulfo, Rudey, Rudi, Rudie, Rudolf, Rudolfo, Rudolphus, Rudy**

RUDYARD Old English. "Red paddock." Rudyard Kipling, 1856–1936, British author of *The Jungle Book* and other works about India, his birthplace. **Rudd, Ruddie, Ruddy, Rudy**

RUFORD Old English. "Rough crossing." **Rufe, Ruferd, Rufert, Rufford**

RUFUS Latin. "Red-haired." **Ruffus, Rufous**

RUGBY Old English. "Rook fortress."

RUMFORD Old English. "Wide river-crossing."

RUPERT Variant of **Robert. Ruperto, Ruprecht**

RURIK Scandinavian variant of **Roderick.** Old German, "renowned ruler."

RUSHFORD Old English. "Crossing with rushes."

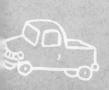

RUSKIN Old French. "Little red-haired one."

RUSSEL French variant of **Rufus**. Latin, "Red-haired." **Rossel, Rossell, Russ, Russell**

RUSTY English. "Red-haired."

RUTHERFORD Old English. "Cattle crossing." **Rutherfurd**

RUTLAND Old Norse. "Land of roots." Also a city in Vermont.

RUTLEY Old English. "Root meadow." **Rutleigh**

RYAN Irish. Disputed meaning. **Ryen, Ryon, Ryun**

RYCROFT Old English. "Rye field." **Ryecroft**

RYDER Old English variant of **Rider**. "Horseman."

RYLAND Old English. "Land where rye is grown." **Ryeland**

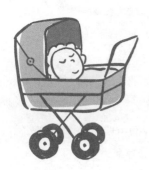

SABATH Hebrew. "Rest." **Sabat, Shabbet, Shabbetai**

SABER French. "Sword." **Sabre**

SABIN Latin. "Sabine," a member of an ancient tribe that inhabited the Apennines. **Sabino**

SACHA Russian variant of **Alexander**. Greek, "defender of mankind." **Sascha, Sash, Sasha, Sashe**

SADLER Old English. "Harness maker." **Saddler**

SAFFORD Old English. "Willow river-crossing." **Safferd**

SAGI Aramaic. "Mighty." **Saggai**

SAID Arabic. "Happy." **Saeed, Sayed, Sayeed, Sayid**

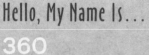 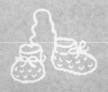

SALATHIEL Hebrew. "Requested of God." **Sealtiele, Shaltiel**

SALIM Arabic. "Tranquility." **Saleem, Salem**

SALTON Old English. "Salt town."

SALVADOR Spanish. "Savior." Salvador Dali, twentieth-century Spanish surrealist painter. **Salvidor**

SALVATORE Italian. "Savior." **Sal, Salvator, Salvatori, Salvetor**

SAM Short form of **Samson, Samuel. Sahm, Sami, Samm, Sammi, Sammey, Sammie, Sammy, Samy**

SAMI Arabic. "Exhalted one."

SAMIR Arabic. "Entertainer."

SAMORI Mandinka. A Mandinka king.

SAMOSET Algonquin. "Traveler."

SAMSON Hebrew. "Sun." **Sam** et al., **Sampson, Sansom, Sanson, Sansone**

SAMUEL Hebrew. "Told by God." **Sam** et al., **Samuele, Samuello**

SAN Chinese. "Three" or "third."

SANBORN Old English. "Sandy stream." **Sanborne, Sanbourn, Sanbourne, Sanburn, Sanburne, Sandborn, Sandborne, Sandbourne, Sandburn, Sandburne**

SANCHO Spanish. "Sincere." **Sanchez, Sauncho**

SANDER Variant of **Alexander**. Greek, "defender of mankind." **Sandero, Sandor, Sandore, Sandro, Saunder**

SANDERS Middle English. "Son of Alexander." **Sanderson, Sandersson, Sanson, Saunders, Saunderson**

SANDITON Old English. "Sandy town."

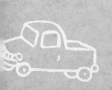

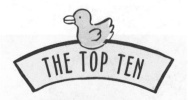

THE TOP TEN

FRENCH NAMES OF 2001

BOYS

Thomas
Lucas
Théo
Hugo
Maxime
Antoine
Quentin
Clément
Alexandre
Nicolas

GIRLS

Léa
Manon
Chloé
Camille
Emma
Océane
Sarah
Marie
Laura
Julie

SANDOR Hungarian variant of **Alexander.** Greek, "defender of mankind." **Sandore**

SANDY Shorter form of **Alexander.** Greek. "Defender of mankind." **Sandey, Sandi, Sandie**

SANFORD Old English. "Sandy ford." **Sandford, Sandfurd, Sanferd, Sanfred**

SANTIAGO Spanish. "St. James."

SANTO Italian, Spanish. "Holy" or "saint." **Santos**

SAPHIR Sanskrit. "Sapphire." **Safir, Saffir**

SARGENT Old French. "Officer." **Sargant, Sarge, Sargeant, Sarjeant, Sergant, Sergent**

SARTO Italian. "Tailor."

SATURN Roman. The god of sowers and seeds and the father of Jupiter. Also the sixth planet from the sun. **Saturnin, Saturnino, Saturno, Saturnus.** St. Saturnino.

SAUL Hebrew. "Asked for." **Saule, Saulo, Shaul, Sol, Sollie, Solly, Zaul, Zol**

SAUVEUR French. "Savior."

SAVILLE French. "Willow town." **Savil, Savile, Savill, Savylle, Sevil, Seville**

SAWYER Middle English. "One who saws." **Sawyere**

SAXON Middle English. "Of the Saxons," a Germanic tribe that entered England in the fifth century, or "from Saxony." **Sax, Saxe, Saxen, Saxin**

SAYER Welsh. "Victorious." **Saer, Say, Sayers, Sayre, Sayrrs**

SCANLON French. "Little trapper." **Scanlan, Scanlen, Skanlen, Skanlon**

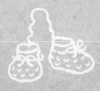

SCHUYLER Dutch. "Protection." **Schuylar**

SCIPIO Latin. "Staff." **Sipio**

SCOTT Old English. "Scotsman." **Schott, Scot, Scoti, Scottie, Scotto, Scotty**

SEABERN Old English "Stream near the sea." **Seaberne, Seabourn, Seabourne, Seaburn, Seaburne**

SEABERT Old English. "Shining sea." **Seabright, Sebert, Seibert**

SEABROOK Old English. "Stream near the sea." **Seabrooke**

SEAMUS Irish variant of **James.** Hebrew, "he who supplants." **Seumas, Seumus, Shamus**

SEAN Irish variant of **John.** Hebrew, "God is gracious." **Cian, Shane** et al., **Seann, Shaughn, Shaun, Shawn**

SEARLE Old English. "Battle." **Sear, Searl, Sears, Serel, Serill, Serle**

SEATON Old English. "Town near the sea." **Seeton, Seton**

SEBASTIAN Latin. "Revered." **Basti, Bastin, Bastian, Bastiano, Bastien, Sabastian, Sabastino, Seb, Sebastiano, Sebastien, Sebestyen, Sebo, Steb**

SEDGLEY Old English. "Sedge meadow." **Sedgeley, Sedgely, Seggley**

SEDGWICK Old English. "Sedge place." **Sedgewick, Sedgewyck, Sedgwyck, Seggwick**

SEELEY Old English. "Blessed." **Sealey, Seely**

SEFTON Old English. "Town in the rushes."

SEGEL Hebrew. "Treasure." **Segal**

SEGER Old English. "Sea fighter." **Seagar, Seager, Segar, Seeger**

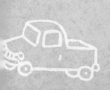

SEGEV Hebrew. "Regal."

SEGUNDO Spanish. "Second."

SEIJI Japanese. "Lawful."

SELBY Old English. "Village by the willows."

SELDON Old English. "Willow valley." **Selden, Sellden**

SELIG Old German. "Holy." **Zelig, Zelik**

SELIGMAN Old German. "Holy man." **Seligmann**

SELWYN Old English. "Friend of the house." **Selwin, Selwinn, Selwynn, Selwynne, Win, Wyn, Wynne**

SENIOR Old French. "Older."

SENNETT French. "Elderly." **Sennet**

SEPTIMUS Latin. "Seventh." **Sept**

SEQUOYAH Cherokee. "Sparrow." Cherokee leader, 1766–1843, who created a written Cherokee language, published a newspaper in that language, taught thousands to read and write, and helped to unite the Cherokee. The redwoods of California, *Sequoia sempervirens* and *Sequoiadendron,* are named for him. **Sequoia, Sequoiah**

SERAPHIM Hebrew. "Ardent." In the Bible, the fiery six-winged angels who guard God's throne. **Seraf, Serafin, Serafino, Seraph, Seraphimus**

SERENO Latin. "Tranquil." **Ceren, Cereno**

SERGE Latin. "Servant." **Sergei, Sergey, Sergi, Sergio, Sergios, Sergiu, Sergiusz, Serguei, Sirge, Sirgio, Sirgios**

SETH Hebrew. "Appointed." **Set, Sethe**

SETON Old English. "Sea town." **Seaton**

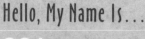

SEVERIN Latin. "Severe." **Severino, Severo, Severus, Seweryn** Septimius Severus, Roman emperor, 193–211. St. Severo.

SEVERN Old English. "Boundary." **Severne**

SEVILEN Turkish. "Beloved."

SEWALL Old English. "Sea strong." **Sewal, Sewald, Sewall, Sewel, Sewell**

SEWARD Old English. "Sea guardian." **Seaward, Seawerd, Seawert, Sewerd, Sewert**

SEXTON Middle English. "Church custodian."

SEXTUS Latin. "Sixth." **Sixtus**

SEYMOUR Old French. "From St. Maur." **Seamor, Seamore, Seamour, Seymore**

SHADRACH Babylonian. "Commanded by God." **Shadrack**

SHAFER Hebrew. "Handsome." **Schafer, Shafir**

SHAHEEN Persian. "Royal falcon."

SHAIMING Chinese. "Sunshine."

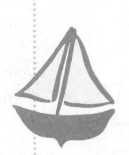

SHAKA Zulu. "Great king." A nineteenth-century Zulu king who led wars against neighboring tribes. **Chaka**

SHALOM Variant of **Solomon.** Hebrew, "peace." **Sholom**

SHAMIR Hebrew. "Strong."

SHANAHAN Irish. "Wise, clever."

SHANDY Old English. "Boisterous, high-spirited." **Shandey, Shandi, Shantey, Shanti**

SHANE Variant of **Sean,** Irish variant of **John.** Hebrew, "God is gracious." **Shaine, Shayn, Shayne**

SHANLEY Irish. "Small and ancient." **Shannley**

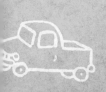

SHANNON Irish. "Ancient." **Shaanan, Shanan, Shannan, Shannen, Shanon**

SHAQUILLE Arabic. "Handsome." Shaquille O'Neal, contemporary professional basketball player. **Shakil, Shakile, Shaquil, Shaquile**

SHARIF Arabic. "Honest." **Shareef**

SHAW Old English. "Wood."

SHAWNEE Native American. "Southern people." An Algonquin tribe of the eastern woodlands.

SHAYAAN Arabic. "Intelligent."

SHAYAN Persian. "Suitable."

SHEEHAN Irish. "Small and tranquil." **Sheen, Shehen, Shennan**

SHEFFIELD Old English. "Crooked meadow."

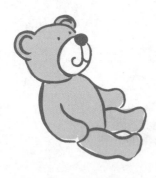

SHEL Short form of **Shelby, Sheldon, Shelley, Shelton.** Shel (Sheldon Allan) Silverstein, 1930–1999, American writer of mostly humorous songs, poems, and children's stories.

SHELBY Old English. "Farm on the ledge." **Shel, Shelbey, Shelbie**

SHELDON Old English. "Steep valley." **Shel, Shelden, Sheldin**

SHELLEY Old English. "Ledge meadow." **Shel, Shell, Shellie, Shelly**

SHELTON Old English. "Ledge town."

SHEM Hebrew. "Name."

SHEPHERD Old English. "Shepherd." **Shep, Shepard, Sheperd, Shephard, Shepp, Sheppard, Shepperd**

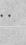

SHEPLEY Old English. "Sheep meadow." **Shapleigh, Shapley, Sheplea, Shepleigh, Shepply, Ship, Shipley, Shipp**

SHERBORN Old English. "Bright stream." **Sherborne, Sherbourn, Sherburn, Sherburne**

SHERIDAN Irish. "Seeker." **Sherdan, Sherdon, Sheredan, Sheredon, Sheridon, Sherridan, Sherridon**

SHERILL Old English. "Countryside." **Sherril, Sherrill**

SHERIRA Arabic. "Strong."

SHERLOCK Old English. "Wooded enclosure." Sherlock Holmes, fictional detective created by Sir Arthur Conan Doyle. **Sherlocke**

SHERMAN Old English. "Shearing man." **Scherman, Schermann, Shearman, Shermann, Shurman**

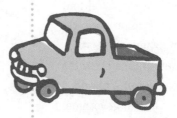

SHERWIN Middle English. "Friend to the community." **Sherwind, Sherwinn, Sherwyn, Sherwynn, Sherwynne, Win, Winnie, Winny**

SHERWOOD Old English. "Community forest." **Sherwoode, Shurwood, Wood, Woodie, Woody**

SHIPLEY Variant of **Shepley.** Old English. "Sheep meadow." **Ship, Shipp**

SHIPTON Old English. "Ship town."

SHLOMO Variant of **Solomon.** Hebrew, "peace." **Shelomo**

SHOLTO Scottish. "Propagator."

SIDNEY Old English. "From St. Denis." **Sid, Syd, Sydney**

SIEGFRIED Old German. "Victory peace." **Siffe, Siffre, Sigfed, Sigfrid, Sigfried, Sigfryd, Sigge, Sygfied, Zig, Ziggie**

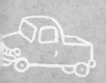

The curious case of President Truman's S

When Harry Truman was born, his parents could not agree on which of his grandfathers' names they should give him—*Shipp* or *Solomon*—so they gave the child an S instead of a middle name. Through the years, persnickety persons and publications have insisted that the S should have no period after it, but examinations of Truman's autographs show that he occasionally put a period after the S. Official government publications referring to the thirty-third president contain the period, as does the name of the Harry S. Truman Library.

SIGMUND Old German. "Victorious protector." Sigmund Freud, inventor of psychoanalysis. **Siegmund, Sig, Sigismond, Sigismondo, Sigismund, Sigismundo, Sigismundus, Sigmond, Sigsmond, Szygmond**

SIGWALD Old German. "Victorious leader." **Siegwald, Sigvard, Sigwalde, Sigwold**

SILAS Greek. "Wood." **Cilas, Cilus, Sillas, Sillus, Silo, Silus**

SILVANUS Latin. "Wood dweller." **Silvain, Silvan, Silvano, Silvio, Sylvan, Sylvanus, Sylvio**

SILVESTER Latin. "Wooded." **Silver, Silvestor, Silvestr, Silvestre, Silvestro, Sly, Sy, Sylvere, Sylvester, Vester**

SIMBA Swahili. "Lion."

SIMON Hebrew. "One who listened." St. Simon, one of the twelve disciples of Jesus. Simon Peter (St. Peter), the most prominent of the twelve disciples. **Cimon, Jímen** et al., **Shimon, Shimone, Si, Sim, Simen, Simeon, Simi, Simie, Simmie, Simmonds, Simmons, Simms, Simón, Simone, Sims, Simu, Sy, Symms, Symon, Szymon, Ximenes** et al.

SIMPSON English. "Son of Simon." **Simpsen, Simsen, Simson**

SINBAD Arabic. Sinbad the Sailor, a hero in the *Arabian Nights*. **Sindbad**

SINCLAIR Old French. "St. Clair." Sinclair Lewis, 1885–1951, American novelist, author of *Main Street*. **Sinclare, St. Clair, Synclair**

SIRAJ Arabic. "Light, beam."

SIRO Italian variant of **Syrus**. Latin, "Syrian."

SKELLY Irish. "Bard." **Scully**

SKERRY Old Norse. "Stony isle."

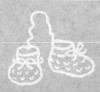

SKIP Scandinavian. "Ship captain." **Skipp, Skipper, Skippy**

SKYLAR Dutch. "Protection." **Skuyler, Skyler**

SLADE Old English. "Valley." **Slaide, Slayde**

SLAVIN Irish. "Mountain man." **Slawin, Sleven**

SLOAN Irish. "Man of arms." **Sloane, Slone**

SMEDLEY Old English. "Flat meadow." **Smedleigh, Smedly**

SMITH Old English. "Blacksmith." **Smit, Smithy, Smitty, Smyth, Smythe**

SNOWDEN Old English. "Snowy hill." **Snowdenn, Snowdin, Snowdon**

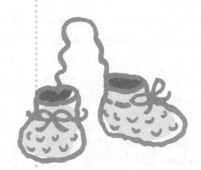

SOCRATES Greek. Ancient philosopher of Athens, Plato's teacher. **Sokrates**

SOL Latin. "Sun." Also short form of **Solomon,** variant of **Saul.**

SOLOMON Hebrew. "Peace." **Salamon, Salmen, Salmon, Salo, Saloman, Salome, Salomo, Salomon, Salomone, Shalom, Shelomo, Shlomo, Sholom, Shomo, Sol, Solaman, Sollie, Solmon, Soloman, Zalman** et al., **Zadok** et al.

SOMERSET Old English. "Summer settlement." **Sommerset, Summerset**

SOMERTON Old English. "Summer town."

SOMERVILLE Old English. "Summer town." **Somervile**

SORRELL Old French. "Red-brown." **Sorell**

SOUTHWELL Old English. "South well." **Sothel**

SPALDING Old English. "Divided field." **Spaulding**

SPEAR Old English. "Spear." **Speare, Spears, Speer, Spier**

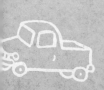

Native American dancers

Across the country, Native Americans gather every year to compete in various kinds of dance. The dancers named below come from three tribes of the Ute Nation—the Northern Ute Tribe, the Southern Ute Tribe, and the Mountain Ute Tribe—all of which gather annually in Delta, Colorado, for the Council Tree Pow Wow and Cultural Festival. These dancers were winners in 2001.

Junior Girls Fancy/Jingle Dancing
1st Symone Paskemin
2nd Alexandra Aldrich
3rd Taylor Anderson
4th Mayla Manning
5th Tia Kane

Junior Boys Traditional
1st Dwayne Iron
2nd Michael Grant
3rd Jamon Paskemin
4th Montie Long Hair
5th Seth Rouibideaux

Junior Boys Fancy/Grass Dance
1st Willie Tapoof
2nd Johnnie "DJ" Johnson
3rd Jo Jo Sammaripa
4th Lanson Manning
5th Austin Ridley

Teen Girls Traditional
1st Michelle Allrunner
2nd Ricki Snatistevan
3rd Snow Wing
4th Martine Root

Teen Girls Fancy Dance
1st Jolynn Begay
2nd Cecily Yankton
3rd Sierrah Lofton-Bearrobe
4th Serenity Foote
5th Lindsay Box

Women's Northern Traditional
1st Tavia Natchees
2nd Daisy Frost
3rd Tetona Kanip
4th Joetta Bitsuie
5th Paula Rouillard

Women's Fancy Dance
1st Raelene Whiteshield
2nd Amber Windy Boy
3rd Sancha Paskemin
4th Tiffany Phelps
5th Gracie Foote

Men's Northern Traditional
1st Parris Leighton-Greene
2nd Asay No Braid
3rd Josh Williamson
4th Frances Sherwood
5th Lynn Burson

Men's Grass Dance
1st Randall Paskemin
2nd Bart Pawaukee
3rd J. R. McCabe
4th Jeremiah Little Soldier
5th Lionel Bel

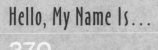

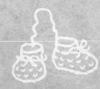

SPENCER Middle English. "Provisioner." **Spence, Spens, Spense, Spenser**

SPIKE Contemporary American, from Middle English. "Large nail."

SPIRIDON Greek. "Of the soul or spirit." **Spiridion, Spiro, Spiros, Spyridon, Spyros.** Spiro Agnew, U.S. vice president during the Nixon administration.

SQUIRE Middle English. "Knight's attendant."

STACY Irish. "Bountiful." **Stacey**

STAFFORD Old English. "From the ford by the landing place." **Staferd, Stafferd, Stafforde, Staford**

STANBURY Old English. "Stone fortification." **Stanbar, Stanber, Stanberry, Stanbery**

STANDISH Old English. "Stony parkland."

STANFELD Old English. "Stony field." **Stanfield, Stansfield**

STANFORD Old English "Stony ford." **Stamford, Standford**

STANISLAS Slavic. Disputed meaning. **Stan, Stanislao, Stanislaus, Stanislav, Stanislaw, Stanislus, Stannes**

STANLEY Old English. "Stony field." **Stan, Stanlea, Stanleigh, Stanly**

STANTON Old English. "Stony village." **Stanten, Stantin, Staunton**

STANWAY Old English. "Stony path." **Stanaway, Stannaway, Stannway**

STANWICK Old English. "Rocky village." **Stanviche, Stanvish, Stanwicke, Stanwyck**

STANWOOD Old English. "Stony woods." **Stanwoode**

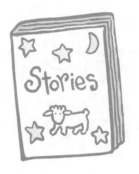

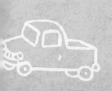

STARR Middle English "Star." **Star, Starre**

STASIUS Short form of **Anastasius.** Greek, "resurrection." **Stasio**

STAVROS Greek. "Crowned."

STEADMAN Old English. "Farmstead occupant." **Steadmann, Stedman**

STEEL Old English. "Steel." **Steal, Steele**

STEIN German. "Stone." **Steen**

STEPHEN Greek. "Crowned." **Estéban** et al., **Estienne, Estvan, Etienne, Staffan, Stefan, Stefano, Steffen, Stephan, Stephanus, Stephens, Stevan, Steve, Steven, Stevie, Stevy**

STEPHENSON Old English. "Son of Steven." **Stephens, Stevens, Stevenson**

STERLING Old English. "High quality." **Stirling**

STERNE Middle English. "Unyielding." **Stearn, Stearne, Stearns, Stern**

STEWART Old English. "Steward." **Stew, Steward, Stu, Stuart**

STILLMAN Old English. "Silent man." **Stillmen, Stillmin, Stilman, Stilmen, Stilmin**

STOCKLEY Old English. "Field by fallen trees." **Stockly**

STOCKTON Old English. "Town by fallen trees." **Stocktin**

STOCKWELL Old English. "Well near fallen trees."

STODDARD Old English. "Horse guard."

STORM Old English. "Storm."

STORR Old Norse. "Great one."

STRAHAN Irish. "Minstrel." **Strachan, Streahan**

STRATFORD Old English. "Street river-crossing."

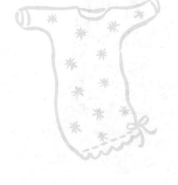

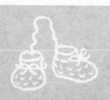

STROM Greek. "Bed."

STRONG Old English. "Powerful."

STRUTHERS Irish. "Near the brook." **Struther**

STUART Old English. "Steward." **Steward, Stewart, Stu**

STYLES Old English. "Stiles." **Stiles**

SUFFIELD Old English. "Southern field." **Suffeld**

SULAMAIN Arabic. "Peaceable." **Sulayman, Suleiman, Suleyman, Sulimein.** Under Sulayman I, the Ottoman Empire reached the height of its power.

SULLIVAN Irish. "Dark eyes." **Sullavan, Sullevan, Sully**

SULLY Old English. "South meadow." Also short form of **Sullivan. Sulleigh, Sulley**

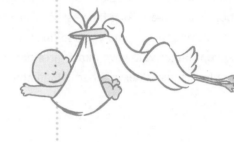

SULTAN Arabic. "Monarch."

SUTCLIFF Old English. "Southern cliff." **Sutcliffe**

SUTHERLAND Scandinavian. "Southern land." **Southerland**

SUTTON Old English. "Southern settlement."

SVEN Scandinavian. "Youth." **Svein, Svend, Swen**

SWEENEY Irish. "Small hero." **Sweeny**

SWENSON Scandinavian. "Son of Swen." **Svensen, Svenson**

SWINBURNE Old English. "Swine stream." **Swinbern, Swinborn, Swinbourne, Swinburn, Swinbyrn, Swynborne**

SWINFORD Old English. "Swine crossing." **Swynford**

SWINTON Old English. "Swine town."

SYLVESTER Variant of **Silvester.** Latin. "Wooded."

SYRUS Latin. "Syrian."

SYSHE Hebrew. "Street."

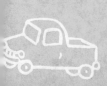

The Real Boy Named Sue

Shel Silverstein, the poet and author of children's books, is famous in country-music circles for penning one of Johnny Cash's most popular songs, "A Boy Named Sue." Released in 1969 on the album *Johnny Cash at San Quentin,* the song reached Number One on the country chart and Number Two on the pop chart. In a talking-blues style, Cash told the story of a boy who vows to find and kill the absent father who gave him a girl's name. Sue confronts his father in a bar in Gatlinburg, Tennessee; the two have an epic fight and become reconciled.

The inspiration for the song was a real man, Sue K. Hicks, who was named by his father after his mother died at his birth. He was one of the prosecuting attorneys in the 1925 Scopes trial in Dayton, Tennessee, where Clarence Darrow and William Jennings Bryan clashed over the theory of evolution. Hicks later became a judge, tried hundreds of murder cases, and survived all the other attorneys in the Scopes trial.

TAB Short form of **David.** Hebrew. "Beloved." **Tabb, Taber, Tabor**

TABBAI Arabic. "Good."

TABIB Turkish. "Doctor." **Tabeeb**

TABOR Middle English. "Drum." **Tab, Tabb, Taber, Tabour, Taibor, Tayber, Taybor**

TADEO Spanish variant of **Thaddeus.** Greek, "gift of God." **Taddeo, Tadio, Tadyo**

TADOKA Variant of **Dakota.** Sioux, "friend."

TAFT Old English. "River."

TAGGERT Irish. "Son of the priest." **Taggart**

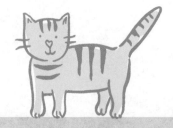

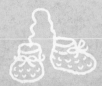

TAHIR Arabic. "Pure." **Taheer, Taher**

TAI Chinese. "Very big."

TAIT Old Norse. "Happy." **Tate, Tayte**

TAIZO Japanese. "Third son."

TAL Hebrew. "Rain." **Talor**

TALBOT Disputed origin. **Talbert, Talbie, Talbott, Talby, Tallbot, Tallbott**

TALMAN Aramaic. "To oppress."

TANASE Cherokee. "Tennessee River." **Tanasi, Tennessee**

TANCRED Old German. "Counselor." **Tancret**

TANNER Old English. "Leather tanner." **Tan, Tann, Tanney, Tannie, Tanny**

TARLETON Old English. "Thor's town." **Tarlton**

TARO Japanese. "Strong first son."

TARRANT Old Welsh. "Thunder." **Tarrent**

TATE Middle English. "Happy." **Tayte**

TAUTON English. A town in England. **Tanton**

TAVI Hebrew. "Good." **Tov, Tova, Tovi**

TAVISH Irish. "Twin." **Tav, Tavis, Tev, Tevis**

TAYLOR Middle English. "Tailor." **Tailer, Tailor, Tayler**

TEAGUE Irish. "Poet." **Teagan, Teige**

TECUMSEH Shawnee. "Panther passing across." Tecumseh, Shawnee military leader who planned a confederacy of tribes to resist U.S. encroachment and fought with the British against the Americans in the War of 1812. William Tecumseh Sherman, Union general in the U.S. Civil War.

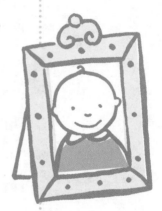

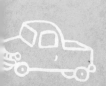

TED Short form of **Tedmund, Theobald, Theodore. Tedd, Teddey, Teddie, Teddy**

TEDMUND Old English. "Protector of the land." **Ted, Tedmond, Tedmundo**

TELFORD Old French. "Iron piercer." **Telfer, Telferd, Telfor, Telfour**

TEMAN Hebrew. "To the right." **Temani**

TEMPEST French. "Storm."

TEMPLETON Old English. "Temple town." **Temp, Temple, Templeten**

TENNANT Old English. "Tenant." **Tenant, Tennent**

TENNESSEE Variant of **Tanase.** Cherokee, "Tennessee River." Also a U.S. state. Tennessee Williams, twentieth-century American playwright.

TENNYSON Middle English. "Son of Dennis." **Tennis, Tenny**

TERENCE Latin. Clan name. **Tarrance, Terencio, Terrance, Terrence, Terris, Terry** et al., **Torrance, Torrence, Torrey, Torry**

TERRELL Old French. "One who pulls." **Terel, Terrall, Terrel, Terrill, Terry** et al., **Terryl, Terryll, Tirrel, Tirrell, Tyrel, Tyrell, Tyrrell**

TERRY Short form of **Terence, Terrell. Terrey, Terri, Terree**

TEXAS Contemporary American, from Spanish. "Roof tiles." A U.S. state. **Tex**

THADDEUS Greek. "Gift of God." **Tad, Tadd, Taddeus, Taddeusz, Tadeo** et al., **Tadzio, Thad, Thaddaus, Thadeus**

THANE Old English. "Man." **Thain, Thaine, Thayne**

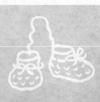

THATCHER Old English. "Roof thatcher." **Thacher, Thatch, Thaxter**

THAW Old English. "Melt."

THELMUS Greek. "Will." **Tel, Tell, Thel**

THEOBALD Old German. "Courageous people." **Dietbald, Dietbold, Tebald, Ted** et al., **Teobaldo, Thebault, Theo, Thibaud, Thibaude, Thibault, Thibaut, Tibald, Tibalt, Tibbald, Tibold, Tiebold, Tiebout, Tybald, Tybalt, Tybault**

THEODORE Greek. "Gift of God." **Fedor** et al., **Tad, Tadore, Teador, Ted** et al., **Tedor, Telli, Telly, Teo, Teodoor, Teodor, Teodoro, Teodosie, Theo, Theodor, Theodoro, Theodorus, Theodosios, Tod, Todd, Todor, Tudor, Tutor**

THEODORIC Old German. "People's ruler." **Derek** et al., **Dietrich** et al., **Dirk** et al., **Rich, Rick, Rik, Ted, Tedd, Teodorico, Thedric, Thedrick, Thierry** et al.

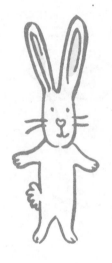

THEOPHILUS Greek. "Loved by God." **Teofilo, Teolil, Théophile, Theophillus**

THERON Greek. "Beast." **Tharon**

THIERRY French variant of **Theodoric.** Old German, "people's ruler." **Therri, Therry**

THOMAS Greek. "Twin." **Tam, Tamas, Tamlane, Tamsen, Tamson, Thom, Tip, Tom, Tomás, Tomaso, Tomasso, Tomasz, Tome, Tomek, Tomey, Tomie, Tomin, Tomislaw, Tomkin, Tomlen, Tomlin, Tommaso, Tommey, Tommie, Tommy**

THOMPSON English. "Son of Thomas." **Thomasen, Thomason, Thomassen, Thomson**

THOR Old Norse. "Thunder." The god of thunder, for whom Thursday is named. **Thorin, Tor, Tore, Torin, Torre**

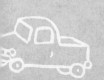

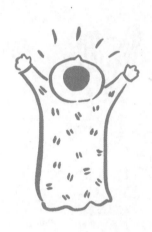

THORALD Old Norse. "Follower of Thor." **Thorold, Torald**

THORBERT Old Norse. "Thor's brightness." **Thorburt, Torbert, Torburt**

THORBURN Old Norse. "Thor's bear." **Thorbjorn, Thorburne, Toburn, Torburn**

THORLEY Old Norse. "Thor's meadow." **Thorlea, Thorlee, Thorleigh, Thorli, Thorly, Torley, Torly**

THORMOND Old English. "Defended by Thor." **Thormonde, Thurmond, Thurmund**

THORNDIKE Old English. "Thorny bank." **Thorndik, Thorndyck, Thorndyke**

THORNE Old English. "Thorn bush." **Thorn**

THORNLEY Old English. "Thorny meadow." **Thornlea, Thornlee, Thornleigh, Thornly**

THORNTON Old English. "Thorny town." **Thorntin, Torin**

THORPE Old English. "Village." **Thorp**

THORSON Old Norse. "Son of Thor."

THORVALD Old Norse. "Thor's power."

THRON Greek. "Throne." **Throne**

THURLOW Old English. "Thor's hill."

THURMAN Old English. "Servant of Thor." **Thorman, Thormen, Thurmen**

THURSTON Scandinavian. "Thor's stone." **Thorstan, Thorstein, Thorsten, Thurstain, Thurstan, Thursten, Torsten, Torston**

TIBERIUS Latin. "The Tiber River." **Tiberus**

TIBOR Slavic. "Holy place."

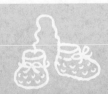

TIERNAN Irish. "Lord." **Tierney**

TIGER Old English. "Tiger." **Tige, Tigger**

TILDEN Old English. "Fertile valley." **Tildon, Tillden, Tilldon, Tilly**

TILFORD Old English. "Fertile ford." **Tilferd**

TILL German. "People's ruler." **Thilo, Tillman, Tilmann**

TILTON Old English. "Fertile estate."

TIMON English variant of **Timothy.** Greek, "reverent." In Shakespeare's *Timon of Athens,* a misanthrope. **Timone, Tymone**

TIMOTHY Greek. "Reverent." **Tim, Timmie, Timmothy, Timmy, Timo, Timofei, Timofeo, Timofey, Timon** et al., **Timoteo, Timoteus, Timothé, Timothee, Timotheo, Timotheus, Timothey, Tymmothy, Tymoteusz, Tymothee, Tymothy**

TITAN Greek. One of the elder gods of ancient Greece.

TITUS Latin. "Defender." **Tito, Titos, Toto, Totus**

TOBIAS Hebrew. "The Lord is good." **Tobe, Tobey, Tobia, Tobiah, Tobie, Tobin, Tobit, Toby, Tobyn**

TODD Middle English. "Fox." **Tad, Toddi, Toddie, Toddy, Tody**

TOMLIN Old English. "Little Tom." **Tomin, Tomlen**

TOMLINSON Old English. "Son of Little Tom."

TOR Norwegian variant of **Thor.** Old Norse, "thunder." Also variant of **Torr.**

TORBERT Old English. "Stony hill." **Tober, Topher, Topper**

TORQUIL Old Norse. "Thor's kettle." **Torquill**

TORR Old English. "Tower." Also short form of **Torrance. Tor**

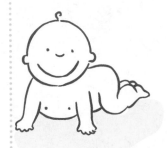

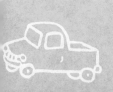

TORRANCE Irish. "Little hills." **Tore, Torey, Torin, Torr, Torrence, Torrey, Torrin, Torry**

TOWNLEY Old English. "Town meadow." **Townlea, Townlee, Townleigh, Townlie, Townly**

TOWNSEND Old English. "End of town." **Tonsend, Tonsin, Tonzen, Tonzin**

TRACY Irish. "Warlike." **Trace, Tracey, Treacy**

TRAHERN Welsh. "Strength of iron." **Traherne**

TRAVIS Old French. "Toll taker." **Traver, Travers, Travys**

TREMAIN Cornish. "Stone house." **Tremaine, Tremayne**

TRENT A river in England.

TRENTON English. "Trent town." **Trenten, Trentin**

TREVOR Welsh. "Large homestead." **Trefor, Trev, Treva, Trevar, Trever**

TREY Middle English. "Three." **Tre**

TRINIDAD Spanish "(Holy) Trinity." Trinidad (Trini) Lopez III, contemporary Latino pop singer. **Trini**

TRINITY English, from Latin. "(Holy) trinity."

TRISTAN Welsh. In legend, a knight of King Arthur's court and lover of Isolde. **Drystam, Drystan, Tris, Tristam, Tristram, Tristen**

TROTH Middle English. "Loyalty."

TROWBRIDGE Old English. "Bridge by the tree."

TROY Irish. "Foot soldier." **Troi, Trove**

TRUMAN Old English. "Trustworthy." **Trueman, Trumaine, Trumann**

TUCKER Old English. "Fabric pleater." **Tuck**

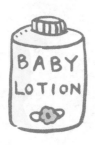

TUDOR Welsh variant of **Theodore**. Greek, "gift of God." **Tutor**

TULLEY Latin. "Honored name." **Tule, Tull, Tullis, Tully, Tulos**

TURNER Middle English. "Woodworker."

TWAIN Middle English. "Divided in two." **Twaine, Twayn, Twin, Twine**

TWYFORD Old English. "Double river crossing."

TYBALT A fiery young Capulet in Shakespeare's *Romeo and Juliet,* who slays Mercutio and is slain by Romeo.

TYDEUS Greek. In legend, one of five Athenians killed in battle with Thebes.

TYLER Old English. "Maker of tiles." **Tilar, Ty, Tylar**

TYNAN Irish. "Dark, dusky."

TYRESE Contemporary American. **Tyreece, Tyreese**

TYRONE Irish. "Land of Owen." **Tyron**

TYSON Old French. "Wild one."

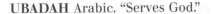

UBADAH Arabic. "Serves God."

UBALDO Old German. "Courageous."

UBERTO Italian variant of **Hubert**. Old German, "shining intellect."

UDELL Old English. "Valley of yew trees." **Del, Dell, Eudel, Udal, Udale, Udall, Udel, Yudale, Yudell**

UDO Variant of **Eudo**. Greek, "well-being."

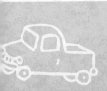

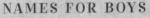

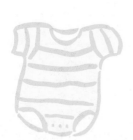

UDOLF Old English. "Wolf-wealth." **Udolfo, Udolph**

UGO Italian variant of **Hugh.** Old German, "intellect."

UILLIAM Irish variant of **William.** Old German, "determined protector."

ULF Old German. "Wolf."

ULL Old Norse. "Magnificent hunter."

ULMER Old English. "Fame of the wolf." **Ullmar, Ulmar**

ULRIC Old German. "Power of the wolf." **Ric, Rick, Ricki, Ullric, Ulrich, Ulrick, Ulrik, Ulu**

ULTAN Irish. "Man from Ulster."

ULTIMUS Latin. "Final." **Ultimo**

ULYSSES Latin variant of **Odysseus.** Greek, "wrathful." **Ulick, Ulises, Ulisse, Uluxe**

UMBERTO Italian variant of **Humbert.** Old German, "famous warrior."

UMED Sanskrit. "Hope."

UNWIN Old English. "Non-friend." **Unwinn, Unwyn, Unwynne**

UPTON Old English. "Upper town."

UPWOOD Old English. "Upper forest."

URANUS Greek. In myth, the Titan god of the sky. Also the seventh planet from the sun.

URBAN Latin. "From the city." A name of popes. Urban II brought about the First Crusade. Urban VI, who murdered cardinals, brought about the Great Schism. **Urbain, Urbaine, Urbane, Urbano, Urbanus**

URIAH Hebrew. "The Lord is my light." **Uri, Uria, Urias, Yuri, Yuria**

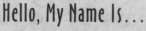
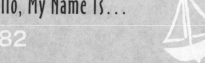

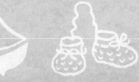

URIAN Welsh. Unknown meaning. **Urean, Uryan**

URIEL Hebrew. "Flame of God."

URSEL Latin. "Bear." **Orsel, Ursell, Urshell**

USAMAH Arabic. "Like a lion." **Osama, Osamah, Usama**

USMAN Arabic. "Serpent."

UWE Old Norse. "Sword's edge."

UZIEL Hebrew. "Strength, power." **Uzi, Uzziah, Uzziel**

VACHEL Old French. "Small cow." **Vachell**

VACLAV Slavic. "Great glory." **Venceslav**

VADA Latin. "Shallow water."

VAIL Old English. "Valley." **Vaile, Vaill, Vale**

VALDEMAR Old German. "Renowned leader." **Valdemoor, Valdemor**

VALENTINE Latin. "Strong." St. Valentine, for whom Valentine's Day is named. **Val, Valentijn, Valentin, Valentino, Valentyn, Vallie**

VALERI Old German. "Foreign power."

VALERIAN Latin. "Healthy." Also a medicinal plant. **Valerien, Valerio, Valerius, Valéry, Valeryan, Walerian.** St. Valerio.

VALI Old Norse. In myth, the son of the highest God. **Valle, Vallie**

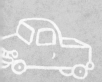

A name to nag about

While the mother of a newly born son rested in the hospital with her baby, her husband offered to go to the records office of Boscotrecase, a small town in southern Italy, to register the boy's name, which she assumed would be *Cristiano.*

When the father returned, the mother learned that he had officially named their son *Varenne Giampaolo.* This name, which sounds reasonable enough to American ears, actually combines the name of Italy's most famous horse with that of his driver. Varenne, considered by many to be the best trotting horse of all time, was voted Italy's athlete of the year in 2001. The famed trotter pulls a sulky driven by Giampaolo Minnucci.

The irate mother had to go to court to change the boy's name.

VAN Dutch. "Of." **Vane, Vann, Vanne, Von**

VANCE Old English. "Marshland."

VANDYKE Dutch. "Of the bank." **Van Dyke**

VANYA Russian variant of **John**. Hebrew, "the Lord is gracious." **Vanek, Vanko, Vania, Vanie, Vanye**

VARDON Old French. "Green knoll." **Varden, Vardin, Verdon, Verdun**

VARICK Old German. "Leader who defends." **Varrick, Warick, Warrick**

VASCO Spanish, from Basque. "Basque." Vasco da Gama, Portuguese navigator, was the first European to travel by sea to India.

VASILIS Greek. "Royal." **Basil** et al., **Vasil, Vasileios, Vasili, Vasilios, Vasily, Vaso, Vasos, Vassili, Vassilie, Vassily, Vasya, Wassily**

VAUGHN Welsh. "Small." **Vagn, Vaughan, Vaun, Vaune, Von, Vonne**

VEDIE Latin. "I saw."

VELIBOR Serbian. "Tall pine."

VENTURO Spanish. "Luck."

VERE Old French. "Springtime."

VERED Hebrew. "Rose."

VERMONT French. "Green mountain." A New England state.

VERNER Scandinavian. "Defender." **Werner** et al.

VERNON Old French. "Alder grove." **Vern, Verne, Vernee, Vernen, Verney, Vernie, Vernin, Verny**

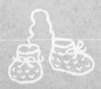

VERRILL Old German. "Masculine." **Verill, Verrall, Verrell, Verroll, Veryl**

VIBERT French. "Flourishing life."

VICTOR Latin. "Conqueror." **Vic, Vick, Victorien, Victorin, Vidor, Viktor, Vitor, Vitorio, Vittorio, Vittorios**

VIDAR Old Norse. God of silence and revenge.

VILMOS Hungarian. "Determined fighter."

VINCE Short form of **Vincent.** Latin, "conquering."

VINCENT Latin. "Conquering." **Vicente, Vicenzio, Vicenzo, Vin, Vince, Vincens, Vincentius, Vincents, Vincenty, Vincenz, Vincenzio, Vincenzo, Vincien, Vine, Vinicent, Vinnie, Vinny, Vinson, Vinzenz**

VINE Old English. "Wine."

VINNY Diminutive of **Vincent.** Latin, "conquering." **Vinnie**

VINSON Old English. "Son of Vincent."

VIRGIL Latin. Clan name. Virgil, 70–19 B.C., great Roman poet. **Verge, Vergil, Vergilius, Virge, Virgie, Virgilio**

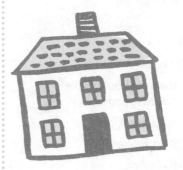

VITUS Latin. "Alive." **Vidal, Viel, Vital, Vitale, Vitalis, Vito, Witold**

VIVIAN Latin. "Full of life." **Bibian, Bibien, Vivion, Vivyan, Vyvian, Vyvyan**

VLADIC Slavic. "To rule." **Vlad, Vladek, Vladik.** Vlad Dracula, fifteenth-century prince of Wallachia, inspiration for the fictional vampire Count Dracula.

VLADIMIR Slavic. "Renowned prince." Vladimir Ilyich Lenin, founder of the Soviet state. **Vlad, Vladamir, Vladimeer, Volodymyr, Wladimir, Wladimyr**

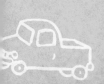

Names with the blues

Many blues performers have wonderful names. Some carry their original names, some bear names that other people have given to them, and others have names they have created for themselves.

Pink Anderson

Kokomo Arnold

Howard "Louie Bluie" Armstrong

Barbecue Bob

Blind Blake

Black Ace

Scrapper Blackwell

Pillie Bolling

Wee Bea Booze (Muriel Nicholls)

Ishmon Bracey

Big Bill (Broonzy) DeLuxe

Buster Brown

Gabriel Brown

Bumble Bee Slim

Gus Cannon

Bo Carter

Ford "Snooks" Eaglin

Dave "Honeyboy" Edwards

Sleepy John Estes

Bud Ezell

Blind Boy Fuller

Arvella Grey

Buddy Guy

"Hacksaw" Harney

Buddy Boy Hawkins

Son House

Peg Leg Howell

Howling Wolf

Mississippi John Hurt

James "Bo Weavil" Jackson

Elmore James

Homesick James

Skip James

Mager Johnson

McKinney Jones

B. B. King

Leadbelly

Furry Lewis

Mance Lipscombe

Robert Jr. Lockwood

Maxwell Street Jimmie

Brownie McGhee

Memphis Minnie

Hammie Nixon

Washington Phillips

Yank Rachell

Spark Plug Smith

Roosevelt Sykes

Tampa Red

Sister Rosetta Tharpe

Rambling Thomas

Muddy Waters

Curley Weaver

Peetie Wheatstraw

Bukka White

Josh White

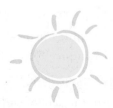

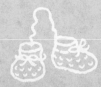

VLADISLAV Old Slavic. "Splendid ruler." **Ladislav, Vlad, Wladyslaw**

VOLKER German. "People's defender."

VOLNEY Old German. "Spirit of the folk."

VON Old Norse, "hope." German, "of."

WADE Old English. "River ford." **Wayde**

WADELL Old English. "Wade." **Waydel, Wydel, Wydell**

WADLEY Old English. "Ford meadow." **Wadleigh, Wadly**

WADSWORTH Old English. "Homestead near the ford." **Waddsworth, Wadswort**

WAGNER German. "Wagon driver." **Waggoner**

WAINWRIGHT Old English. "Wagon builder." **Wainright, Wayneright, Waynewright, Waynright**

WAITE Middle English. "Watchman." **Waits, Wayte**

WAKEFIELD Old English. "Damp field."

WAKELEY Old English. "Damp meadow." **Wakelea, Wakeleigh, Wakely**

WAKEMAN Old English. "Watchman." **Wake**

WALBERT Old English. "Well bright." **Walber**

WALCOTT Old English. "Cottage by the wall." **Wallcot, Wallcott, Wolcott**

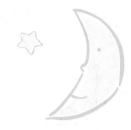

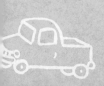

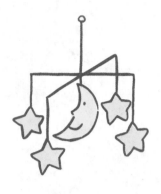

WALDEMAR Old German. "Renowned ruler." **Valdemar, Valdmar, Waldmar**

WALDEN Old English. "Wooded valley." **Waldi, Waldon**

WALDO Old German. "Ruler."

WALFRED Old German. "Ruler of peace."

WALKER Old English. "One who cleans and thickens cloth by treading on it."

WALLACE Old English. "Welshman." **Wal, Wall, Wallach, Wallache, Wallas, Wallie, Wallis, Wally, Walsh, Welch, Welsh**

WALTER Old German. "Ruler of the people." **Gauthier** et al., **Valter, Valther, Walder, Wally, Walt, Walther, Wat, Watley, Watly, Wolly, Wolter, Wolther**

WALTON Old English. "Walled town." **Walley, Wallie, Wally, Walt**

WALWORTH Old English. "Walled farm." **Wallworth**

WALWYN Old English. "Welsh friend." **Walwin, Walwinn, Walwynn, Walwynne, Welwyn**

WARBURTON Old English. "Fortress town." **Warbert, Warberton, Warburt**

WARD Old English. "Guard." **Warde, Warden, Worden**

WARDELL Old English. "Watchman's hill."

WARDLEY Old English. "Watchman's meadow." **Wardlea, Wardleigh**

WARE Old English. "Watchful." **Waring**

WARFIELD Middle English. "Field by the weir." **Warfeld, Werfeld, Werfield**

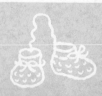

WARFORD Middle English. "Crossing at the weir."

WARLEY Middle English. "Meadow near the weir." **Warly**

WARNER Old German. "Defender." **Werner** et al., **Varner**

WARREN Old English. "Game preserve." **Warrin**

WARRENER Old English. "Officer of a game preserve."
Warriner

WARTON Old English. "Town near the dam."

WARWICK Old English. "Building near the dam." **Warick,
Warrick**

WASHBURN Old English. "Flooding stream." **Warbourn,
Warbourne, Washburne**

WASHINGTON Old English place name. Also the forty-second
U.S. state. Washington Irving, 1783–1859, American writer of
tales such as *Rip Van Winkle* and *The Legend of Sleepy
Hollow.* **Wash**

WATKIN Middle English. "Little Walter."

WATLEY Old English. "Wall." **Watlie, Watly**

WATSON Old English. "Son of Walter." **Watsin, Wattson**

WAVERLY Old English. "Meadow of quivering aspens."
Waverlie, Waverley

WAYLAND Old English. "Land by the road." **Walen, Way,
Waylan, Waylen, Waylin, Waylon, Weylin.** Waylon Jennings,
American country singer and guitar player.

WAYNE Old English. "Wagon." **Wain, Waine, Wayn**

WEAVER Old English. "Weaver."

WEBB Old English. "Weaver." **Web, Weber, Webster**

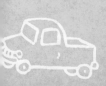

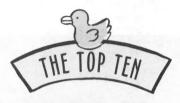

THE TOP TEN

NORWEGIAN NAMES OF 2003

BOYS

Mathias
Tobias
Andreas
Martin
Kristian
Jonas
Markus
Sander
Kristoffer
Daniel

GIRLS

Emma
Ida
Thea
Sara
Julie
Nora
Emilie
Maria
Ingrid
Hanna

WEBLEY Old English. "Weaver's meadow." **Webbley, Webbly, Webly**

WELBORNE Old English. "Spring-fed stream." **Welborn, Welbourne, Welburn, Wellborn, Wellbourn, Wellbourne, Wellburn**

WELBY Old English. "Farm by the spring." **Welbey, Welbie, Wellbey, Wellby**

WELDON Old English. "Hill by the spring." **Welden, Welldon**

WELFORD Old English. "Ford by the spring." **Wellford**

WELLINGTON Old English. Disputed meaning; possibly "town where the water surges." The name of towns in Kansas, New Zealand, and Australia.

WELLS Old English. "Springs." **Welis, Well, Wellis**

WELTON Old English. "Spring town." **Wellton, Wilton**

WENCESLAUS Old Slavic. "Glorious garland." Wenceslaus, 1378–1400, Holy Roman emperor and German king. **Wenceslas, Wenzel, Wiencyslaw**

WENDELL Old German. "Wanderer." **Wendall, Wendel**

WENTWORTH Old English. "Winter stronghold."

WERNER Old German. "Defender." **Verner, Warner, Wernhar, Wernher**

WESLEY Old English. "Western meadow." **Wes, Wesely, Wesly, Wessely, Wessley, Wessly, West, Westleigh, Westley, Westly**

WESTBROOK Old English. "Western stream." **Brook, Brooke, Wes, Wesbrook, Wesbrooke, West, Westbrooke**

WESTBY Old English. "Western farmstead." **Westbey**

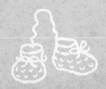

WESTCOTT Old English. "Western cottage." **Wescot, Wescott, Westcot**

WESTON Old English. "Western town." **Westen, Westin**

WETHERBY Old English. "Sheep farm." **Weatherbey, Weatherbie, Weatherby, Wetherbey, Wetherbie**

WETHERELL Old English. "Sheep corner." **Weatherell, Weatherill, Wetherill, Wethrell, Wethrill**

WETHERLY Old English. "Sheep meadow." **Weatherley, Weatherly, Wetherleigh, Wetherley**

WHARTON Old English. "Shore town." **Warton**

WHEATLEY Old English. "Wheat field." **Weatley, Wheatlea, Wheatleigh, Wheatly**

WHEATON Old English. "Wheat town."

WHEELER Old English. "Wheel maker." **Wealer, Whealer**

WHISTLER Old English. "Piper."

WHITBY Old English. "White farm." **Whitbey, Whitbie**

WHITCOMB Old English. "White valley." **Whitcom, Whitcombe**

WHITELAW Old English. "White hill." **Whitlaw**

WHITFIELD Old English. "Small field." **Wiffeld**

WHITFORD Old English. "White ford."

WHITLEY Old English. "White meadow." **Witley**

WHITLOCK Old English. "White hair." **Whitelock**

WHITMAN Old English. "White man." **Witman**

WHITMORE Old English. "White moor." **Whitmoor, Whittemore, Witmore, Wittemore**

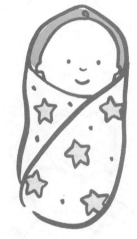

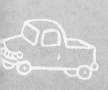

WHITNEY Old English. "White island."

WHITTAKER Old English. "White field." **Whitacker, Whitaker**

WICKHAM Old English. "Village paddock."

WILBERT Old German. "Brilliant and resolute." **Wilburt, Wilburton**

WILBUR Old German. Disputed meaning. **Wilber, Wilburh, Wilburn, Willbur, Wilver**

WILDER Old English. "Wilderness."

WILEY Variant of **William.** Old German, "determined protector." **Willey, Wylie**

WILFORD Old English. "Willow ford."

WILFRED Old English. "Desiring peace." **Wilfredo, Wilfrid, Wilfried, Wilfryd, Will, Willfred, Willfredo, Willfried**

WILKINSON Old English. "Son of Will." **Wilkins, Willkins, Willkinson**

WILLARD Old German. "Bold will."

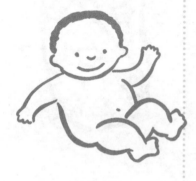

WILLIAM Old German. "Determined protector." **Bill, Billie, Billy, Guillaume** et al., **Guillemot, Liam, Uilliam, Vilhelm, Villem, Wil, Wilek, Wilem, Wiley, Wilhelm, Wilhelmus, Wilkes, Wilkie, Will, Willem, Willey, Willhelmus, Willi, Willie, Willis, Willkie, Wills, Willy, Wilmot, Wilmott, Wim**

WILLIAMSON Old English. "Son of William."

WILLOUGHBY Old English. "Farm by the willows." **Willoughbey, Willoughbie**

WILMER Old German. "Determined fame." **Willmer, Wilmar, Wylmer**

WILSON Old English. "Son of Will." **Willson**

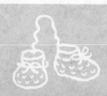

WILTON Old English. "Well town." **Wellton, Welton**

WINDSOR Old English. "Riverbank with a winch." **Wyndsor**

WINFIELD Old English. "Friend's field." **Winnfield, Wynfield, Wynnfield**

WINFRED Welsh. "Good friend." **Winfrid, Winfried**

WINGATE Old English. "Winding gate."

WINSLOW Old English. "Friend's hill."

WINSTON Old English. "Friend's town." **Winsten, Winstonn, Wynstan, Wynston**

WINTHROP Old English. "Friend's village." **Winthrope**

WINTON Old English. "Friend's town." **Wynton.** Wynton Marsalis, contemporary jazz musician.

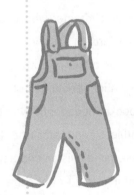

WITT Old English. "Fair-skinned." **Witter, Wittie, Witty**

WOLCOTT Old English. "Cottage." **Wolcotte**

WOLFE Old English. "Wolf." **Wolf, Wolfie, Wolfy, Woolf, Wulf**

WOLFGANG Old German. "Traveling wolf."

WOODBURN Old English. "Stream in the wood." **Woodie, Woody**

WOODROW Old English. "Hedgerow." **Wood, Woodie, Woody**

WOODWARD Old English. "Facing the woods." **Woodard, Woodie, Woody**

WOODY English diminutive of **Elwood, Garwood, Haywood, Sherwood, Woodburn, Woodrow, Woodward. Woodie**

WORTH Old English. "Valuable." **Worthey, Worthy**

WORTHINGTON Old English. "Worthy town."

WRIGHT Old English. "Carpenter."

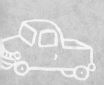

Ixnay the Osama: Boys' names to avoid

As they say, it's a free country, but a boy with any of the following names will have a miserable time growing up in the United States. Some of these are names of real bad guys; others are strongly associated with a fictional character.

Adolf—leader of Nazi Germany

Beavis—cartoon character whose sidekick had an even worse name

Cain—first murderer in history

Draco—blond foe of Harry Potter

Elvis—mid-twentieth-century king

Fagin—pickpocket pedagogue who taught Oliver to twist out wallets from victims

Genghis—ruthless conqueror from the East

Gilligan—moronic television character never voted off the island

Hagrid—giant in Harry Potter saga

Herod—Jewish king who massacred all young boys in hopes of killing Jesus

Judas—disciple who sold out Jesus

Narcissus—young Greek who loved himself to death

Nero—cruel Roman emperor and amateur violinist

Oedipus—Greek with misguided family values

Onan—Biblical figure whose coitus interruptus led to his death

Osama—infamous terrorist

Quasimodo—deformed bell-ringer at Notre Dame Cathedral

Saddam—former leader of Iraq

Satan—Biblical prince of darkness

Sherlock—genius detective

Shylock—Shakespeare's merciless moneylender

Frightful females: Girls' names to avoid

Perhaps because women tend not to be as monstrous as their male counterparts, their list of names to avoid is shorter.

Agrippina—poisoned her husband to land the job of emperor for her son Nero

Barbie—doll with impossible figure and bimbo accoutrements

Cruella—Disney character who loved dogs for the wrong reasons

Delilah—Biblical temptress of Samson

Elvira—busty movie hostess, a.k.a. "Mistress of the Dark"

Goneril—treacherous daughter in King Lear

Medea—vengeful woman in Greek tragedy

Medusa—Greek mythological figure for whom every day was a bad hair day

Morgan or **Morgana**—King Arthur's wicked fairy half-sister

Pandora—in Greek mythology, she opened a box and released the world's evil

Salome—her dance of the seven veils cost John the Baptist his head

WYATT Old English. "Strong and courageous." Wyatt Earp, 1848–1929, American gambler and lawman. **Wiatt, Wyatte, Wyeth, Wyte**

WYCLIFF Old English. "White cliff." **Wycliffe**

WYLIE Old English. "Clever." **Wiley, Wye**

WYNDHAM Old English. "Winding village." **Windham**

WYNN Welsh. "White." Also short form of **Selwynn**. Old English, "friend of the house." **Win, Winn, Wynne**

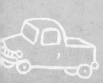

XAN Short form of **Alexander.** Greek, "defender of mankind."

XANTHUS Greek. "Golden-haired." **Xanthos**

XAVIER Basque. "New house." **Javier, Xever, Zavier**

XENOPHON Greek. "Foreign voice." **Xeno, Zeno**

XENOS Greek. "Hospitality." **Zeno, Zenos**

XERXES Persian. "King."

XIA Chinese. "China" or "summer."

XIMENES Spanish variant of **Simon.** Hebrew. "One who listened." **Gímen, Jímen, Jimenes, Jimenez, Xímen, Ximenez**

XYLON Greek. "Forest."

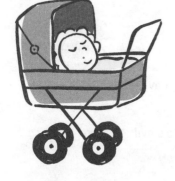

YAAKOV Variant of **Jacob.** Hebrew, "he who supplants." **Yaacob, Yachov, Yacov, Yago, Yakob, Yakov**

YAEL Variant of **Jael.** Hebrew, "mountain goat."

YAKIR Hebrew. "Precious."

YALE Old English. "Fertile moor."

YANCY Unknown origin. **Yance, Yancey, Yantsey**

YANKEE American. "American" or "New Englander." **Yank**

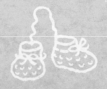

YANNIS Greek variant of **John**. Hebrew, "the Lord is gracious." **Ioannis, Yannakis, Yanni, Yanno**

YAO West African. "Boy born on Thursday." **Kwaw, Kwo, Yaw, Yawo**

YAPHET Hebrew. "He expands." **Japhet, Japheth, Yafet, Yapheth**

YARDEN Hebrew. "Descend." **Jordan** et al.

YARDLEY Old English. "Fenced meadow." **Lee, Leigh, Yard, Yardlea, Yardlee, Yardleigh, Yardly**

YASAHIRO Japanese. "Serene."

YASIR Arabic. "Well-to-do." **Yaseer, Yasser.** Yasser Arafat, Palestinian leader, 1929–2004.

YATES Middle English. "The gates." **Yeats**

YAVIN Hebrew. "God will judge." **Jabin, Yadin, Yadon, Yediel, Yekutiel, Yoram**

YEHEZEKEL Variant of **Ezekiel**. Hebrew, "strength of God."

YEHUDI Variant of **Judah**. Hebrew, "praise." Yehudi Menuhin, contemporary American violinist. **Yechudi, Yechudit, Yehuda, Yehudah, Yehudit**

YEN Vietnamese. "Tranquil."

YEOMAN Middle English. "Attendant." **Youman**

YITZHAK Variant of **Isaac**. Hebrew, "laughter." Yitzhak Rabin, 1922–1995, Israeli military general and politician. He was twice the prime minister of Israel. **Itzak, Izaak, Yitzchak**

YORA Hebrew. "Teach." **Jorah**

YORK Old English. "Boar settlement." **Yorick, Yorrick, Yorke**

YOTAM Hebrew. "God is perfect."

Madam, I'm Adam

Palindromic names are those that read the same way spelled forwards or backwards: *Ada, Ala, Ana, Anna, Anona, Asa, Ava, Aya, Bob, Ebbe, Ele, Elle, Eve, Hannah, Lal, Lil, Nan, Natan, Odo, Otto, Pip, Sabas, Savas, Viv,* and *Vyv*. A harder feat is having a palindromic first and last name. Lon Nol, the former premier of Cambodia, had such a name, as did Revilo P. Oliver, a founder of the John Birch Society. Then there was the Ohio couple who gave each of their eleven children a first and middle name that together form a palindrome. Examples of their children's names are *Noel Leon, Lledo Odell, Laur Rual, Loneva Avenol, Lebanna Annabel,* and *Leah Hael.*

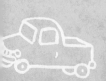

YOURI Dutch variant of **George.** Greek, "farmer."

YUCEL Turkish. "Sublime."

YUKI Variant of **Jacob.** Hebrew, "he who supplants."

YUKIO Japanese. "Snow boy."

YULE Old English. "Winter solstice." **Euell, Ewell, Yul**

YUMA Yuma. A Native American nation of the Southwest United States and its language.

YURI Russian variant of **George.** Greek, "farmer." Also a variant of **Uriah. Yurii, Yury**

YUSUF Variant of **Joseph.** Hebrew, "the Lord increases." **Yosef, Yoseff, Yusef, Yusuff**

YVES French variant of **Evan.** Welsh, "young warrior."

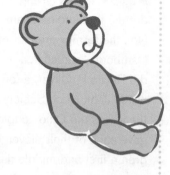

ZACHARIAH Hebrew. "The Lord has remembered." **Zacaria, Zacarias, Zacaríus, Zacary, Zaccaria, Zaccariah, Zacchaeus, Zaccheus, Zach, Zachaios, Zacharia, Zachariah, Zacharias, Zacharie, Zachary, Zachery, Zacheus, Zack, Zackariah, Zackerias, Zackery, Zak, Zakarias, Zakarie, Zakariyyah, Zakery, Zecharia, Zechariah, Zecharias, Zekariah, Zeke, Zekeriah**

ZADOK Variant of **Solomon.** Hebrew, "peace." **Zadoc, Zaydok**

ZAHID Arabic. "Ascetic."

ZAHIR Arabic. "Brilliant." **Zayyir**

ZAIN Arabic. "Friend" or "beloved."

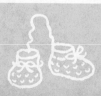

ZALE Greek. "Sea-strength." **Zayle**

ZALMAN Variant of **Solomon.** Hebrew, "peace." **Salman, Zalmon, Zaloman, Zalomon**

ZAMIR Hebrew. "Song."

ZANE English variant of **John.** Hebrew, "the Lord is gracious." **Zayne**

ZARED Hebrew. "Trap."

ZEBADIAH Hebrew. "Gift of Jehovah." **Zeb, Zebedee, Zebediah**

ZEBULON Hebrew. "To give honor to." **Zebulen, Zebulun, Zevulon, Zevulun**

ZEDEDIAH Hebrew. "The Lord is just." **Zed, Zedechiah, Zedelias**

ZEIRA Arabic. "Small."

ZEKE Short form of **Ezekiel, Zachariah.**

ZELIG Yiddish. "Holy." **Selig, Zelik**

ZELIGMAN Yiddish. "Holy man." **Seligman, Seligmann, Zeligmann**

ZENAS Greek. "Hospitable." **Zeno, Zenon, Zenón, Zenus.** Zeno, Roman emperor of the East, 474–491. Zeno of Elea, Greek philosopher, fifth century B.C. St. Zenon.

ZENOPHON Variant of **Xenophon.** Greek, "foreign voice." **Zeno**

ZENOS Variant of **Xenos.** Greek. "Hospitality." **Zeno**

ZEPHANIAH Hebrew. "Precious to the Lord." **Zeph, Zephan**

ZEPHYR Greek. "West wind." **Zephi, Zephy**

ZEPPELIN German. "Airship." **Zeppi, Zeppie, Zeppy**

ZERO Arabic. "Void."

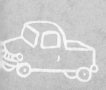

ZEUS Greek. In myth, the lord of the skies and supreme ruler.

ZHIAN Persian. "Strong."

ZINDEL Yiddish variant of **Alexander.** Greek, "defender of mankind." **Zindil**

ZION Hebrew. The mythical City of David, the Jewish Promised Land.

ZIV Hebrew. "Full of life." **Ziven, Zivon**

ZOLTÁN Hungarian. "Life."

ZUHAYR Arabic. "Brilliant."

ZURIEL Hebrew. "The Lord, my rock."

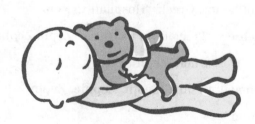

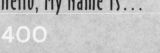

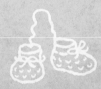

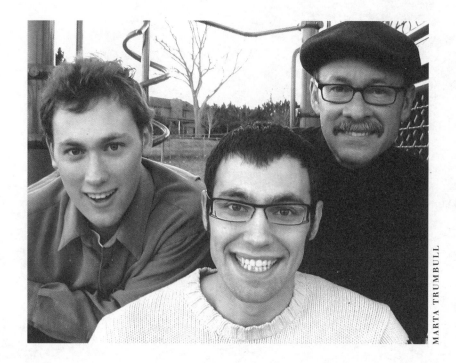

MARTA TRUMBULL

About the Authors

Jeff Bradley, the author of five books, has written for numerous newspapers and magazines and taught writing at Harvard University for eight years. This is the first book he has written with his sons, Truman and Walker. **Truman Bradley,** who lives in Denver, Colorado, writes as well as competes in swing dance events across the nation. **Walker Bradley** is a student at the University of Colorado in Boulder. A man of the outdoors, he enjoys scuba diving and backpacking. In helping to choose his sons' names, Jeff Bradley was mindful that one day they will select his nursing home.